Prion Diseases

Prion Diseases

Edited by

JOHN COLLINGE

and

MARK S. PALMER

Department of Biochemistry and Molecular Genetics,
St Mary's Hospital Medical School, London

OXFORD   NEW YORK   TOKYO

OXFORD UNIVERSITY PRESS

1997

Oxford University Press, Great Clarendon Street, Oxford OX2 6DP

Oxford New York

Athens Auckland Bangkok Bogota Bombay Buenos Aires
Calcutta Cape Town Dar es Salaam Delhi Florence Hong Kong
Istanbul Karachi Kuala Lumpur Madras Madrid Melbourne
Mexico City Nairobi Paris Singapore Taipei Tokyo Toronto

and associated companies in
Berlin Ibadan

Oxford is a trade mark of Oxford University Press

Published in the United States
by Oxford University Press Inc., New York

© Oxford University Press, 1997

Chapter 4 © (British) Crown copyright 1997. Published with the permission of the
Controller of Her (Britannic) Majesty's Stationery Office. The views expressed are those of
the author and do not necessarily reflect those of the HMSO or the Central Veterinary
Laboratory or any other (British) government department.

A catalogue record for this book is available from the British Library

Library of Congress Cataloging in Publication Data
Prion diseases / edited by John Collinge and Mark S. Palmer.
Includes bibliographical references.
1. Prion diseases. 2. Prion diseases in animals. I. Collinge,
John, MD. II. Palmer, Mark S.
[DNLM: 1. Prion Diseases—physiopathology. WL 300 P9585 1996]
QR201.P737P742 1996 616.8′047—dc20 96–30984
ISBN 0 19 854789 7

Typeset by EXPO Holdings, Malaysia

Printed in Great Britain by
Bookcraft (Bath) Ltd
Midsomer Norton, Avon.

Contents

Contributors

Jeanne E. Bell,   National CJD Surveillance Unit, Neuropathology Department, Western General Hospital, Edinburgh EH4 2XU.

Ray Bradley,   Central Veterinary Laboratory, Woodham Lane, New Haw, Addlestone, Surrey KT15 3NB.

Anthony R. Clarke,   Department of Biochemistry, School of Medical Sciences, University of Bristol, University Walk, Bristol BS8 1TD.

John Collinge,   Prion Disease Group, Department of Biochemistry and Molecular Genetics, St Mary's Hospital Medical School, Norfolk Place, London W2 1PG.

James W. Ironside,   National CJD Surveillance Unit, Neuropathology Department, Western General Hospital, Edinburgh EH4 2XU.

John G. R. Jefferys, Neuronal Networks Group, Department of Physiology and Biophysics, St Mary's Hospital Medical School, Imperial College of Science, Technology and Medicine, Norfolk Place, London W2 1PG.

Mark S. Palmer,   Prion Disease Group, Department of Biochemistry and Molecular Genetics, St Mary's Hospital Medical School, Norfolk Place, London W2 1PG.

Stanley B. Prusiner,   Department of Neurology HSE 781, University of California, San Francisco, CA 94143-0518, USA.

Corinne Smith,   MRC Laboratory of Molecular Biology, Hills Road, Cambridge CB2 2QH.

1 Prion diseases: an introduction

MARK S. PALMER AND JOHN COLLINGE

The transmissible spongiform encephalopathies

The first records of what have become known as prion diseases date back to the early 18th century (reported in McGowan 1922), with the mention of disorders of sheep in France with trembling disease (*la tremblante*), and in Germany with itching disease (*Gnubberkrankheit*) or trotting disease (*Traberkrankheit*) (Leopoldt 1759). This descriptive terminology reflects the variation in clinical features associated with the disease, which is now more generally known by the Scottish term 'scrapie', itself a word describing the tendency of afflicted animals to scrape their fleece against trees and bushes. Sheep have been central to the prosperity of the British Isles for the past 2000 years. The fine quality of British wool was recognized throughout continental Europe from Roman times and remained the principal export until superseded by woollen cloth in the late middle ages. By the turn of this century the impact of scrapie was of such economic importance that the Government included funds for scrapie research in its first grant to the Royal Veterinary College in London in 1910. The long-standing commitment to scrapie research of the Moredun Institute in Edinburgh (now the Neuropathogenesis Unit at the Institute for Animal Health, Edinburgh) and later the Institute for Animal Health laboratories at Compton, Oxfordshire, was reinforced by the ban imposed by many countries during the 1940s and 1950s on the import of sheep from Britain until they could be shown to be scrapie-free.

For many years the aetiology of scrapie was far from obvious and research was conducted in the context of a folk lore of scrapie causes, including sexual excess and being struck by lightning. The concept of slow viruses was not well established before the middle of the 20th century and when two French workers, Cuillé and Chelle (1936) reported transmission of scrapie by inoculation of healthy sheep with spinal cord from affected sheep, their work was received with scepticism because of the long incubation periods of 14 to 22 months. The success rate for transmission to sheep was also only about 25%. The repetition of these transmission studies elsewhere and the demonstration in 1939 of transmissibility of scrapie to goats with a 100% success rate (Cuillé and Chelle 1939; Pattison *et al.* 1959) convinced the research community that this was an infectious disease and the search began for the transmissible agent. An important advance was the transmission of scrapie to mice, and subsequently to hamsters, with much reduced incubation times (Chandler 1961, 1963); the time-scale for experiments and the costs could now be substantially reduced while the number of possible experiments could be expanded.

During the 1950s, while scrapie research was gathering momentum, there was a growing interest in kuru, an epidemic disease amongst the Fore-speaking people of the Eastern Highlands of Papua New Guinea, which was characterized by ataxia, tremor and behavioural changes, and associated neuropathologically with degeneration of the olivo-ponto-cerebellar system and marked atrophy of the cerebellar vermis (Zigas and Gajdusek 1957; Klatzo *et al.* 1959; Alpers 1970). Kuru is the Fore word for shaking or tremors. Because of the emotional lability which accompanies kuru, the disease was also called *negi nagi*, meaning a silly or foolish person. It has not been possible to determine when kuru first arose in New Guinea though anthropologists have found evidence of kuru emerging in local consciousness between 1900 and 1920 with many people in the late 1950s giving accounts of kuru cases that they had seen 30 or 40 years earlier (Glasse and Lindenbaum 1992). The pathology of kuru was strikingly similar to that of scrapie, with little spongiosis of the grey matter. This similarity, together with the comparable clinical features of kuru and scrapie, was particularly noted by W. J. Hadlow who was working on scrapie at Compton. In a letter to the *Lancet* he suggested that kuru might also prove to be a transmissible disease and that it might be 'profitable...to examine the possibility of the experimental induction of kuru in a laboratory primate' (Hadlow 1959). Within the next few years such studies were initiated and Gajdusek and colleagues (1966*a*,*b*) reported the transmission of kuru to chimpanzees with an incubation time of 18 to 21 months.

The transmissibility of kuru to experimental animals supported the idea that the route of transmission was ritualistic cannibalism which was performed as a mark of respect for their deceased relatives. Although cannibalism implies the transmission by an oral route, other possible routes of exposure in women and children, who were involved with the preparation of the feast, were skin inoculation associated with scratching insect bites or conjunctival exposure by rubbing their eyes.

By this period, interest in slow virus infections had intensified with the recognition that a delayed response to measles infection caused type-A inclusion encephalopathy or subacute sclerosing panencephalitis, and there was a belief that virus-induced slow infections might be more generally responsible for progressive degenerative diseases of the central nervous system. The experimental transmission studies performed at this time were therefore widened to include a range of neurodegenerative diseases including amyotrophic lateral sclerosis-parkinsonism dementia of Guam, Alzheimer's disease, Pick's disease, multiple sclerosis, and Creutzfeldt–Jakob disease (CJD) (Gajdusek *et al.* 1965). The pathological lesions observed in the brains of CJD patients had been recognized to be strikingly similar to those seen in kuru patients (Klatzo *et al.* 1959) and the relatedness of these two diseases was established when transmission of CJD to chimpanzees was reported (Gibbs *et al.* 1968). Other neurodegenerative diseases were not transmitted. This key work established the idea of the transmissible spongiform encephalopathies, or transmissible dementias.

The human transmissible spongiform encephalopathies encompass kuru, CJD, and Gerstmann–Sträussler syndrome (GSS). GSS is also called Gerstmann–

Sträussler–Scheinker disease. CJD has been known by many other names including disseminated encephalopathy, spastic pseudosclerosis, cortico-pallido-spinal degeneration, cortico-striatal-spinal degeneration, Jakob's syndrome, presenile dementia with cortical blindness, Heidenhain's syndrome, subacute vascular encephalopathy with mental disorder, subacute presenile spongiosis atrophy, Nevin–Jones disease, and Brownell–Oppenheimer syndrome. The new diagnostic method of experimental transmissibility allowed existing clinicopathological diagnostic criteria for CJD, until then fairly loosely defined, to be revised and refined. CJD is recognized today by the occurrence of a rapidly progressive dementia with myoclonus often accompanied by pyramidal signs, cerebellar ataxia, or extrapyramidal features. The clinical course of CJD is rapid with a mean duration of four to five months. Patients are generally affected in the 45–75 year age range. CJD is a sporadic disease with a uniform worldwide incidence of about 0.4–1 case per million per year (Brown *et al.* 1987). About 15% of cases, however, are familial and show an autosomal dominant pattern of disease segregation. GSS, which is nearly always seen as a familial disease, has a much longer duration with a mean of more than five years. Classically, GSS presents with cerebellar ataxia, and dementia occurs much later in the disease. The incidence of GSS is about one-tenth that of CJD. Experimental transmission of GSS to primates was reported by Masters *et al.* (1981).

Familial forms of CJD and GSS are all associated with mutations in the same gene, the prion protein gene, and can be reclassified using aetiological criteria as subtypes of inherited prion disease. They show a range of clinical and pathological presentations which extend beyond the classical phenotypes of CJD and GSS to include a much wider spectrum (see Chapter 2). The neuropathology of human prion diseases, discussed in detail in Chapter 3, shows a number of features that are also found in the pathology of the animal diseases. These characteristically include the spongiform degeneration of the neuropil of the grey matter, neuronal loss, astrocytosis, and amyloid plaque formation. The plaques of these diseases are congophilic and show the gold-green birefringence under polarizing light that is characteristic of amyloid. However, the protein deposited in these plaques is distinct from the amyloid of Alzheimer's disease. Laboratory tests are unhelpful for diagnosing human prion disease, though classical CJD often presents with a characteristic electroencephalogram (EEG) which shows pseudoperiodic sharp-wave activity (Beck and Daniel 1969; Field 1970).

The spectrum of human disease has been further extended in recent years by the inclusion of the disease fatal familial insomnia (FFI). This disorder, first described in 1986, is an autosomally dominant inherited sleep disorder, presenting as progressive untreatable insomnia and autonomic dysfunction (Lugaresi *et al.* 1986). The main histopathological finding in FFI is thalamic atrophy. The anterior-ventral and medial dorsal thalamic nuclei are consistently affected, while the cortex shows moderate astrocytosis. Two patients who had widespread spongiosis, and also had periodic EEG, were subsequently found to also have mutations in the prion protein gene (Medori *et al.* 1992*a,b*; Gambetti *et al.* 1993). Surprisingly, the mutation was identified as being at a position (codon 178), which had previously been identified in patients with CJD. FFI has now also been transmitted to laboratory animals (Collinge *et al.* 1995; Tateishi *et al.* 1995).

Although most human prion diseases are sporadic or inherited, the group of acquired diseases, which includes kuru, also includes a number of patients in whom the disease has been transmitted by accidental inoculation with the transmissible agent. Such iatrogenic transmission, covered in Chapter 2, has arisen from a number of sources including intracerebral electrodes, dura mater and corneal grafts, and human pituitary-derived hormones. It is possible that kuru arose originally following cannibalism of an individual who developed sporadic CJD many generations earlier and that the human agent was then propagated through these ritualistic practices (Dickinson *et al.* 1967; Pattison and Jones 1968).

As well as the spongiform encephalopathies of sheep and humans, two other related animal diseases have been recognized for some years as transmissible encephalopathies. These are chronic wasting disease (CWD) of mule deer and elk, and transmissible mink encephalopathy (TME) in ranched mink. CWD has been reported in zoological parks in North America and a 12-year history of disease experience was reported in 1980 (Williams and Young 1980). The source of infectivity for this disease is unclear. TME, by contrast, is prevalent among caged mink in North America, and appears to be caused by contaminated feed. The first outbreaks occurred on two commercial mink ranches in Wisconsin and Minnesota in 1947 (Hartsough and Burger 1965) but it has subsequently been identified on ranches in Idaho, Finland, East Germany, and Russia. TME has been found to be transmissible to many other animals, including European ferrets, skunks, racoons, martins, hamsters, and monkeys, but not to mice (reviewed in Marsh 1992). More recently the epidemic of a new animal spongiform encephalopathy—bovine spongiform encephalopathy (BSE)—in the UK has refocused attention on these diseases and has led to concerns that transmission to humans may occur via dietary exposure. Furthermore, a number of new animal spongiform encephalopathies have been identified which have probably arisen from dietary exposure to the BSE agent (Bruce *et al.* 1994) (see Chapter 4).

The infectious agent

Most of the experimental approaches to the nature of the infectious agent in these diseases, until recently, have come from studies of the scrapie agent propagated in mice or hamsters. Early studies on the scrapie agent showed that, while there was a decrease in biological activity upon heating, some of the infectivity survived boiling. Prolonged autoclaving above 120°C was necessary to eliminate the activity (Gordon 1946). The agent was more resistant to dry heat and survived temperatures above 120°C for considerable periods in the absence of water. However, most scrapie workers believed that the agent must be a virus. There were no sound reasons to think otherwise and the main thrust of research was to isolate this putative virus. The agent, which concentrated in microsomal and plasma membrane fractions of infected brain homogenates, would not pass through 30 nm pore diameter filters but would pass through filters of larger pore size, and had an exclusion size similar to the small RNA viruses (Hunter *et al.* 1969). The biochemistry of the agent proved elusive as infectivity could not be dissociated from the membranous components (Gibbons and Hunter 1967). Virologists failed to find evidence for viral particles under the electron microscope and immunological studies failed to find any immune response during infection. Immune-suppressed mice developed scrapie in the same way as normal mice (Delahousse *et al.* 1971).

Studies on dry preparations exposed to ionizing radiations suggested, from the dose required to give one inactivating event per macromolecule, that the agent was at least 10 times smaller than any known virus, with an apparent molecular mass of 100 000 kDa (Alper *et al.* 1966; Alper 1985). Exposure of dried preparations to wavelengths of 254 nm from a low-pressure mercury lamp (which is usually fully germicidal because it is close to the peak absorption of nucleic acids) was incapable of inactivating the agent even after enormous doses were used. Irradiation with other wavelengths suggested that shorter wavelengths around 237 nm were more effective at inactivating the agent, although this corresponds to the region of absorption thought to be characteristic of lipopolysaccharide–protein complexes. In the presence of ionizing radiation, proteins and nucleic acids are usually protected by the addition of oxygen to the solution. However, for the scrapie agent the presence of oxygen enhanced the inactivating effect. This was believed to be due to lipid peroxidation, suggesting that the agent contained a vital membrane component (Alper *et al.* 1978).

The unusual properties of the scrapie agent, in particular its resistance to reagents such as formalin (Pattison 1965) and its resistance to ionizing radiation (Adams *et al.* 1969), cast doubt on whether the agent was a virus after all. There was general agreement that the agent could not be a conventional virus, although the term unconventional virus (Stamp 1967) served primarily to disguise the fact that the macromolecular nature of the infectious agent was no better characterized than when research began. Over the years a number of hypotheses about the chemical nature of the scrapie agent have been put forward. These include: a self-replicating protein (Griffiths 1967; Pattison and Jones 1967); small DNA virus (Kimberlin and Hunter 1967); replicating protein or replicating abnormal polysaccharide within membranes (Gibbons and Hunter 1967); provirus consisting of recessive genes generating RNA particles (Parry 1962); naked nucleic acid-like plant viroids (Diener 1973); and nucleic acids associated with and protected by host protein—the 'virino hypothesis' (Dickinson and Outram 1988). In a review of the properties of the scrapie agent, Millson *et al.* (1976) compared data from different laboratories which indicated that, while infectivity was selectively decreased by treatment with proteases, there was no significant reduction in titre following treatment with nucleases, lipases, or glycosidases. This not only argued against a virus, but also suggested that a protein might be critical for infectivity.

By the early 1980s it was clear that hypotheses about the nature of the agent would have to accommodate a number of diverse observations. They would have to account for the infectious, familial, and sporadic forms of the disease and explain the physicochemical properties of the agent. Such hypotheses would also have to explain the occurrence of multiple strains or isolates of infectious agent.

Strain variation, which has been demonstrated in natural scrapie in sheep, experimental scrapie in mice and hamster, and TME, is the property of experimentally passaged isolates to produce distinctly different, but stable, phenotypes in the same recipient (Pattison and Millson 1961; Dickinson and Meikle 1971; Kimberlin and Walker 1978; Foster and Dickinson 1988; Mori *et al.* 1989). Different strains may result, for example, in different clinical syndromes, incubation periods, and regional brain pathology. Much of the work on strain diversity was initiated by Dickinson and colleagues, and some of the original strains established in the 1970s are still in use today. In general, when scrapie is transmitted from sheep into mice there is an initial long incubation period and some mice may not succumb. However, repeated passage within the same inbred mouse strain results in a fall in incubation period and usually all inoculated mice succumb to disease. Scrapie strain isolates usually have shorter incubation times when transmitted into mice of the same strain as those in which they were propagated. Kimberlin and co-workers (1987) demonstrated that some scrapie strains that had been initiated in mice, such as ME7 and 22A, retained their characteristics even when passaged through hamsters then back into mice. However, other strains, for example 139A and 22C, change their characteristics markedly when passaged through hamsters and then mice. Host effects can therefore also alter the stability of scrapie strains.

It has been proposed that the only way that strain differences can be accounted for is to assume that there is nucleic acid associated with the agent (Dickinson and Outram 1988), despite the biochemical evidence to the contrary. The virino hypothesis suggests that a nucleic acid, not yet detected because of the limitations of current methods, may be closely associated with host-encoded proteins, and encode the information necessary to account for strain differences. Theoretical calculations based on radiation studies suggest that such a nucleic acid could only be around 100–1000 base pairs. Studies using structure-independent methods for detection have further indicated that a nucleic acid-encoded genome, if present, would have to be of 76 base pairs or less, as larger molecules are not present in infectious preparations at concentrations above one molecule per infectious unit (Kellings *et al.* 1994).

The prion protein and prions

Despite early suggestions that the infectious agent of prion disease might be accounted for by a protein-only model (Griffiths 1967), it was not until the early 1980s that progress was made in furthering this hypothesis. A 3000-fold enrichment for the scrapie agent showed that infectivity was associated with a protein which was partially resistant to proteolytic degradation and had a molecular mass of around 27–30 kDa on SDS polyacrylamide gels (Prusiner *et al.* 1982). This protein was associated with infectivity from all scrapie fractions but not from control samples. Since it was the only macromolecule that could be found associated with infectivity, Prusiner proposed the term 'prion' to describe the scrapie agent implying that it was a *pro*teinaceous *in*fectious agent. The prion protein that had been isolated was found to be the product of a cellular gene on the short arm of chromosome 20 in humans and in a syntenic region of chromosome 2 in mice (Chesebro *et al.* 1985; Oesch *et al.* 1985; Robakis *et al.* 1986). The normal product of the gene was found to be expressed on most cell types but expression was predominantly in the brain as a glycosylphosphatidyl inositol-anchored glycoprotein on the outer cell membrane (Baldwin *et al.* 1990; Stahl *et al.* 1990, 1992). It is now clear that the protease-resistant form of the prion protein (designated PrP^{Sc}) produced during disease is derived from the normal protein (designated PrP^{C}) by a post-translational event (Borchelt *et al.* 1990; Caughey and Raymond 1991). No differences in the primary structure of the two isoforms have been identified (Stahl *et al.* 1993) and the difference appears to be conformational rather than covalent (Pan *et al.* 1993) (see Chapter 6).

While arguments for the provocative notion that the transmissible agent may be an abnormal isoform of a host-encoded protein rested largely on the inability of workers to demonstrate significant co-purifying nucleic acids, they obviously remained controversial. A key advance came in 1989 from advances in the molecular genetics of familial CJD and GSS. Given that familial CJD and GSS showed a clear autosomal dominant pattern of disease segregation, the prion protein gene (designated *PRNP* in humans) on the short arm of chromosome 20 was an obvious candidate gene for genetic linkage studies. A 144-base-pair insertional mutation into the coding region of *PRNP* was first identified in a UK family with familial CJD (Owen *et al.* 1989) and a missense mutation at codon 102 (resulting in a proline to leucine substitution in PrP) was identified in two GSS kindreds (from the UK and USA) and shown to be genetically linked to GSS (Hsiao *et al.* 1989). An extensive family of *PRNP* mutations has since been documented in families with these conditions (see Chapter 2). These mutations are seen only in at-risk or affected individuals from these families and have not been seen in the normal population. Strong statistical evidence therefore supported the idea that these were pathogenic mutations. Prusiner and colleagues were able to demonstrate in 1990 that an analogous mutation to that identified in GSS produced spontaneous neurodegeneration in transgenic mice, establishing directly the pathogenicity of this DNA variant (Hsiao *et al.* 1990). Transmission of disease from these mice to wild-type hamsters and to transgenic mice with lower copy numbers of the same transgene has been reported (Hsiao *et al.* 1994). The familial forms of these diseases are therefore autosomal dominant mendelian disorders in addition to being horizontally transmissible to experimental animals by inoculation; these diseases are biologically unique to date in this respect. Such appreciation that PrP mutations produce spontaneous neurodegeneration in humans which is then transmissible by inoculation (and the modelling of this phenomenon in transgenic mice) argues persuasively that PrP, or rather an abnormal isoform of PrP, is the central component of the infectious agent.

The 'protein only' hypothesis argues that PrP^{Sc} is itself the infectious agent and propagates by promoting the conversion of the normal host PrP^C into the disease-related isoform. Recent work in transgenic mice and human molecular genetic studies strongly supports a model based on the importance of direct interaction between PrP molecules (Prusiner *et al.* 1990; Weissmann 1991; Palmer *et al.* 1991). The idea is that PrP^{Sc} may, by dimerization or more complex interaction with PrP^C, act as a template, thereby catalysing the conversion of PrP^C to PrP^{Sc} (Fig. 1.1A). When inoculated into a recipient, PrP^{Sc} sets off a chain reaction with progressively more of the cellular PrP^C being sequestered into the abnormal, protease-resistant isoform which accumulates and may form amyloid. It is argued that the effect of PrP mutations is to render the mutant PrP^C inherently unstable so that the conversion to PrP^{Sc} occurs spontaneously at some time during the lifetime of the individual, setting off the chain reaction of conversion as before (Fig. 1.1B). Once initiated, brain tissue from such inherited cases could then pass on this process to a normal individual by inoculation. Such a disease model, although unprecedented, does not challenge fundamental biological principles. The prion does not need an independent genome; rather, prion replication occurs by catalytic modification of cellular PrP.

A key piece of supporting evidence for the above model is the finding that the large majority of cases of classical sporadic CJD are homozygous with respect to a

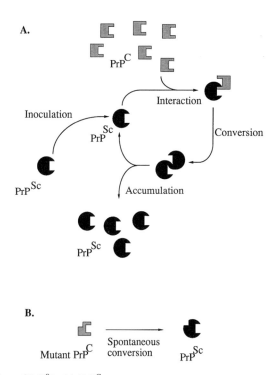

Fig. 1.1   Interaction of PrP^{Sc} with PrP^C.

common protein polymorphism in PrP (Palmer *et al.* 1991). Residue 129 of PrP can be either methionine or valine and nearly all classical sporadic CJD cases are either methionine or valine homozygotes, while in the normal Caucasian population the gene frequencies are estimated as 38% methionine homozygotes, 11% valine homozygotes and 51% heterozygotes. This importance of PrP sequence homology is further emphasized by the observation in some families with inherited prion diseases that the age at onset is later in individuals heterozygous at codon 129 than in homozygotes (Baker *et al.* 1991; Dlouhy *et al.* 1992; Poulter *et al.* 1992).

A 'unified theory' of prion propagation has been proposed to accommodate both the proteinaceous nature of the infectious agent and the existence of strain variation (Weissmann 1991*b*). This model assumes that the proteinaceous component (designated the apoprion), while capable of mediating the infectious process independently, can also associate with a small nucleic acid within the host cell (the co-prion). This co-prion could confer strain-specific information to the combined infectious agent (the holoprion). Infection of an animal with the holoprion of a particular strain type could give rise to a new host-modified strain by the coupling of newly generated apoprions with a new co-prion from the host. A prediction of this model is that removal of the co-prion from holoprions would result in loss of strain-specific properties. Similarly, the strain-specific properties of one strain could be conferred on another by substitution of its co-prion by that of the other strain. According to this model, infectivity would be resistant to treatments which inactivated nucleic acids, but strain-specific properties would not. No such studies have yet been published but the observation of the acquisition of strain-specific features of PrP^{Sc} *in vitro* (Bessen *et al.* 1995) (see Chapter 6) suggests that strain-specific information may be carried within the protein itself and may not require additional nucleic acids.

In 1992, Weissmann and colleagues reported the successful 'knockout' of the mouse PrP gene (Bueler *et al.* 1992). In view of the high degree of evolutionary conservation of PrP and its expression during early development in the mouse (Manson *et al.* 1992), it was widely anticipated that mice lacking PrP would have a severe phenotype. In fact, these mice both developed and behaved normally (Büeler *et al.* 1992). However, the viability of these PrP null mice allowed a key experiment to be performed, namely the challenge of the mice with scrapie. Such PrP null mice are entirely resistant to scrapie (Büeler *et al.* 1993; Prusiner *et al.* 1993).

Overexpression in transgenic mice of normal hamster or murine prion proteins to very high levels results in a necrotizing myopathy involving skeletal muscle, a demyelinating polyneuropathy, and focal vacuolation of the central nervous system (Westaway *et al.* 1994) and transmission from such mice has been achieved in a few cases. These and other transgenic models are described in Chapter 5.

The cell biology of prion protein has been addressed in a number of tissue culture systems. Mouse neuroblastoma cells can be infected with hamster scrapie and maintain infectivity *in vitro* indefinitely (Caughey *et al.* 1989; Borchelt *et al.* 1990, 1992). Metabolic labelling studies demonstrate that PrP^{Sc} derives from PrP^{C}, though whether all PrP^{C} is available for conversion or only a subset can be converted remains unclear (Borchelt *et al.* 1990; Caughey and Raymond 1991). The site of conversion is also unknown but there is evidence that protease resistance may be acquired in the endocytic pathway following the recycling of normal PrP^C from the cell surface (Lazlo *et al.* 1992). It has been possible to transfect neuroblastomas that are infected with mouse scrapie with mutant PrP transgenes to determine which components of the molecule are required for conversion to a protease-resistant phenotype (Rogers *et al.* 1993). Modifications including removal of the glycosylation sites, the glycosylphosphatidyl inositol anchor or the amino-terminal residues that include an octapeptide repeat region, have not prevented the formation of protease-resistant protein, suggesting that many truncated or variant constructs may be converted.

Attempts to catalogue post-translational modifications between PrP^{Sc} and PrP^C have failed to show any consistent covalent differences; PrP^C and PrP^{Sc} are therefore assumed to be conformational isomers and much work is focusing on determining the tertiary structures of these isoforms. Such studies have been limited by the high degree of insolubility of PrP^{Sc} and the difficulty obtaining large quantities of PrP^C in its native state. Studies so far have used synthetic peptide fragments corresponding to regions of PrP that are predicted, from secondary structure prediction algorithms, to adopt α-helical structures (Gasset *et al.* 1992; Goldfarb *et al.* 1993). Four regions are thought from sequence alignment predictions to adopt an α-helix, but the synthetic peptides corresponding to three of these adopt a β-sheet conformation as determined by infrared spectroscopy and their affinity for Congo red. Additionally, secondary structure content of PrP^C and PrP^{Sc} has been studied by spectroscopic methods. These studies provide support for a conformational difference between the two isoforms, since PrP^C is rich in α-helical structure whereas, as would be expected from its propensity to form amyloid, PrP^{Sc} contains largely β-sheet structure (Pan *et al.* 1993). It will be of considerable importance to determine high-resolution tertiary structures of PrP to further understand the molecular basis of prions and prion propagation.

For many, a direct proof of the protein-only hypothesis would require demonstration of production of infectivity *in vitro* from highly purified recombinant-derived PrP. The production of protease-resistant PrP *in vitro* has now been reported (Kocisko *et al.* 1994). However, since a large excess of PrP^{Sc} was required to drive this conversion reaction, it has not been possible to determine whether infectivity has been generated in such experiments. The biophysics of the prion protein is reviewed in Chapter 7.

Despite the wealth of evidence indicating the central role of PrP in these diseases, the normal cellular function remains unclear. Mice homozygous for PrP null alleles appear to develop and behave normally (Büeler *et al.* 1992). However, electrophysiological studies have demonstrated impaired $GABA_A$-mediated synaptic inhibition in hippocampal brain slices maintained *in vitro* and reduced long-term potentiation (Collinge *et al.* 1994; Manson *et al.* 1995). These abnormalities of synaptic inhibition are reminiscent of the neurophysiological abnormalities seen in patients with CJD and in scrapie-infected mice (Jeffreys *et al.* 1994), raising the possibility that prion neurodegeneration may be, at least in part, due to loss of PrP function rather than to a deleterious effect of PrP^{Sc} (Collinge *et al.* 1994). The relative normality of PrP null mice, which do not develop progressive neurodegeneration, may be the result of adaptive changes during neurodevelopment.

The prion hypothesis has been seen by some as a challenge to the central dogma of 20th century biology, namely that the informational molecule for replicating organisms is nucleic acid. However, it is clear from the account presented in this short introduction that while the properties of these diseases are certainly bizarre, being both inherited and transmissible, and while the physicochemical properties of the infectious agent are most unusual, the mechanism by which a protein might replicate itself, by acting as a template for the conversion of a less stable conformation into this same conformation, is consistent with established biochemical principles.

Over the last few years, research on prions has led to the spongiform encephalopathies becoming probably the best understood of the neurodegenerative diseases. What then is a prion disease and how is it best defined? The understanding of the biology of these conditions is advancing quickly and it is important not to be dogmatic in such definitions. In the case of the human inherited prion diseases, the identification of a pathogenic PrP mutation represents the clearest etiological marker, however these constitute only a minority of cases. In most of the prion diseases, protease-resistant PrP can be demonstrated either by immunohistochemical identification of PrP amyloid or by immunoblotting of brain homogenates. However, apparent exceptions have been described (for example Collinge *et al.* 1995). It also appears that uncoupling of protease resistance and infectivity may occur (Xi *et al.* 1992). It has been suggested for this reason that infectious PrP be designated PrP*, while PrP^{Sc} refers to protease-resistant material which may or may not contain PrP* (Weissmann 1991*b*).

The process hypothesized to account for prion propagation may not be unique to PrP. Two other possible examples have been considered. First, the p53 protein associated with many tumours is known to adopt a different conformation when it possesses activating mutations lacking normal growth-suppressor function (Milner and Medcalf 1991). It has been demonstrated that mutant p53 can drive co-translated wild-type p53 into the mutant conformation. These different mutant forms can be distinguished by conformation-specific antibodies, which unfortunately do not exist for the prion protein. A second area of possible interest comes from yeast genetics in which two unrelated yeast phenotypes are recognized that are inherited in a non-mendelian fashion apparently as a cytoplasmic factor (Wickner 1994). In the case of the [URE3] mutant genetic crosses show that persistence of this phenotype is dependent upon the normal product of the Ure2 gene. Although there is not yet any direct protein evidence, a plausible explanation is that, like PrP^{Sc}, the [URE3] product is an abnormal conformation of the Ure2 product but propagates itself by converting the Ure2 product from the wild-type to the abnormal conformation. It is possible therefore that the mechanism proposed for the prion diseases may be of much wider relevance in pathobiology. However, to be as transmissible, such proteins, like PrP^{Sc}, would need to be sufficiently stable in the environment (and in the gastrointestinal tract) to reach their cellular target in another host. The detection of other hypothetical prion diseases may therefore only be possible in specific experimental conditions.

Once the precise molecular mechanism of the production of PrP^{Sc} is determined it may be possible to produce a more precise definition of prion disease based on principles that may be of significance for other neurological and non-neurological disorders. Whether inherited, sporadic, or iatrogenic, prion diseases appear to be diseases of protein folding and protein interaction. Ultimately our understanding of the mechanism of conformational change and prion interactions should make it possible to design ligands that will interfere with this process and provide a basis for novel therapeutic strategies. This bizarre group of rare diseases may become the first neurodegenerative disorders for which rational pharmacological treatments become available.

References

Adams, D. H., Caspary, E. A., and Field, E. J. (1969). Susceptibility of scrapie agent to ionizing radiation. *Nature*, **221**, 90–91.

Alper, T. (1985). Scrapie agent unlike viruses in size and susceptibility to inactivation by ionizing or ultraviolet radiation. *Nature*, **317**, 750.

Alper, T., Haig, D. A., and Clarke, M. C. (1966). The exceptionally small size of the scrapie agent. *Biochemical and Biophysical Research Communications*, **22**, 278–284.

Alper, T., Haig, D. A., and Clarke, M. C. (1978). The scrapie agent: evidence against its dependence for replication on intrinsic nucleic acid. *Journal of General Virology*, **41**, 503–516.

Alpers, M. (1970). Kuru in New Guinea: its changing pattern and etiologic elucidation. *American Journal of Tropical Medicine and Hygiene*, **19**, 133–137.

Baker, H. E., Poulter, M., Crow, T. J., Frith, C. D., Lofthouse, R., Ridley, R. M., and Collinge, J. (1991). Aminoacid polymorphism in human prion protein and age at death in inherited prion disease. *Lancet*, **337**, 1286.

Baldwin, M. A., Stahl, N., Reinders, L. G., Gibson, B. W., Prusiner, S. B., and Burlingame, A. L. (1990). Permethylation and tandem mass spectrometry of oligosaccharides having free hexosamine: analysis of the glycoinositol phospholipid anchor glycan from the scrapie prion protein. *Analytical Biochemistry*, **191**, 174–182.

Beck, E. and Daniel, P. M. (1969). EEG changes in subacute encephalopathy (Creutzfeldt–Jakob disease). *Electroencephalography and Clinical Neurophysiology*, **27**, 217.

Bessen, R. A., Kocisko, D. A., Raymond, G. J., Nandan, S., Lansbury, P. T., and Caughey, B. (1995). Non-genetic propagation of strain-specific properties of scrapie prion protein. *Nature*, **375**, 698–700.

Borchelt, D. R., Scott, M., Taraboulos, A., Stahl, N., and Prusiner, S. B. (1990). Scrapie and cellular prion proteins differ in their kinetics of synthesis and topology in cultured cells. *Journal of Cell Biology*, **110**, 743–752.

Borchelt, D. R., Taraboulos, A., and Prusiner, S. B. (1992). Evidence for synthesis of scrapie prion proteins in the endocytic pathway. *Journal of Biological Chemistry*, **267**, 16188–16199.

Brown, P., Cathala, F., Raubertas, R. F., Gajdusek, D. C., and Castaigne, P. (1987). The epidemiology of Creutzfeldt–Jakob disease: conclusion of a 15-year investigation in France and review of the world literature. *Neurology*, **37**, 895–904.

Bruce, M. E. (1993). Scrapie strain variation and mutation. *British Medical Bulletin*, **49**, 822–838.

Bruce, M., Chree, A., McConnel, I., Foster, J., Pearson, G., and Fraser, H. (1994). Transmission of bovine spongiform encephalopathy and scrapie to mice: strain variation and the species barrier. *Philosophical Transactions of the Royal Society, London*, Series B, **343**, 405–411.

Büeler, H., Fischer, M., Lang, Y., Bluethmann, H., Lipp, H. P., DeArmond, S. J., et al. (1992). Normal development and behaviour of mice lacking the neuronal cell-surface PrP protein. *Nature*, **356**, 577–582.

Büeler, H., Aguzzi, A., Sailer, A., Greiner, R. A., Autenried, P., Aguet, M., et al. (1993). Mice devoid of PrP are resistant to scrapie. *Cell*, **73**, 1339–1347.

Caughey, B. and Raymond, G. J. (1991). The scrapie-associated form of PrP is made from a cell surface precursor that is both protease- and phospholipase-sensitive. *Journal of Biological Chemistry*, **266**, 18217–18223.

Caughey, B., Race, R. E., Ernst, D., Buchmeier, M. J., and Chesebro, B. (1989). Prion protein biosynthesis in scrapie-infected and uninfected neuroblastoma cells. *Journal of Virology*, **63**, 175–181.

Chandler, R. (1961). Encephalopathy in mice produced by inoculation with scrapie brain material. *Lancet*, **i**, 1378–1379.

Chandler, R. (1963). Experimental scrapie in the mouse. *Research in Veterinary Science*, **4**, 276–285.

Chesebro, B., Race, R., Wehrly, K., Nishio, J., Bloom, M., Lechner, D., et al. (1985). Identification of scrapie prion protein-specific mRNA in scrapie-infected and uninfected brain. *Nature*, **315**, 331–333.

Collinge, J., Whittington, M., Sidle, K., Smith, C., Palmer, M., Clarke, A. et al. (1994). Prion protein is necessary for normal synaptic function. *Nature*, **370**, 295–297.

Collinge, J., Palmer, M., Sidle, K., Gowland, I., Medori, R., Ironside, J. et al. (1995). Transmission of fatal familial insomnia to laboratory animals. *Lancet*, **346**, 569–570.

Cuillé, J. and Chelle, P. -L. (1936). La maladie dite tremblante du mouton, est-elle inoculable? *Comptes rendu de l'Academie des Sciences*, **203**, 1552–1554.

Cuillé, J. and Chelle, P. (1939). Transmission expérimental de la tremblante chez la chévre. *Comptes rendu de l'Academie des Sciences*, **208**, 1058–1060.

Delahousse, J., Petit, H., and Warot, P. (1971). Scrapie in immunologically deficient mice. *Nature*, **233**, 336.

Dickinson, A. and Meikle, V. (1971). Host-genotype and agent effects in scrapie incubation change in allelic interaction with different strains of agent. *Molecular and General Genetics*, **72,** 595–603.

Dickinson, A. G. and Outram, G. W. (1988). Genetic aspects of unconventional virus infections: the basis of the virino hypothesis. *Ciba Foundation Symposium*, **135**, 63–83.

Dickinson, A. G., Young, G. B., Stamp, J. T., and Renwick, C. C. (1967). Cannibalism in the Kuru region of New Guinea. *Transactions of the New York Academy of Sciences*, **29**, 748–754.

Diener, T. O. (1973). Kuru and Creutzfeldt–Jakob disease: experimental models of noninflammatory degenerative slow virus disease of the central nervous system. *Annals of Clinical Research*, **5**, 254–261.

Dlouhy, S. R., Hsiao, K., Farlow, M. R., Foroud, T., Conneally, P. M., Johnson, P., et al. (1992). Linkage of the Indiana kindred of Gerstmann–Sträussler–Scheinker disease to the prion protein gene. *Nature Genetics*, **1**, 64–67.

Field, E. J. (1970). EEG differential diagnosis of Jakob–Creutzfeldt disease. *Electroencephalography and Clinical Neurophysiology*, **28**, 327.

Foster, J. D. and Dickinson, A. G. (1988). The unusual properties of CH1641, a sheep-passaged isolate of scrapie. *Veterinary Record*, **123**, 5–8.

Gajdusek, D., Gibbs, C., and Alpers, M. (1965). Slow, latent and temperate viral infections. *NINDB Monograph No 2, Public Health Service Publication No 1378*, US Government Printing Office, Washington DC.

Gajdusek, D. C., Gibbs, C. J., and Alpers, M. (1966a). Experimental 'kuru' in chimpanzees: a pathological report. *Lancet*, **ii**, 1056–1059.

Gajdusek, D. C., Gibbs, C. J., and Alpers, M. (1966b). Experimental transmission of a kuru-like syndrome to chimpanzees. *Nature*, **209**, 794–796.

Gambetti, P., Petersen, R., Monari, L., Tabaton, M., Autilio, G. L., Cortelli, P., et al. (1993). Fatal familial insomnia and the widening spectrum of prion diseases. *British Medical Bulletin*, **49**, 980–994.

Gasset, M., Baldwin, M. A., Lloyd, D. H., Gabriel, J.-M., Holtzman, D. M., Cohen, F., et al. (1992). Predicted α-helical regions of the prion protein when synthesized as peptides from amyloid. *Proceedings of the National Academy of Sciences of the USA*, **89**, 10940–10944.

Gibbons, R. and Hunter, G. (1967). Nature of the scrapie agent. *Nature*, **215**, 1041–1043.

Gibbs, C. J., Gajdusek, D. C., Asher, D. M., Alpers, M. P., Beck, E., Daniel, P. M. et al. (1968). Creutzfeldt–Jakob disease (spongiform encephalopathy): transmission to the chimpanzee. *Science*, **161**, 388–389.

Glasse, R. and Lindenbaum, S. (1992). Fieldwork in the South Fore: the process of ethno-geographic inquiry. In *Prion diseases in humans and animals* (ed. S. Prusiner, J. Collinge, J. Powell, and B. Anderton), pp. 77–91. Ellis Horwood, London.

Goldfarb, L. G., Brown, P., Haltia, M., Ghiso, J., Frangione, B., and Gajdusek, D. C. (1993). Synthetic peptides corresponding to different mutated regions of the amyloid gene in familial Creutzfeldt–Jakob disease show enhanced in vitro formation of morphologically different amyloid fibrils. *Proceedings of the National Academy of Sciences of the USA*, **90**, 4451–4454.

Gordon, W. (1946). Advances in veterinary research. *Veterinary Research*, **58**, 516–520.

Griffiths, J. (1967). Self replication and scrapie. *Nature*, **215**, 1043–1044.

Hadlow, W. J. (1959). Scrapie and kuru. *Lancet*, **ii**, 289–290.

Hartsough, G. and Burger, D. (1965). Encephalopathy of mink. I. Epizootiologic and clinical observations. *Journal of Infectious Diseases*, **115**, 387–392.

Hsiao, K., Baker, H. F., Crow, T. J., Poulter, M., Owen, F., Terwilliger, J. D., et al. (1989). Linkage of a prion protein missense variant to Gerstmann–Sträussler syndrome. *Nature*, **338**, 342–345.

Hsiao, K. K., Scott, M., Foster, D., Groth, D. F., DeArmond, S. J., and Prusiner, S. B. (1990). Spontaneous neurodegeneration in transgenic mice with mutant prion protein. *Science*, **250**, 1587–1590.

Hsiao, K. K., Groth, D., Scott, M., Yang, S., Serban, H., Rapp, D., et al. (1994). Serial transmission in rodents of neurodegeneration from transgenic mice expressing mutant prion protein. *Proceedings of the National Academy of Sciences of the USA*, **91**, 9126–9130.

Hunter, G. D., Gibbons, R. A., Kimberlin, R. H., and Millson, G. C. (1969). Further studies of the infectivity and stability of extracts and homogenates derived from scrapie affected mouse brains. *Journal of Comparative Pathology*, **79**, 101–108.

Jefferys, J., Empson, R., Whittington, M., and Prusiner, S. (1994). Scrapie infection of transgenic mice leads to network and intrinsic dysfunction of cortical and hippocampal neurones. *Neurobiology of Disease*, **1**, 25–30.

Kellings, K., Prusiner, S. B., and Riesner, D. (1994). Nucleic acids in prion preparations: unspecific background or essential component. *Philosophical Transactions of The Royal Society of London (Biology)*, **343**, 425–430.

Kimberlin, R. H. and Hunter, G. D. (1967). DNA synthesis in scrapie-affected mouse brain. *Journal of General Virology*, **1**, 115–124.

Kimberlin, R. H. and Walker, C. A. (1978). Evidence that the transmission of one source of scrapie agent to hamsters involves separation of agent strains from a mixture. *Journal of General Virology*, **39**, 487–496.

Kimberlin, R. H., Cole, S., and Walker, C. A. (1987). Temporary and permanent modifications to a single strain of mouse scrapie on transmission to rats and hamsters. *Journal of General Virology*, **68**, 1875–1881.

Klatzo, I., Gajdusek, D. C., and Zigas, V. (1959). Pathology of kuru. *Laboratory Investigations*, **8**, 799–847.

Kocisko, D., Come, J., Priola, S., Chesebro, B., Raymond, G., Lansbury, P. *et al.* (1994). Cell free formation of protease-resistant prion protein. *Nature*, **370**, 471–474.

Laszlo, L., Lowe, J., Self, T., Kenward, N., Landon, M., McBride, T., *et al.* (1992). Lysosomes as key organelles in the pathogenesis of prion encephalopathies. *Journal of Pathology*, **166**, 333–341.

Leopoldt, J. (1759). *Nützliche und auf die Erfahrung gegründete Einleitung zu der Landwirtshaft*, Part 5, Chapter 12, pp. 344–360. Glogau, Berlin.

Lugaresi, E., Medori, R., Baruzzi, P. M., Cortelli, P., Lugaresi, A., Tinuper, P., *et al.* (1986). Fatal familial insomnia and dysautonomia, with selective degeneration of thalamic nuclei. *New England Journal of Medicine*, **315**, 997–1003.

Manson, J., West, J. D., Thomson, V., McBride, P., Kaufman, M. H., and Hope, J. (1992). The prion protein gene: a role in mouse embryogenesis? *Development*, **115**, 117–122.

Manson, J. C., Hope, J., Clarke, A. R., Johnston, A., Black, C., and MacLeod, N. (1995). PrP gene dosage and long term potentiation. *Neurodegeneration*, **4**, 113–114.

Marsh, R. (1992). Transmissible mink encephalopathy. In *Prion diseases of humans and animals* (ed. S. Prusiner, J. Collinge, J. Powell, and B. Anderton), pp. 300–307. Ellis Horwood, London.

Masters, C. L., Gajdusek, D. C., and Gibbs, C. J., Jr (1981). Creutzfeldt–Jakob disease virus isolations from the Gerstmann–Sträussler syndrome with an analysis of the various forms of amyloid plaque deposition in the virus-induced spongiform encephalopathies. *Brain*, **104**, 559–588.

McGowan, J. (1922). Scrapie in sheep. *Scottish Journal of Agriculture*, **5**, 365–375.

Medori, R., Montagna, P., Tritschler, H. J., LeBlanc, A., Cortelli, P., Tinuper, P., *et al.* (1992*a*). Fatal familial insomnia: a second kindred with mutation of prion protein gene at codon 178. *Neurology*, **42**, 669–670.

Medori, R., Tritschler, H. J., LeBlanc, A., Villare, F., Manetto, V., Chen, H. Y., *et al.* (1992*b*). Fatal familial insomnia, a prion disease with a mutation at codon 178 of the prion protein gene. *New England Journal of Medicine*, **326**, 444–449.

Millson, G. C., Hunter, G. D., and Kimberlin, R. H. (1976). The physico-chemical nature of the scrapie agent. *Frontiers in Biology*, **44**, 243–266.

Milner, J. and Medcalf, E. A. (1991). Cotranslation of activated mutant p53 with wild type drives the wild type p53 protein into the mutant conformation. *Cell*, **65**, 765–774.

Mori, S., Hamada, C., Kumanishi, T., Fukuhara, N., Ichihashi, Y., Ikuta, F., *et al.* (1989). A Creutzfeldt–Jakob disease agent (Echigo-1 strain) recovered from brain tissue showing the 'panencephalopathic type' disease. *Neurology*, **39**, 1337–1342.

Oesch, B., Westaway, D., Walchli, M., McKinley, M. P., Kent, S. B., Aebersold, R., *et al.* (1985). A cellular gene encodes scrapie PrP 27–30 protein. *Cell*, **40**, 735–746.

Owen, F., Poulter, M., Lofthouse, R., Collinge, J., Crow, T. J., Risby, D., *et al.* (1989). Insertion in prion protein gene in familial Creutzfeldt–Jakob disease. *Lancet*, **i**, 51–52.

Palmer, M. S., Dryden, A. J., Hughes, J. T., and Collinge, J. (1991). Homozygous prion protein genotype predisposes to sporadic Creutzfeldt–Jakob disease. *Nature*, **352**, 340–342.

Pan, K. M., Baldwin, M., Nguyen, J., Gasset, M., Serban, A., Groth, D., *et al.* (1993). Conversion of alpha-helices into beta-sheets features in the formation of the scrapie prion proteins. *Proceedings of the National Academy of Sciences of the USA*, **90**, 10962–10966.

Parry, H. (1962). Scrapie, a transmissible and hereditary disease of sheep. *Heredity*, **17**, 75–105.

Pattison, I. (1965). Resistance of the scrapie agent to formalin. *Journal of Comparative Pathology*, **75**, 159–164.

Pattison, I. and Millson, G. (1961). Scrapie produced experimentally in goats with special reference to the clinical syndrome. *Journal of Comparative Pathology*, **71**, 101–108.

Pattison, I. H. and Jones, K. M. (1967). The possible nature of the transmissible agent of scrapie. *Veterinary Record*, **80**, 2–9.

Pattison, I. H. and Jones, K. M. (1968). A medical hazard of cannibalism. *Canadian Medical Association Journal*, **99**, 866.

Pattison, I., Gordon, W., and Millson, G. (1959). Experimental production of scrapie in goats. *Journal of Comparative Pathology*, **69**, 300–312.

Poulter, M., Baker, H. F., Frith, C. D., Leach, M., Lofthouse, R., Ridley, R. M., *et al.* (1992). Inherited prion disease with 144 base pair gene insertion: I: Genealogical and molecular studies. *Brain*, **115**, 675–685.

Prusiner, S. B. (1982). Novel proteinaceous infectious particles cause scrapie. *Science*, **216**, 136–144.

Prusiner, S. B., Bolton, D. C., Groth, D. F., Bowman, K. A., Cochran, S. P., and McKinley, M. P. (1982). Further purification and characterization of scrapie prions. *Biochemistry*, **21**, 6942–6950.

Prusiner, S. B., Scott, M., Foster, D., Pan, K. M., Groth, D., Mirenda, C., *et al.* (1990). Transgenetic studies implicate interactions between homologous PrP isoforms in scrapie prion replication. *Cell*, **63**, 673–686.

Prusiner, S. B., Groth, D., Serban, A., Koehler, R., Foster, D., Torchia, M., *et al.* (1993). Ablation of the prion protein (PrP) gene in mice prevents scrapie and facilitates production of anti-PrP antibodies. *Proceedings of the National Academy of Sciences of the USA*, **90**, 10608–10612.

Robakis, N. K., Devine, G. E., Jenkins, E. C., Kascsak, R. J., Brown, W. T., Krawczun, M. S., *et al.* (1986). Localization of a human gene homologous to the PrP gene on the p arm of chromosome 20 and detection of PrP-related antigens in normal human brain. *Biochemical and Biophysics Research Communications*, **140**, 758–765.

Rogers, M., Yehiely, F., Scott, M., and Prusiner, S. B. (1993). Conversion of truncated and elongated prion proteins into the scrapie isoform in cultured cells *Proceedings of the National Academy of Sciences of the USA*, **90**, 3182–3186.

Stahl, N., Baldwin, M. A., Burlingame, A. L., and Prusiner, S. B. (1990). Identification of glycoinositol phospholipid linked and truncated forms of the scrapie prion protein. *Biochemistry*, **29**, 8879–8884.

Stahl, N., Baldwin, M. A., Hecker, R., Pan, K. M., Burlingame, A. L., and Prusiner, S. B. (1992). Glycosylinositol phospholipid anchors of the scrapie and cellular prion proteins contain sialic-acid. *Biochemistry*, **31**, 5043–5053.

Stahl, N., Baldwin, M. A., Teplow, D. B., Hood, L., Gibson, B. W., Burlingame, A. L., *et al.* (1993). Structural studies of the scrapie prion protein using mass-spectrometry and amino-acid sequencing. *Biochemistry*, **32**, 1991–2002.

Stamp, J. T. (1967). Nature of the scrapie agent. *Nature*, **215**, 1041–1043.

Tateishi, J., Brown, P., and Kitamoto, T. (1995). First experimental transmission of fatal familial insomnia. *Nature*, **376**, 434–435.

Weissmann, C. (1991*a*). Spongiform encephalopathies: the prion's progress. *Nature*, **349**, 569–571.

Weissmann, C. (1991*b*). A 'unified theory' of prion propagation. *Nature*, **352**, 679–683.

Westaway, D., DeArmond, S. J., Cayetano, C. J., Groth, D., Foster, D., Yang, S. L., *et al.* (1994). Degeneration of skeletal muscle, peripheral nerves, and the central nervous system in transgenic mice overexpressing wild-type prion proteins. *Cell*, **76**, 117–129.

Wickner, R. B. (1994). [URE3] as an altered URE2 protein: evidence for a prion analog in *Saccharomyces cerevisiae*. *Science*, **264**, 566–569.

Wilesmith, J. W. (1993). Epidemiology of bovine spongiform encephalopathy and related diseases. *Archives of Virology*, Supplement **7**, 245–254.

Williams, E. and Young, S. (1980). Chronic wasting disease of captive mule deer: a spongiform encephalopathy. *Journal of Wildlife Diseases*, **16**, 89–98.

Xi, Y. G., Ingrosso, L., Ladogana, A., Masullo, C., and Pocchiari, M. (1992). Ampothericin B treatment dissociates *in vivo* replication of the scrapie agent from PrP accumulation. *Nature*, **356**, 598–601.

Zigas, V. and Gajdusek, D. C. (1957). Kuru: clinical study of a new syndrome resembling paralysis agitans in natives of the Eastern Highlands of Australian New Guinea. *Medical Journal of Australia*, **2**, 745–754.

2 Human prion diseases

JOHN COLLINGE AND MARK S. PALMER

Introduction

The human prion diseases, previously known as the subacute spongiform encephalopathies, slow virus diseases, or transmissible dementias, have been traditionally classified into Creutzfeldt–Jakob disease (CJD), Gerstmann–Sträussler syndrome (GSS) (also known as Gerstmann–Sträussler–Scheinker disease), and kuru. They are rare neurodegenerative disorders affecting about one person per million world-wide per annum. Although this equates to only 50 or so new cases in the United Kingdom each year, remarkable attention has recently been focused on these diseases. This is because of their unique biology and also because of the fears that an epidemic of a newly recognized bovine prion disease—bovine spongiform encephalopathy (BSE)—among UK cattle could pose a threat to public health through dietary exposure to infected tissues.

Transmissibility of the human diseases to experimental animals was demonstrated with the transmission, by intracerebral inoculation with brain homogenates into chimpanzees, of first kuru and then CJD in 1966 and 1968, respectively (Gajdusek et al. 1966; Gibbs et al. 1968). Transmission of GSS followed in 1981 (Masters et al. 1981). The prototypic prion disease is the naturally occurring disease scrapie of sheep and goats, which has been recognized in the UK for over 200 years (McGowan 1922). Scrapie was demonstrated to be transmissible by inoculation in 1936 (Cuillé and Chelle 1936) and it was the recognition that histopathologically kuru, and then CJD, resembled scrapie that led to suggestions that these diseases may also be transmitted by inoculation (Hadlow 1959; Klatzo et al. 1959). Kuru is a neurodegenerative condition characterized principally by a progressive cerebellar ataxia, which reached epidemic proportions amongst the Fore linguistic group in the eastern highlands of Papua New Guinea and which was transmitted by cannibalism. Since the cessation of cannibalism in the 1950s the disease has declined but a few cases still occur as a result of the long incubation periods in this condition (Alpers 1987). The term Creutzfeldt–Jakob disease was introduced by Spielmeyer (1922), bringing together the case reports published by Creutzfeldt (1920) and Jakob (1921 a, b, c). Several of these cases would not meet modern diagnostic criteria for CJD and indeed it was not until the demonstration of transmissibility allowed diagnostic criteria to be reassessed and refined that a clear diagnostic entity developed. All these diseases share common histopathological features. The classical triad of spongiform vacuolation (affecting any part of the cerebral grey matter), astrocytic proliferation, and neuronal loss may be accompanied by the deposition of amyloid plaques (Beck and Daniel 1987).

Many of the key advances in understanding the pathogenesis of the prion diseases have come from study of the various forms of human prion disease. In particular, the recognition that the familial forms of the human diseases are autosomally dominantly inherited conditions, associated with coding mutations in the prion protein gene on chromosome 20p, as well as being transmissible to laboratory animals by inoculation, strongly supported by the contention that the transmissible agent, or prion, was composed principally of an abnormal isoform of prion protein. The epidemiology of the human prion diseases encompasses the three aetiological types of prion disease: inherited, sporadic, and acquired. Inherited cases constitute around 15% of cases, acquired cases are rare and include iatrogenic CJD as well as the now nearly extinct prion disease kuru. Most human cases are sporadic, and their precise aetiology is still unclear. The advances in understanding the molecular biology of these diseases, and in particular the availability of molecular genetic diagnostic markers has allowed appreciation of their remarkable phenotypic diversity at both the clinical and the histopathological levels and has extended the recognized disease spectrum beyond the classically syndromes of CJD, GSS, and kuru to what can now be defined as the human prion diseases.

Aetiology

The transmissible agent, or prion, seems to consist principally of an abnormal isoform of a host-encoded protein, the prion protein (PrP), designated PrP^{Sc}. PrP^{Sc} is known to be derived from the cellular isoform, PrP^{C}, by a post-translational mechanism and evidence is mounting that this change may be conformational rather than covalent (Gasset *et al.* 1993; Pan *et al.* 1993) (Fig. 2.1). While PrP^{C} is fully sensitive to proteolysis, PrP^{Sc}, which accumulates in the brain in disease (and may form amyloid), is partially protease resistant. The human PrP gene (*PRNP*) is a single-copy gene located on the short arm of chromosome 20 (Robakis *et al.* 1986) in a region syntenic with the murine PrP gene (*Prnp*) on chromosome 2; it spans 16 kb and contains two exons (Oesch *et al.* 1985; Kretzschmar *et al.* 1986). The complete open reading frame of 759 nucleotides is contained within the larger second exon which comprises the majority of the 2.4 kb mRNA. The PrP gene was an obvious candidate for genetic linkage studies in the familial forms of CJD and GSS, which both showed an autosomal dominant pattern of disease segregation. A turning point in understanding the human prion diseases was the identification of mutations in the prion protein gene in familial CJD and GSS in 1989. The first mutation to be identified in *PRNP* was in a family with CJD and involved a 144 bp insertion into the coding sequence (Owen *et al.* 1989). A second mutation was reported in two families with GSS and genetic linkage was confirmed between this missense variant at codon 102 and GSS, confirming that GSS was an autosomal dominant Mendelian disorder (Hsiao *et al.* 1989). This genetic variant was not present in the normal population but was rapidly identified in numerous other

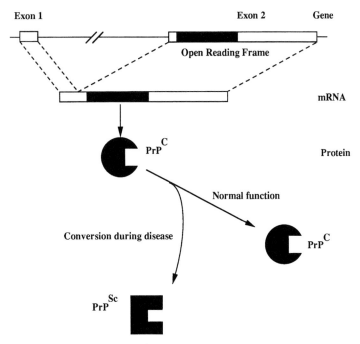

Fig. 2.1 Human prion protein gene expression. The coding sequence contained in a single open reading frame in exon 2. PrP^C, represented by the round symbol, is converted during the disease process to PrP^Sc, represented by the square symbol. The precise nature of this post-translational modification of PrP is unclear, but appears to involve a conformational change. PrP, prion protein; PrP^C, normal cellular isoform of PrP; PrP^Sc, disease related isoform of PrP; mRNA, messenger RNA.

unrelated GSS kindreds (Doh ura *et al.* 1989, 1990; Brown *et al.* 1991; Kretzschmar *et al.* 1991, 1992; Speer *et al.* 1991). On statistical grounds therefore it seemed likely that this mutation was causal for GSS in these families. Uniquely, these diseases are therefore both inherited and infectious. A whole family of PrP mutations was rapidly described by a number of groups (Figs 2.2 and 2.3). The availability of such direct gene markers allowed molecular diagnosis of cases and the identification of cases expressing phenotypes that differed markedly from CJD and GSS (Collinge *et al.* 1989, 1990). Indeed CJD- and GSS-like syndromes could co-exist in the same family and it was appreciated that they form part of a more extensive disease spectrum better referred to as inherited prion disease (Collinge *et al.* 1992). The combined LOD scores in these conditions now exceeds 30, confirming the initial suggestions that these are indeed inherited conditions, in addition to their transmissibility to experimental animals by inoculation.

Experimental confirmation of the pathogenicity of the codon 102 mutation was provided in 1990 by the demonstration that transgenic mice which overexpressed a murine prion protein with an analogous mutation spontaneously developed spongi-

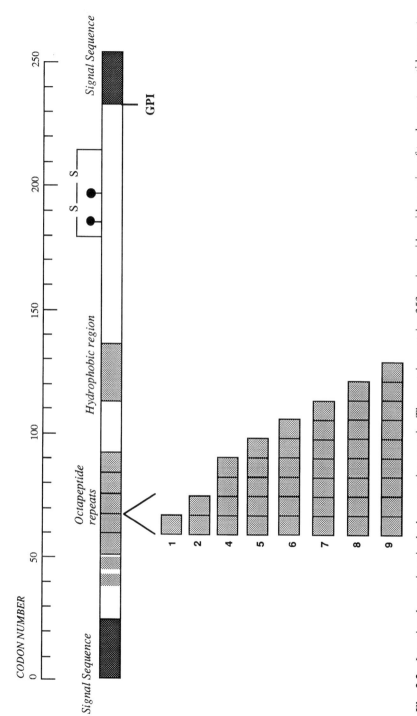

Fig. 2.2 Insertional mutations in the human prion protein. The protein contains 253 amino acids, with a series of tandem octapeptide repeats near the N terminal. Insertions of additional integral numbers of repeat elements are associated with some of the inherited prion diseases.

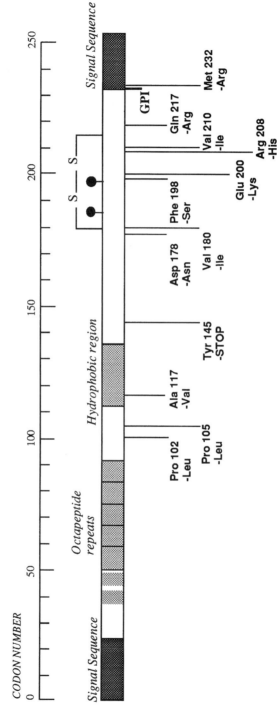

Fig. 2.3 Disease-related point mutations in the human prion protein. The complete protein of 253 amino acids is illustrated, the signal sequences are removed during processing and addition of the glycosylphosphatidylinositol anchor (GPI), which attaches the protein to the outer surface of the cell membrane. There is a single disulphide bond, indicated by –S–S–. The stick and ball symbols indicate glycosylation sites. Amino acid substitutions are indicated by three letter code.

form neurodegeneration (Hsiao *et al.* 1990). Further, brain tissue from such spontaneously sick transgenic animals can transmit the disease to wild-type hamsters and
transgenic mice with lower copy numbers of the same mutant transgene (Hsiao
et al. 1994). Therefore a transmissible disease has been produced by overexpression of a mutant prion protein.

Current evidence suggests that around 15% of prion diseases are inherited and at
least 18 coding mutations in *PRNP* are recognized. With the exception of the rare
iatrogenic CJD cases mentioned above, most prion disease occurs as sporadic CJD.
While, by definition, there will not be a family history in sporadic cases, mutations
are seen in occasional apparently sporadic cases, because with a late-onset disease
the family history may not be apparent or non-paternity may occur. However, in the
majority of sporadic CJD cases there is neither a coding mutation nor a history of
iatrogenic exposure. Human prion diseases can therefore be subdivided into inherited, sporadic, and acquired forms.

Genetic predisposition is, however, highly relevant to the aetiology of both
acquired and sporadic CJD. Study of seven CJD cases related to human pituitary
hormone revealed a significant excess of a valine 129 homozygous genotype
(Collinge *et al.* 1991*a*). There are two common forms of PrP in humans, with either
methionine or valine encoded at codon 129 (Fig. 2.4). In Caucasians around 51%
are heterozygotes while 38% are methionine homozygotes; the least common genotype is valine homozygous, around 11% of the population falling into this cate-
gory. Four of the seven cases studied were valine homozygotes. This suggested
that this genotype may render an individual more susceptible to prion disease on
challenge with the transmissible agent. Although the original study was based on a
small series (although including all reported UK cases at the time) this finding has
now been replicated in larger studies in the USA (Brown *et al.* 1994*a*) and France
(Laplanche *et al.* 1994).

A study of 22 clearly defined sporadic CJD cases revealed that all but one was a
homozygote either to methionine or valine (Palmer *et al.* 1991). While 51% of the
Caucasian population are heterozygous with respect to this polymorphism it seems
that the vast majority of people who develop classical sporadic CJD are homozygotes. This finding has been borne out in other studies (Laplanche *et al.* 1994;
Salvatore *et al.* 1994) and in a larger UK study (Windl *et al.*, in press).

In 1990, Prusiner and colleagues demonstrated that the species barrier to transmission of prion disease from hamsters to mice could be overcome by overexpressing normal hamster prion protein in transgenic mice (Prusiner *et al.* 1990).
Although prion diseases can be transmitted between mammalian species by inoculation, in practice it is difficult to do so. Typically, transmission occurs in only a
small proportion of inoculated animals and then only after prolonged incubation
periods. When such transgenic mice were challenged with mouse-derived prions,
the infectivity they produced was fully pathogenic for mice but not hamsters, while
on challenge with hamster-derived prions they produced prions fully pathogenic
for hamsters but not mice. The interpretation of this finding is that a direct interaction between PrP molecules occurs at some stage in the process of prion propaga-

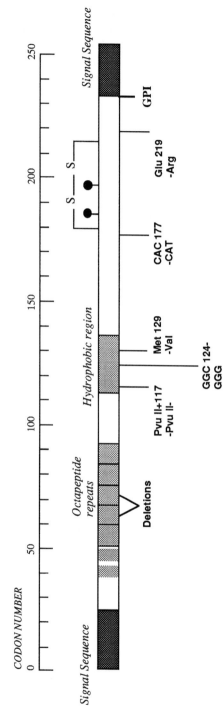

Fig. 2.4 Non-coding and coding polymorphisms in the human prion protein. Amino acid changes are indicated by three letter code (see text for details). The residue 129 polymorphism plays an important part in genetic susceptibility to prion diseases. The other changes appear at the same frequency in patients and controls and have not been clearly linked with susceptibility to disease or modification of disease phenotype.

tion and that such interaction occurs most easily if the interacting PrP molecules are identical. Since there are a number of amino acid differences between murine and hamster PrP, interaction between the two different forms would be less favoured. Such work has led to the idea that replication of prions may occur by the abnormal isoform of PrP, PrP^{Sc}, interacting directly with the normal cellular isoform, PrP^C to PrP^{Sc}. (Prusiner *et al.* 1990; Weissmann 1991) (see Chapter 1, Fig. 1.1(a)). Such an effect could then lead to a chain reaction with the progressive conversion of increasing amounts of PrP^C to PrP^{Sc}. This could then produce disease either by progressive loss of PrP function or alternatively by cellular damage resulting from accumulation of PrP^{Sc}.

Clearly, the implication is that the pathogenic mutations in the prion protein result in the production of a protein that may convert spontaneously to PrP^{Sc} in individuals with inherited prion diseases (see Chapter 1, Fig. 1.1(b)). This PrP^{Sc} will then produce the same catalytic chain reaction as hypothesized in cases where PrP^{Sc} is inoculated. Such a model provides an explanation of how a disease can be simultaneously inherited and transmissible. The finding that nearly all sporadic CJD occurs in homozygotes with respect to a common and apparently innocent protein polymorphism lends strong support to such a mechanism (Palmer *et al.* 1991). Again, prion protein interaction would occur most favourably in individuals with two identical copies of the prion protein. Heterozygotes, producing two different proteins, would be somewhat protected, as if by an internal 'species barrier'. It is possible that the occasional individuals heterozygous at codon 129 who do develop sporadic CJD have a more prolonged illness, but more detailed studies are required to investigate this further. Additional evidence for this model is provided by the observation that in one of the inherited prion diseases, onset of the disease occurs one to two decades later in individuals heterozygous at codon 129 (Baker *et al.* 1991). This effect has now also been reported in another inherited prion disease kindred with a different *PRNP* mutation (Dlouhy *et al.* 1992).

PrP valine 129 and PrP methionine 129 would be expected to differ slightly in their propensity to convert to PrP^{Sc}. The excess of PrP valine 129 homozygotes amongst human pituitary hormone related cases suggests that PrP valine 129 may be the more susceptible (Collinge *et al.* 1991*a*).

It is of particular interest that mice heterozygous for a PrP null allele, which produce around 50% of the normal amount of PrP, have very prolonged incubation periods and then develop a much more slowly progressive illness than wild-type mice (Bueler *et al.* 1993, 1995). This finding may be relevant to homozygosity in sporadic CJD where the presence of two different prion proteins, in heterozygotes at codon 129, may result in a similar situation, the disease process occurring only between homologous molecules present at 50% of the normal level.

The aetiology of sporadic CJD remains unclear. It has been speculated that these cases might arise from somatic mutation of *PRNP* or spontaneous conversion of PrP^C to PrP^{Sc} as a rare stochastic event. The alternative hypothesis, that such cases arise as a result of exposure to an environmental source of either human or animal prions, is not supported by epidemiological evidence (Brown *et al.* 1987). Since transgenic mice expressing extremely high levels of wild-type hamster or murine PrP develop a spontaneous neuromuscular disease (Westaway *et al.* 1994), which appears to be transmissible, it has also been suggested that some cases of sporadic CJD may arise as a result of PrP overexpression.

The clinical syndromes of human prion disease

The human prion diseases have been classically divided into Creutzfeldt–Jakob disease (CJD), Gerstmann–Sträussler–Scheinker syndrome (GSS), and kuru. With the advances in our understanding of the aetiology of these conditions it now seems more appropriate to divide the human prion disease into inherited, sporadic, and acquired forms (see Table 2.1) with CJD, GSS, and kuru now seen as clinicopathological syndromes within a wider spectrum of disease.

Kindreds with inherited prion disease have been described with phenotypes of classical CJD, GSS, and with other neurodegenerative syndromes including fatal familial insomnia (Medori *et al.* 1992*a, b*). Some kindreds show remarkable phenotypic variability which can encompass both CJD- and GSS-like cases as well as other cases which do not conform to either CJD or GSS phenotypes (Collinge *et al.* 1992). Cases diagnosed by PrP gene analysis have been reported which are not only clinically atypical but lack the classical histological features entirely (Collinge *et al.* 1990). Significant clinical overlap exists with familial Alzheimer's disease, Pick's disease, frontal lobe degeneration of non-Alzheimer type, and amyotrophic lateral sclerosis with dementia. Although classical GSS is described below it now seems more sensible to designate the familial illnesses as inherited prion diseases

Table 2.1   Human prion diseases

Type	Clinical syndromes	Aetiology
Acquired	Kuru Iatrogenic CJD	Cannibalism Inoculation
Sporadic	CJD Atypical CJD	? Somatic *PRNP* mutation or spontaneous conversion of PrP^C to PrP^{Sc}
Inherited	Familial CJD GSS FFI Various atypical dementias	Germline *PRNP* mutation

CJD, Creutzfeldt–Jakob disease; GSS, Gerstmann–Sträussler–Scheinker disease; FFI, fatal familial insomnia; *PRNP*, human prion protein gene and to then sub-classify these according to mutation (see Figs 2.2 and 2.3). Acquired prion diseases include iatrogenic CJD and kuru. Sporadic prion diseases at present consist of CJD and atypical variants of CJD (which may be classified as CJD on the basis of transmissibility to primates). Cases lacking the characteristic histological features of CJD have been transmitted. As there is at present no equivalent aetiological diagnostic marker for sporadic prion diseases to those for the inherited diseases, it cannot yet be excluded that more diverse phenotypic variants of sporadic prion disease exist which may not be as easily transmissible to primates as cases with classical spongiform encephalopathy.

Sporadic prion disease

Creutzfeldt–Jakob disease

Epidemiology

Extensive epidemiological studies of CJD have been performed in a number of countries and all obtained broadly similar results (Brown *et al.* 1987). The overall annual incidence in most studies was around 0.5–1 case per million. There is no significant case clustering other than in familial clusters. Cases are distributed apparently at random with a frequency related only to local population density. In particular, there is no evidence for case-to-case spread (other than with respect to iatrogenic foci which are discussed below), and no evidence of an association with local scrapie prevalence. For instance, CJD is as common in Australia and New Zealand, which have been scrapie free for many years, as in the UK where scrapie is endemic. Numerous case–control studies have not shown consistent associations with particular occupational groups or dietary components. However, the BSE epidemic has led to renewed interest in this area and since 1990 an attempt has been made to monitor all suspected cases of CJD in the UK by the National CJD Surveillance Unit in Edinburgh (Will 1993). Parallel studies have commenced in a number of other European countries, some of which have recently reported BSE cases in their cattle population, and a co-ordinated study of CJD epidemiology in the EU is in progress (Brown *et al.* 1987). While these large-scale prospective studies have generated an enormous body of experience of this rare disease, overall incidence figures do not appear to have risen more in the UK than in countries which do not have BSE. An overall increase in incidence has been noted in most of these surveillance programmes but this is thought to be due to increased identification of cases as so much attention is now being focused on these diseases. This may be particularly relevant to the increased incidence noted in the elderly, where other dementing illnesses are common. Although occasional weak statistical associations with particular foodstuffs are reported, these have tended to disappear in subsequent years of the study and no consistent new risk factors have emerged. Recently concern has been expressed about the occurrence of CJD in a number of dairy farmers in the UK (Gore 1995; Smith *et al.* 1995), in two teenagers (Britton *et al.* 1995; Bateman *et al.* 1995), and in a 28-year-old woman (Tabrizi *et al.* 1996). While the dairy farmers had a typical clinicopathological picture of sporadic CJD, the young cases had clinical and pathological features that were unusual and in some respects reminiscent of kuru. Further epidemiological surveillance revealed additional young cases early in 1996 and it was realized that these cases shared a previously unrecognized pattern of neuropathology (Will *et al.* 1996), raising the possibility that they were linked to BSE. This newly recognized variant of human prion disease will be discussed later.

Clinical features

The core clinical syndrome of CJD is of a rapidly progressive multifocal dementia usually with myoclonus. The onset is usually in the 45–75 year age group with peak onset between 60 and 65. The clinical progression is typically over weeks progressing to akinetic mutism and death, often within two to three months. Around 70% of cases die in under six months. Prodromal features, present in around a third of cases, include fatigue, insomnia, depression, weight loss, headaches, general malaise, and ill-defined pain sensations. In addition to mental deterioration and myoclonus, frequent additional neurological features include extrapyramidal signs, cerebellar ataxia, pyramidal signs, and cortical blindness. About 10% of cases present initially with cerebellar ataxia. Routine haematological and biochemical investigations are normal although occasional cases have been noted to have raised serum transaminases or alkaline phosphatase. There are no immunological markers and acute-phase proteins are not elevated. Examination of the cerebrospinal fluid is normal although raised neuronal-specific enolase, indicating loss of neurones, has been proposed as a useful marker. Neuroimaging with CT or MRI is useful to exclude other causes of subacute neurological illness but there are no diagnostic features. Cerebral and cerebellar atrophy may be present. The most useful investigation is the electroencephalogram (EEG) which may show characteristic pseudoperiodic sharp-wave activity (Fig. 2.5).

Prospective edpidemiological studies have demonstrated that cases with a progressive dementia and two or more of myoclonus, cortical blindness, pyramidal, cerebellar or extrapyramidal signs, or akinetic mutism with a typical EEG nearly always turn out to be confirmed as histologically definite CJD if neuropathological examination is performed.

Neuropathological confirmation of CJD is by demonstration of spongiform change, neuronal loss, and astrocytosis. PrP amyloid plaques are usually not present in CJD although protease-resistant PrP, seen in all the currently recognized prion diseases, can be demonstrated by immunoblotting of brain homogenates. Genetic susceptibility has been demonstrated in that most cases of classical CJD are homozygous with respect to a common protein polymorphism of PrP (see section on aetiology, above).

Atypical forms of Creutzfeldt–Jakob disease

Atypical forms of Creutzfeldt–Jakob disease are well recognized. Around 10% of cases have a longer clinical course of over two years (Brown *et al.* 1984). These cases may represent the occasional occurrence of CJD in individuals heterozygous for PrP polymorphisms (Collinge *et al.* 1994). Around 10% of CJD cases present

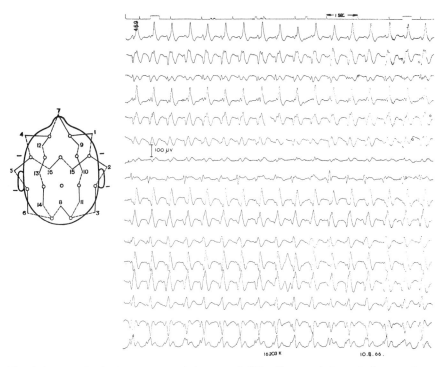

Fig. 2.5 The classical electroencephalogram of CJD. Characteristic periodic complexes occur at the rate of approximately two per second in a markedly abnormal background devoid of normal cerebral rhythms. (Kindly provided by Dr Shelagh Smith, National Hospital for Neurology and Neurosurgery.)

with cerebellar ataxia rather than cognitive impairment, so-called ataxic CJD (Gomori *et al.* 1973). Heidenhain's variant of CJD refers to cases in which cortical blindness predominates with severe involvement of the occipital lobes. The panencephalopathic type of CJD refers to cases with extensive degeneration of the cerebral white matter in addition to spongiform vacuolation of the grey matter and has been predominately reported in Japan (Gomori *et al.* 1973).

Amyotrophic variants of CJD have been described with prominent early muscle wasting. However, most cases of dementia with amyotrophy are not experimentally transmissible (Salazar *et al.* 1983) and their relationship with CJD is unclear. Most cases are probably variants of motor neurone disease with associated dementia. Amyotrophic features in CJD are usually seen in late disease when other features are well established.

Acquired prion diseases

While prion diseases can be transmitted to experimental animals by inoculation, it is important to appreciate that they are not contagious in humans. Documented

case-to-case spread has only occurred by cannibalism (kuru) or following accidental inoculation with prions (iatrogenic CJD).

Kuru

Although now nearly extinct, kuru remains of immense importance to an understanding of these diseases. In particular, studies of the kuru epidemic provide by far
the most extensive clinical experience of acquired prion disease in humans. The
epidemiology of kuru clearly indicates the infectious, but non-contagious, properties of prions and provides extensive evidence that vertical transmission from pregnant woman to child does not occur.

Epidemiology

Kuru reached epidemic proportions amongst a defined population living in the
Okapa district of the eastern highlands of Papua New Guinea. The earliest cases are
thought to date from the early part of the century (Scrimgeour *et al.* 1983). Kuru
affected the people of the Fore linguistic group and neighbours with whom they
had intermarried. The disease began in the north-western part of the region among
the Keiagana people, spread into the north Fore and moved slowly further north,
and more dramatically into the south Fore where it evolved into an epidemic
(Alpers 1987). The highlands were unknown to the outside world until 1930.
Recognition of kuru followed formal administrative contacts with this region in the
1950s and epidemiological surveillance was started in 1957 (Gajdusek and Zigas
1958).

At this stage the annual mortality was around 200, affecting predominantly
women and children (of both sexes), with only 2% of cases in adult males (Alpers
1987). Kuru was the commonest cause of death among women in affected villages.
There was also occasional clustering of cases with four or five clan members in a
village developing kuru within several months of each other. Around 10 years after
the first contacts, although the overall kuru incidence had fallen only slightly, the
disease, which had previously affected children as young as five, had now disap-
peared in children under the age of 10 (Gajdusek *et al.* 1966). This decline continued in the younger age groups with no new cases in those born after 1956. Direct
contacts with Government had occurred at this time, with setting up of the Okapa
patrol post in 1955 and the discouragement of ritual cannibalism. It was the practice
in these communities to engage in consumption of dead relatives as a mark of
respect and mourning. Women and children predominantly ate the brain and internal organs, which is thought to explain the differential age and sex incidence.
Preparation of the cadaver for consumption was performed by the women and children such that other routes of exposure might also have been relevant. Liquefying
brain tissue was scooped by hand into bamboo cylinders and would have been
accompanied by scratching of ubiquitous itching scabies with impetiginous skin
eruptions, insect bites, and sores. As well as wiping their eyes and noses the women
would have eaten with their bare hands without washing, so oral, intradermal, and
possibly conjunctival exposure to tissues would have been common.

The original slow progression of the disease from a single point was consistent with cannibalism as the mode of transmission. Such cannibalistic practices were, however, not confined to those living in the kuru region. It is thought that the epidemic related to a single sporadic CJD case occurring in the region some decades earlier. The clusters of cases within a particular clan could also be explained by this routine of transmission as the same extended family would participate in a particular feast, thereby contracting kuru at the same time but at different ages. Clusters occurring during the later stages of the epidemic, which stood out against the low overall prevalence, could be related to the last, well remembered, cannibalistic feast in the community (Klitzman *et al.* 1984).

Epidemiological studies provided no evidence for vertical transmission, since most of the children born after 1956 and all of those born after 1959 of mothers afflicted with or incubating kuru were unaffected (Alpers 1987). From the age of the youngest affected patient, the shortest incubation period is estimated as 4.5 years, although it may have been shorter, since time of infection was usually unknown. Currently, six to eight cases are occurring annually, all in individuals aged 40 or more, consistent with exposure before 1956 and indicating that incubation periods can be 40 years or more (Alpers, personal communication).

Clinical features

Kuru affects both sexes and onset of disease has ranged from the age of five to over 60. The mean clinical duration of illness is 12 months with a range of three months to three years; the course tends to be shorter in children. The central clinical feature is progressive cerebellar ataxia. In sharp contrast to CJD, dementia is usually absent, even in the latter stages, although in the terminal stages many patients have their faculties obtunded (Alpers 1987). The occasional case in which gross dementia occurs is in marked contrast to the clinical norm. Detailed clinical descriptions have been given by a number of observers and the disease does not appear to have changed in features at different stages of the epidemic (Gajdusek and Zigas 1957; Simpson *et al.* 1959; Hornabrook 1968; Alpers and Raib 1971; Prusiner *et al.* 1982; Scrimgeour *et al.* 1983). A prodrome and three clinical stages are recognized.

1. *Prodromal stage* Kuru typically begins with prodromal symptoms consisting of headache, aching of limbs, and joint pains which can last for several months.

2. *Ambulatory stage* Kuru was frequently self-diagnosed by patients at the earliest onset of unsteadiness in standing or walking, or of dysarthria or diplopia. At this stage there may be no objective signs of disease. Gait ataxia worsens and patients develop a broad-based gait, truncal instability, and titubation. A coarse postural tremor is usually present and accentuated by movement; patients characteristically hold their hands together in the midline to suppress this. Standing with feet together reveals clawing of toes to maintain posture. This marked clawing response is regarded as pathognomonic of kuru. Signs at this stage are therefore those of midline truncal ataxia. This is presumably due to paleocerebellar disease, reflected

pathologically by the only clear macroscopic brain abnormality seen in kuru—atrophy of the cerebellar vermis.

Patients often become withdrawn at this stage and occasionally develop a severe reactive depression. Prodromal symptoms tend to disappear. Astasia and gait ataxia worsen and the patient requires a stick for walking. Signs of neocerebellar disease such as intention tremor, dysmetria, hypotonia, and dysdiadochokinesis develop. Although eye movements are ataxic and jerky, nystagmus is rarely seen. Strabismus, usually convergent, may occur particularly in children. This strabismus does not appear to be concomitant or paralytic and may fluctuate in both extent and type, sometimes disappearing later in the clinical course. Photophobia is common and there may be an abnormal cold sensitivity with shivering and pilo-erection in a warm environment. Tendon reflexes are reduced or normal, and plantar responses are flexor. Dysarthria usually occurs. As ataxia progresses the patient passes from the first (ambulatory) stage to the second (sedentary) stage. The mean clinical duration of the first stage is around eight months and correlates closely with total duration (Alpers 1964).

3. *Sedentary stage*   At this stage patients are able to sit unsupported but are largely confined to the house as they cannot walk. Attempts to walk with support lead to a high steppage, wide-based gait with reeling instability, and flinging arm movements in an attempt to maintain posture. Hyper-reflexia is seen, although usually plantar responses remain flexor and abdominal reflexes intact. Clonus is characteristically short-lived. Athetoid and choreiform movements and parkinsonian tremors may occur. There is no paralysis, although muscle power is reduced. Obesity is common at this stage but may be present in early disease associated with bulimia. Characteristically, there is emotional lability and bizarre uncontrollable laughter, which has led to the disease being referred to as 'laughing death'. There is no sensory impairment. In sharp contrast to CJD, myoclonic jerking is rarely seen. EEG is usually normal or may show nonspecific changes (Cobb *et al.* 1973). This stage lasts around two to three months. When truncal ataxia reaches the point where the patient is unable to sit unsupported, the third or tertiary stage is reached.

4. *Tertiary stage*   Hypotonia and hyporeflexia develop and the terminal state is marked by flaccid muscle weakness. Plantar responses remain flexor and abdominal reflexes intact. Progressive dysphagia occurs and patients become incontinent of urine and faeces. Inanition and emaciation develop. Transient conjugate eye signs and dementia may occur. Primitive reflexes develop in occasional cases. Brainstem involvement and both bulbar and pseudobulbar signs occur. Respiratory failure and bronchopneumonia eventually lead to death. The tertiary stage lasts one to two months.

Iatrogenic Creutzfeldt–Jakob disease
Iatrogenic prion disease is usually referred to as CJD although cases arising as a result of peripheral (rather than intracerebral) inoculation with prions usually have

a clinical picture more reminiscent of kuru, with a prominent cerebellar syndrome. Transmission of CJD from case to case has occurred by a number of routes involving accidental inoculation with human prions as a result of medical procedures. Such iatrogenic routes include the use of inadequately sterilized neurosurgical instruments, dura mater and corneal grafting, and use of human cadaveric pituitary-derived growth hormone or gonadotrophin. The first recognized case of iatrogenic CJD occurred in 1974 in a 55-year-old woman who had received a corneal transplant 18 months earlier from a donor who was subsequently found to have died of CJD (Duffy *et al.* 1974). Homogenates from the deceased recipient's brain were found to be transmissible to chimpanzees. Transmission through neurosurgical procedures has probably occurred for some time (Will and Matthew 1982). The first documented cases of transmission through neurosurgical instruments arose in 1977 when CJD was reported in two patients who had received stereotactic electroencephalographic depth recordings for epileptic conditions some 16 and 20 months earlier (Bernoulli *et al.* 1977). The same electrodes had previously been used for stereotactic exploration of a CJD patient and had been sterilized with 70% alcohol and formaldehyde vapour. Although this procedure is sufficient for conventional agents it is ineffective against prions and one of the electrodes was found to be still capable of transmitting disease to chimpanzees after implantation in the cerebral cortex.

Homograft transmission by implantation of cadaveric dura mater appears to have arisen in the mid-1980s (Thadani *et al.* 1988). A woman who had undergone surgical resection of a cholesteatoma and dura mater repair developed neurological illness 19 months later. A number of cases have subsequently arisen in New Zealand, the UK, Italy, and Japan (Masullo *et al.* 1989; Nisbet *et al.* 1989; Miyashita *et al.* 1991). Dura mater was generally collected from medical school pathology departments and treated with 10% hydrogen peroxide and ionizing radiation (25 kGy) before lyophilization. Although some cases received dura mater supplied by the same manufacturer, a number of manufacturers have provided infectious material. The manufacturing protocol now includes exposure to 1 M NaOH for one hour as a more effective means of inactivating prions. In addition to these cases, in which there seems to be a well established route of infection, there are examples in which the aetiology is less clear. For example a 51-year-old patient who received a pericardial membrane graft for an eardrum perforation developed CJD two years later with a 28-month duration of illness (Tange *et al.* 1990). The donor of the graft died after surgery and a post-mortem was not carried out. There was no personal or familial history of neurological illness in the donor so if this was an iatrogenic case it would have had to have arisen from a preclinical case of CJD. A 55-year-old orthopaedic surgeon who had worked with dura mater from sheep and human sources between 1968 and 1972 developed CJD in 1992 (Weber *et al.* 1993). The specimens that he had worked with had been sent to one of the companies preparing dura mater for clinical purposes and from which six probable cases of CJD transmission have arisen. It cannot be excluded that the surgeon was a sporadic case of CJD.

The first case of CJD in a recipient of human cadaveric pituitary-derived growth hormone was in a 20-year-old man with idiopathic hypopituitarism. The first clinical use of human growth hormone was described in 1958 and it was adopted in a number of countries (Raben 1958). In the UK, 1908 people received this treatment and in the USA there were about 10 000 recipients. Acetone-dried, powdered pituitary tissue was subjected to repeated organic solvent extraction and acid–base precipitations and the final hormone preparation contained many impurities. After 1975, the extraction method was modified to incorporate isoelectric precipitation and chromatography from frozen glands. Each batch of growth hormone was derived from pooled pituitaries and up to 2000 glands were used per batch with the remnants of some batches being mixed with new batches. Thus there is the potential for even a single gland to contaminate many vials of hormone. Many additional cases have now been recorded in the USA, UK, and in particular in France, with around 100 cases now recorded internationally. In addition to the human growth hormone cases there have been a small number of CJD cases amongst recipients of human pituitary-derived gonadotrophin (Cochius *et al.* 1992). So far all cases appear to have arisen in patients treated in Australia.

It is of considerable interest that cases arising from intracerebral or optic inoculation manifest clinically as classical CJD, with a rapidly progressive dementia, while those resulting from peripheral inoculation, most notably following pituitary-derived growth hormone exposure, typically present with a progressive ataxic syndrome, and are in that respect somewhat reminiscent of kuru. Unsurprisingly, the incubation period in intracerebral cases is shorter (19–46 months for dura mater grafts) than in peripheral cases (typically 15 years or more).

There is evidence for genetic susceptibility to iatrogenic CJD, as there is an excess of codon 129 homozygotes, in particular valine 129 homozygotes, in iatrogenic cases arising from pituitary hormone therapy. This finding was reported initially on a study of seven UK cases (Collinge *et al.* 1991*a*) and has subsequently been confirmed on the larger USA and French series (Brown *et al.* 1992*c*; Laplanche *et al.* 1994). The separate origin of the contaminated growth hormone used in the three countries makes it unlikely that this effect is due to contamination of the batches of hormone with CJD material from individuals homozygous for valine at polymorphic residue 129 as this is the least common genotype. It has been argued that valine 129 PrP may be more susceptible to undergoing the conversion to the disease related isoform than methionine 129 PrP and therefore that valine 129 homozygotes may be particularly susceptible to acquired prion diseases (Collinge *et al.* 1991*a*).

Epidemiological studies have not shown increased risks of particular occupations that may be exposed to human or animal prions, although individual CJD cases in two histopathology technicians, a neuropathologist and a neurosurgeon, have been documented.

While there have been concerns that CJD may be transmissible by blood transfusion, extensive epidemiological analysis in the UK has found that the frequency of blood transfusion and donation was no different in over 200 cases of CJD and a matched control population (Esmonde *et al.* 1993). Recipients of blood transfusions who developed CJD had clinical presentations similar to those of sporadic CJD patients and not to the more kuru-like iatrogenic cases arising from peripheral exposure to human prions. Transmission of CJD to rodents following intracerebral inoculation with buffy coat from CJD cases has been reported (Tateishi 1985), but transfusion of 300 ml of blood into a chimpanzee had not effected transmission after eight years (Gajdusek 1990).

New variant of human prion disease

In late 1995 two cases of sporadic CJD were reported in the UK in teenagers (Britton *et al.* 1995; Bateman *et al.* 1995). Only four cases of sporadic CJD had previously been recorded in the literature in teenagers, and one of these cases occurred in the UK. In addition, both cases were unusual in having kuru-type plaques, a finding seen in only around 5% of CJD cases. Soon afterwards a third very young sporadic CJD case occurred (Tabrizi *et al.* 1996). These cases caused considerable concern and the possibility was raised that they might suggest a link with BSE. It was clearly of some importance to see if any further such extraordinarily unusual cases occurred in the UK. By March 1996, further cases were apparent and review of their histology showed a remarkably consistent and unique pattern. These cases were named 'new variant' CJD although it was clear that they were also rather atypical in their clinical presentation; in fact most cases did not meet the accepted clinical diagnostic criteria for probable CJD. Extensive studies of archival cases of CJD or other prion diseases failed to show this picture and it seemed that that did represent the arrival of a new form of prion disease in the UK. The statistical probability of such cases occurring by chance was vanishingly small and ascertainment bias seemed most unlikely as an explanation. It was clear that a new risk factor for CJD had emerged and appeared to be specific to the UK. The UK Government advisory committee on spongiform encephalopathy (SEAC) concluded that, while there was no direct evidence for a link with BSE, exposure to specified bovine offal (SBO) before the ban on its inclusion in human foodstuffs in 1989 was the most likely explanation. A case of the new variant was soon after reported in France (Chazot *et al.* 1996).

The clinical presentation is with behavioural and psychiatric disturbances. These include anxiety, depression, withdrawal, and behavioural change which progresses. Most patients were referred to a psychiatrist before overt neurological features became apparent. Another early feature in some was dysaesthesiae or pain in the limbs or face or pain which was persistent rather than intermittent and unrelated to anxiety levels. After several weeks or months a progressive cerebellar syndrome developed with gait and limb ataxia. Dementia usually developed later in the clinical course with progression to akinetic mutism in most cases. Myoclonus was seen in most patients, in a few cases preceded by choreoathetosis. The age at onset in the initial 10 cases reported ranged from 16 to 39 years and the clinical course was unusually prolonged (7.5–22.5 months, median 12 months). The EEG was atypical, without the pseudoperiodic pattern seen in most sporadic CJD cases. Neuroimaging was normal or showed only mild atrophy. A high signal in the thalamus and basal ganglia, reported in some CJD cases, was present occasionally. PrP gene analysis showed that all cases available for study were homozygous for methionine at codon 129. No known or novel pathogenic mutations were found in coding sequence.

The neuropathological appearances were striking and consistent. There was widespread spongiform change, gliosis, and neuronal loss, most severe in the basal ganglia and thalamus, but the most remarkable feature was the abundant PrP amyloid plaques in the cerebral and cerebellar cortex. These consisted of kuru-like, 'florid' (surrounded by spongiform vacuoles) and multicentric plaque types. The 'florid' plaques, seen previously only in scrapie, were a particularly unusual but highly consistent feature. There was also abundant pericellular PrP deposition in the cerebral and cerebellar cortex. A further highly unusual feature was the extensive PrP deposition in the molecular layer of the cerebellum.

Some of the features of this syndrome are reminiscent of kuru, in which behavioural changes and progressive ataxia predominate; typical kuru plaques are seen in around 70% of cases and are especially abundant in younger cases. The observation that iatrogenic prion disease related to peripheral exposure to human prions has a more kuru-like than CJD-like clinical picture, which is discussed in detail above, may well be relevant and could perhaps suggest that these cases were acquired via peripheral exposure to prions.

If these cases do represent transmission of BSE to humans, as seems most likely, it is unclear why they should occur in this age group and why none of these cases had a pattern of unusual occupational or dietary exposure of BSE. However, very little is known of which foodstuffs contained high-titre bovine offal. It is possible that certain foods containing particularly high titres were eaten predominately by younger people. It cannot be excluded at present, however, that young people have an inherently higher intrinsic susceptibility to the BSE agent following dietary exposure. It is important to appreciate that BSE-contaminated feed was fed to sheep, pigs, and poultry and that although we have no evidence of natural transmission to these species, it would be prudent to remain open-minded about other dietary exposure to novel animal prions.

Inherited prion diseases

Gerstmann–Sträussler–Scheinker disease

The first report by Gerstmann in 1928 was followed by a more detailed report on seven other affected members of the same family in 1936 (Gerstmann 1928; Gerstmann *et al.* 1936). He described it as a 'peculiar heredo-familial disease of the central nervous system'. A detailed clinicopathological report of this family was presented by Seitelberger (1962). The classical presentation of GSS is with a chronic cerebellar ataxia accompanied by pyramidal features, with dementia occurring later in a much more prolonged clinical course than that seen in CJD. The mean duration is around five years, with onset usually in either the third or fourth decades. Histologically, the hallmark is the presence of multicentric amyloid plaques. Spongiform change, neuronal loss, astrocytosis, and white matter loss are also usually present. Numerous GSS kindreds from several countries (including the original Austrian family described by Gerstmann, Sträussler, and Scheinker in 1936) have now been demonstrated to have mutations in the PrP gene (see below). GSS is an autosomal dominant disorder which can now be classified within the spectrum of inherited prion disease.

Mutations in inherited prion diseases

The identification of one of the pathogenic PrP gene mutations in a case with neurodegenerative disease allows not only molecular diagnosis of an inherited prion disease but also its sub-classification according to mutation. Pathogenic mutations reported to date in the human PrP gene fall into two groups:

(1) point mutations within coding sequence resulting in amino acid substitutions in PrP or in one case production of a stop codon resulting in expression of a truncated PrP (see Fig. 2.3);

(2) insertions encoding additional integral copies of an integral copies of an octapeptide repeat present in a tandem array of five copies in the normal protein (see Fig. 2.2).

A suggested notation for these diseases is 'inherited prion disease (PrP mutation)'; for instance inherited prion disease (PrP 144 bp insertion) or inherited prion disease (PrP P102L or Pro–Leu^{102}).

(1) Missense mutations

PrP Pro–Leu^{102}
This mutation was first reported in 1989 (Hsiao *et al.* 1989) in a UK and an American family and has now been demonstrated in many other kindreds in the USA, UK, Germany, Italy, and Japan (Doh ura *et al.* 1989; Hsiao *et al.* 1989; Brown *et al.* 1991; Speer *et al.* 1991; Kretzschmar *et al.* 1992). It has also been demonstrated in the original Austrian family studied by Gerstmann, Sträussler, and Scheinker in 1936 (Kretzschmar *et al.* 1991). Progressive ataxia is the dominant clinical feature, with dementia and pyramidal features. However, marked variability both at the clinical and the neuropathological levels is apparent in some families, and has recently been extensively documented in the original Austrian family (Hainfellner *et al.* 1995). A family with marked amyotrophic features has also been reported (Kretzschmar *et al.* 1992). Cases with severe dementia in the absence of prominent ataxia are also recognized. Histological examination demonstrates PrP-immunoreactive plaques in the majority of cases. Transmissibility to experimental animals has been demonstrated.

PrP Pro–Leu[105]

The Pro–Leu change at codon 105 has been found in four patients from three Japanese families (Kitamoto *et al.* 1993*b*). It has not been reported outside Japan so far. The patients presented with a history of spastic paraparesis and dementia. The clinical duration from onset to the development of akinetic mutism was around five years. There was no periodic synchronous discharge on EEG but MRI scans showed atrophy of the motor cortex. On pathological examination there were plaques in the cerebral cortex and neuronal loss, but no spongiosis. Neurofibrillary tangles were variably present, and no plaques were found in the cerebellum.

PrP Ala–Val[117]

There are two nucleotide changes at codon 117. One is a non-coding third base polymorphism that is found in about 2.5% of the population (Palmer and Collinge, unpublished data). It can be easily detected as it destroys a *Pvu*II restriction site in the open reading frame (Wu *et al.* 1987). The other change is a coding mutation changing an alanine to valine. The mutational event generating the valine encoding sequence seems to have occurred on a *Pvu*II– allele and therefore differs from the normal alanine encoding *Pvu*II+ sequence by two nucleotides. This mutation was first described in a French family (Doh ura *et al.* 1989) and subsequently in a US family of German origin (Hsiao *et al.* 1991*b*). The US family was originally described as having familial Alzheimer's disease, but was reclassified to GSS when PrP-immunostaining amyloid plaques were found. The clinical features are pre-senile dementia associated with pyramidal signs, parkinsonism, pseudobulbar features, and cerebellar signs. PrP-immunoreactive plaques are usually present. This mutation has also been identified in a large family in the UK (Collinge *et al.* in preparation).

PrP Tyr–STOP[145]

This variant has been of considerable research interest as it results in the production of a truncated PrP. The mutation was detected in a Japanese patient who had a clinical diagnosis of Alzheimer's disease. She developed memory disturbance and a slowly progressive dementia at the age of 38. The duration of illness was 21 years. Histological examination revealed typical Alzheimer pathology without spongiform change (Kitamoto *et al.* 1993*a*). Many amyloid plaques were seen in the cortex along with diffuse neuropil threads of paired helical filaments. However, the plaques were immunoreactive with PrP antisera. A4 immunocytochemistry was negative. Kitamoto and colleagues demonstrated not only that the truncated PrP was indeed expressed in affected individuals but that the deposited protein seemed to consist entirely of the mutant truncated protein, and did not contain the wild-type protein produced by the normal allele. Such an observation is in accordance with the model of prion propagation discussed above, namely that the protein–protein interaction will preferentially involve homologous molecules. Transmission to experimental animals has not yet been reported. The clinicopathological findings in this case emphasize the importance of PrP gene analysis in the differential diagnosis of dementias.

PrP AsP –Asn[178]

This mutation was originally described in two Finnish families with a CJD-like phenotype, although without typical EEG appearances (Goldfarb *et al.* 1991*c*) and has since been demonstrated in additional CJD families in Hungary, The Netherlands, Canada, Finland, France (Nieto *et al.* 1991; Goldfarb *et al.* 1992*a*) and the UK. The Finnish pedigree included 15 affected members in four generations. The mean age of onset was 47 and mean duration was 27.5 months. Brain biopsy and autopsy specimens showed spongiform change without amyloid plaques. A review of 43 patients from seven families with this mutation showed that the age of onset is earlier and the duration longer than for sporadic CJD (Brown *et al.* 1992*b*). As with the Finnish families, periodic sharp-wave activity was absent. However, a case has been reported with onset at 57 with a periodic EEG (Laplanche *et al.* 1992).

This mutation was also reported in two unrelated families with fatal familial insomnia (Lugaresi *et al.* 1986; Medori *et al.* 1992*a, b*). The first cases described had a rapidly progressive disease characterized clinically by untreatable insomnia, dysautonomia, and motor signs, and neuropathologically by selective atrophy of the anterior-ventral and medio-dorsal thalamic nuclei. There was marked thalamic astrocytosis. Mild spongiform change was seen in some cases and protease-resistant PrP can be demonstrated, albeit weakly, by immunoblotting. Proteinase K treatment of PrP^{Sc} extracted from FFI cases and from CJD cases gives different-sized PrP bands on Western blots, suggesting that FFI may be related to a different form of PrP^{Sc}, perhaps with a different protease sensitivity (Monari *et al.* 1994).

Goldfarb *et al.* (1992*b*) reported that in all the families they studied with the codon 178 mutation and a CJD-like disease the mutation was on a valine 129 allele, while all FFI kindreds had the same codon 178 mutation on a methionine 129 allele. They suggested that the genotype at codon 129 determines phenotype. However, they have not demonstrated that the families they describe are unrelated, and therefore their comparison may only be based on two extended families. Insomnia is not uncommon in CJD patients and FFI and CJD may represent extremes of a spectrum of related disease phenotypes. Recently an inherited case with the codon 200 lysine mutation, which is normally associated with a CJD-like phenotype, has been reported with an FFI phenotype (Chapman *et al.* 1996). It is of interest that the CJD-like codon 178 cases have frequently transmitted to experimental animals while the FFI type did not transmit to laboratory primates (Brown *et al.* 1994*c*). Recently, transmission of FFI to mice has been reported, although this case was unusual in that a single octapeptide repeat deletion was present on the same allele (Tateishi *et al.* 1995). This individual came from an extensive kindred in which other family members with the same *PRNP* genotype had a CJD-like phenotype (Bosque *et al.* 1992). However, two cases of FFI, one British and the second Italian, both with the usual FFI genotype of codon 178 Asn / codon 129

Met, transmitted to transgenic mice expressing human prion protein (Collinge *et al.* 1995*a*).

Prp Val–Ile[180]

This mutation was identified in two Japanese patients with subacute dementia and myoclonus (Farlow *et al.* 1989; Ghetti *et al.* 1989; Kitamoto *et al.* 1993*b*). The period from onset to akinetic mutism was six to 10 months. No family history was noted. EEG did not show pseudoperiodic sharp-wave activity. Neuropathological examination demonstrated spongiform change, neuronal loss, and astrocytosis. Interestingly, one of the patients with PrP Ile 180 also had PrP Arg 232 (see later). These were on different alleles. This disease has not been transmitted to laboratory animals (Tateishi *et al.* 1995).

PrP Phe–Ser[198]

A variant form of GSS was described in a large Indiana kindred which has been traced back to 1792 (Farlow *et al.* 1989). Unlike other GSS patients with presenile onset of neurological disability, the Indiana kindred had widespread Alzheimer-like neurofibillary tangles composed of paired helical filaments in the cortex and subcortical nuclei in addition to amyloid plaques. The amyloid plaques were composed of PrP and not βA4 (Ghetti *et al.* 1989). Affected individuals in this kindred have a codon 198 T–C transition resulting in a phenylalanine to serine conversion (Dlouhy *et al.* 1992). There is an apparent codon 129 effect with this mutation, in that individuals who were heterozygous at codon 129 had a later age of onset than homozygotes. Transmission of this disease to laboratory animals has not yet been reported.

PrP Glu–Lys[200]

This mutation was first described in families with CJD. Affected individuals develop a rapidly progressive dementia with myoclonus and pyramidal, cerebellar, or extrapyramidal signs, and a duration of illness usually less than 12 months. The average age of onset for the disease is 55. Histologically, these patients are typical of CJD. Plaques are absent but PrP[Sc] can be demonstrated by immunoblotting. In marked contrast to other variants of inherited prion disease, the EEG usually shows the characteristic pseudoperiodic sharp-wave activity seen in sporadic CJD. Interestingly, this mutation accounts for the three reported ethnogeographic clusters of CJD where the local incidence of CJD is around 100-fold higher than elsewhere (among Libyan Jews, in a region of Slovakia, and in a region of Chile) (Goldfarb *et al.* 1990*a, b*; Hsiao *et al.* 1991*a*; Korczyn *et al.* 1991; Brown *et al.* 1992*a*).

Now that cases can be diagnosed by PrP gene analysis, atypical forms of this condition are being detected with phenotypes other than that of classical CJD. Of interest also are reports that peripheral neuropathy can occur in this disease (Neufeld *et al.* 1992). This mutation also shows incomplete penetrance. Elderly unaffected carriers of the mutation have been reported. Chapman *et al.* (1994) have made a detailed analysis of 52 mutation-carrying patients with definite or probable CJD and 34 unaffected mutation carriers. They conclude that the cumulative penetrance reaches 50% at the age of 60 and 80% by the age of 80. However, there was a group of patients, of ages 69 to 82, with possible CJD containing five proven and two obligate carriers of the mutation. That is to say the patients were demented but did not fulfil the clinical criteria for probable CJD. If the analysis was carried out assuming that these possible cases were actually CJD then the penetrance reaches 100% by the age of 80. Individuals homozygous for the mutation have been identified and are phenotypically indistinguishable from heterozygotes, indicating that this condition is a fully dominant disorder (Hsiao *et al.* 1991*a*). Patients with this condition have now been reported in several other countries outside the recognized clusters, including the UK. At least one of the UK cases does not appear to be related to the ethnogeographic clusters mentioned above, suggesting a separate UK focus for this type of inherited prion disease (Collinge *et al.* 1993). Goldfarb *et al.* (1991*b*) have found this mutation in 46 out of 55 CJD affected families studied at the National Institutes of Health. These families contain 89 affected patients and originate from seven different countries: Slovakia, Poland, Germany, Tunisia, Greece, Libya, and Chile. The codon 129 genotype does not appear to affect age onset of this disorder. Transmission to experimental animals has been demonstrated.

PrP Arg–His^{208}

This has been identified in a single patient with CJD confirmed at autopsy. No details of the family history or phenotypic details are yet published (Mastrianni *et al.* 1995).

PrP Val–Ile^{210}

This mutation has been reported only in a single case in France (Davies *et al.* 1993) with a rapidly progressive dementia, cerebellar signs, and myoclonus, and age at onset of 63. EEG showed pseudoperiodic sharp-wave activity. The clinical duration was four months and neuropathological examination showed spongiform change, neuronal loss, and astrocytosis. No amyloid plaques were seen. The patient's parents had died at the ages of 60 and 66 without dementia. A sister with the mutation had died of colon cancer at age 67. It is possible that this mutation produces a very late onset disease or is incompletely penetrant. Transmission to experimental animals has not been reported.

PrP Gln–Agr^{217}

Reported to date only in a single Swedish family, the presentation is with dementia followed by gait ataxia, dysphagia, and confusion (Hsiao *et al.* 1992*a*). As with the inherited prion disease with codon 198 serine mutation (Indiana kindred) there are prominent neurofibrillary tangles. Transmissibility to experimental animals has not yet been demonstrated in this condition.

PrP Met–Arg^{232}

This mutation was first found on the opposite allele to a codon 180 mutation in a Japanese patient with prion disease (Kitamoto *et al.* 1993*b*). It was further demonstrated in two additional Japanese patients with dementia. Both of the latter cases appeared to present as sporadic cases with no family history of neurological disease. Both patients had progressive dementia, myoclonus, and periodic synchronous discharges in the EEG. The mean duration of illness was three months. Neuropathology showed spongiform change, neuronal loss, and astrocytosis. PrP immunostaining revealed diffuse grey matter staining, but no plaques.

(2) Insertional mutations

PrP 24 bp insertion (one extra repeat)

A single octapeptide repeat insertion has been reported in a single French patient who presented at age 73 with dizziness (Laplanche *et al.* 1995). He later developed visual agnosia, cerebellar ataxia, and intellectual impairment, and diffuse periodic activity was noted on EEG. Myoclonus and cortical blindness developed and he progressed to akinetic mutism. Disease duration was four months. The patient's father had died at 70 from an undiagnosed neurological disorder. No neuropathological information is available.

PrP 48 bp insertion (two extra repeats)

This mutation has been reported in a single family from the USA (Goldfarb *et al.* 1993). The proband had a CJD-like phenotype both clinically and pathologically with a typical EEG and an age at onset of 58. However, the proband's mother had onset of cognitive decline at age 75 with a slow progression to a severe dementia over 13 years. The maternal grandfather had a similar late onset (at age 80) and slowly progressive cognitive decline over 15 years. The codon 129 status of these cases is not stated.

PrP 96 bp insertion (four extra repeats)

A 96-base-pair insertional mutation, encoding four octapeptide elements was first reported in a patient who died aged 63 of liver cirrhosis (Goldfarb *et al.* 1991*a*). There was no history of neurological illness and it is unclear if this finding indicates incomplete penetrance of this mutation. This is the only recorded case of a *PRNP* insertional mutation other than in an affected individual with a prion disease or an at-risk individual from an affected kindred. Two separate four octapeptide repeat mutations have been reported in affected individuals, each differing in the DNA sequence from the original four-repeat insertion, although all three of the mutations encode the same PrP. Laplanche *et al.* (1995) reported a 96 bp insertion in an 82-year-old French woman who developed progressive depression and behavioural changes. She progressed over three months to akinetic mutism with pyramidal signs and myoclonus. EEG showed pseudoperiodic complexes, and the duration of illness was four months. There was no known family history of neurological illness. Another 96 bp insertional mutation was seen in a patient with classical clinical and pathological features of CJD with the exception of the unusual finding of pronounced PrP immunoreactivity in the molecular layer of the cerebellum

(Campbell *et al.* 1996). No family history was apparent in this case but there was non-paternity and details of the biological father were unavailable.

PrP 120 bp insertion (five extra repeats)
A five additional octapeptide repeat mutation was reported in a US family with an illness characterized by progressive dementia, abnormal behaviour, cerebellar signs, tremor, rigidity, hyper-reflexia, and myoclonus. The age at onset was 31–45 with a clinical duration of 5–15 years (Goldfarb *et al.* 1991*a*). EEG showed diffuse slowing only. Histological features were of spongiosis, neuronal loss, and gliosis. Transmission to squirrel and spider monkeys has been demonstrated.

Prp 144 bp insertion (six extra repeats)
This was the first PrP mutation to be reported and was found in a small UK family with familial CJD (Owen *et al.* 1989). The diagnosis in the family had been based on an individual who died in the 1940s with a rapidly progressive illness characteristic of CJD (Meyer *et al.* 1954). The reported duration of illness was six months. Pathologically, there was gross status spongiosis and astrocytosis affecting the entire cerebral cortex, and this case is used to illustrate classic CJD histology in Greenfield's *Neuropathology*. However, other family members had a much longer duration GSS-like illness. Histological features were also extremely variable. This observation led to screening of various case of neurodegenerative disease and to the identification of a case classified on clinical grounds as familial Alzheimer's disease (Collinge *et al.* 1989). More extensive screening work identified further families with the same mutation which were then demonstrated by genealogical studies to form part of an extremely large kindred (Collinge *et al.* 1992; Poulter *et al.* 1992). Clinical information has been collected on around 50 affected individuals over seven generations. Affected individuals develop in the third or fourth decade a progressive dementia associated with a varying combination of cerebellar ataxia and dysarthria, pyramidal signs, myoclonus, and occasionally extrapyramidal signs, chorea, and seizures. The dementia is often preceded by depression and aggressive behaviour. A number of cases have a long-standing personality disorder, characterized by aggression, irritability, antisocial and criminal activity, and hypersexuality which may be present from early childhood, long before overt neurodegenerative disease develops. The histological features vary from those of classical spongiform encephalopathy (with or without PrP amyloid plaques) to cases lacking any specific features of these conditions (Collinge *et al.* 1990). Age at onset in this condition can be predicted according to genotype at polymorphic codon 129. Since this pathogenic insertional mutation occurs on a methionine 129 PrP allele, there are two possible codon 129 genotypes for affected individuals—methionine 129 homozygotes, or methionine 129/valine 129 heterozygotes. Heterozygotes have an age at onset which is about a decade later than homozygotes (Poulter *et al.* 1992). Limited studies of transmission to marmosets were unsuccessful. Transmission to transgenic mice expressing human prion protein has been achieved (Collinge *et al.*

in preparation). Further families with 144 bp insertions nucleotide sequence, have now been reported in the UK (Nicholl *et al.* 1995) and Japan (Oda *et al.* 1995).

PrP 168 bp insertion (seven extra repeats)

This mutation has been reported in a US family. The clinical features described include mood change, abnormal behaviour, confusion, aphasia, cerebellar signs, involuntary movements, rigidity, dementia, and myoclonus. The age at onset was 23–35 years and the clinical duration from 10 to over 13 years. EEG showed diffuse slowing in two cases; a third showed slow-wave burst suppression. Neuropathological examination showed spongiform change, neuronal loss, and gliosis to varying degrees (Goldfarb *et al.* 1991*a*). Experimental transmission to the chimpanzee has been demonstrated.

PrP 192 bp insertion (eight extra repeats)

This mutation has been reported in a French family with clinical features which include abnormal behaviour, cerebellar signs, mutism, pyramidal signs, myoclonus tremor, intellectual slowing, and seizures. The disease duration ranged from three months to 13 years. The EEG findings included diffuse slowing, slow-wave burst suppression, and periodic triphasic complexes. Neuropathological examination revealed spongiform change, neuronal loss, gliosis, and multicentric plaques in the cerebellum (Goldfarb *et al.* 1991*a*; Guiry *et al.* 1993). Experimental transmission to the chimpanzee has been reported.

PrP 216 bp insertion (nine extra repeats)

The finding of a nine octapeptide insertional mutation was first reported in a single case from the UK (Owen *et al.* 1992). The clinical onset was around 54 years with falls, axial rigidity, myoclonic jerks, and progressive dementia (Tagliavini *et al.* 1993). Although there was no clear family history of a similar illness, the mother had died at age 53 with a cerebrovascular event. The maternal grandmother died at age 79 with senile dementia. EEG was of low amplitude but did not show pseudo-periodic sharp-wave activity. Neuropathological examination showed no spongiform encephalopathy but marked deposition of plaques, which in the cerebellum and the basal ganglia showed immunoreactivity with PrP antisera (Tagliavini *et al.* 1993). In the hippocampus there were neuritic plaques positive for both β-amyloid protein and tau. Some neurofibrillary tangles were also seen. In some respects therefore the pathology resembled Alzheimer's disease. Experimental transmission studies have not been attempted. A German family with a nine-octapeptide repeat insertion of different sequence has now been reported (Krasemann *et al.* 1995).

Other polymorphic variation in PRNP

PrP Met–Val^{129}

The role of this important polymorphism in determining susceptibility to acquired and sporadic prion disease, and in affecting age at onset in some kindreds with inherited prion disease has been discussed above, in the aetiology section.

PrP GGC–GGG[124]

This third base change of a glycine codon from GGC to GGG was found on the normal allele of an individual with codon 217 mutation (Hsiao *et al.* 1992*a*). The frequency of this polymorphism is not known, but in a screen of over 700 samples of both normal controls and patients with neurological disease we have only found one instance of it, in an individual with amyotrophic lateral sclerosis who also had a 24 bp deletion.

PrP GCA–GCG[117]

A non-coding third base change seen in around 2.5% of Caucasians (see PrP Ala–Val[117] above).

PrP CAC–CAT[177]

This non-coding third base change was found in an 88-year-old control subject by Ripoll *et al.* (1993).

PrP Glu–Lys[219]

Originally found in a Japanese patient with schizophrenia, this variation has been found to be a fairly common polymorphism in the Japanese population with an allele frequency of 6%. However, it has not yet been reported in Caucasian populations (Furukawa *et al.* 1995).

PrP 24 bp deletion (one less octapeptide repeat)

Deletions in the repeat region of the prion protein are now known to be polymorphisms with a frequency of about 1%. Because of the nature of the repeat region it is not possible to say precisely where the excision point for these 24-base-pair deletions lies. However, three different nucleotide sequences are recognized to be associated with the deletions. All these deleted alleles encode the same amino acid sequence so they are not distinguishable at the protein level (Laplanche *et al.* 1990; Palmer *et al.* 1993).

Presymptomatic and antenatal testing

Since a direct gene test has become available it has been possible to provide an unequivocal diagnosis in patients with inherited forms of the disease. This has also led to the possibility of performing pre-symptomatic testing of unaffected but at-risk family members, as well as antenatal testing (Collinge *et al.* 1991*b*). Because codon 129 genotype affects the age of onset of disease associated with some mutations, it is possible to determine within a family whether a carrier of a mutation will have an early or late onset of disease. Most of the mutations so far found, with the notable exception of the codon 200 mutation, appear to be fully penetrant, but experience with many of the mutations is extremely limited. In codon 200 families there are examples of elderly unaffected gene carriers who appear to have escaped the disease.

Genetic counselling in prion diseases resembles that of Huntington's disease in many respects, and protocols established for Huntington's disease can be adapted for prion disease counselling. PrP gene analysis may have very important consequences for family members other than the individual tested, and it is preferable to discuss all the issues with the whole family before testing commences. Following the identification of a mutation the family should be referred for genetic counselling. Testing of asymptomatic individuals should only follow adequate counselling, and requires their full informed consent.

Prognosis

All forms of prion diseases that are currently recognized are invariably fatal, following a relentlessly progressive course. No treatment alters the clinical course of the disease and all that can be offered at present is general supportive care for the patient and family with hospitalization in the later stages. The duration of illness in sporadic patients is very short with a mean duration of three to four months. However, in some of the inherited cases the duration can be 20 years or more (Collinge *et al.* 1990).

Transmission studies

Experimental transmission studies of the human prion diseases have until recently largely involved transmission to laboratory primates, in particular chimpanzees and squirrel monkeys. The NIH group has reported over 300 successful transmissions (Brown *et al.* 1994*b*). However, transmission studies in primates are severely limited by their expense and by ethical concerns. Attempts by most laboratories to transmit human prions to rodents have been fairly unsuccessful, with only occasional transmissions occurring and then at prolonged incubation periods, close to the natural lifespan of the mice. Some groups have, however, reported more frequent transmissions (Tateishi *et al.* 1981). Recently transgenic mice have become available which have increased susceptibility to human prions. Mice expressing a chimaeric human–mouse PrP were susceptible to three CJD isolates after short incubation periods (Telling *et al.* 1994). It has now become clear that transgenic mice expressing wild-type human PrP, but not mouse PrP, are highly susceptible to CJD, with all inoculated mice succumbing at short incubation periods usually in the range of 180–220 days (Collinge *et al.* 1995*b*; Telling *et al.* 1995). Such mice appear to lack a species barrier to human prions and can now be used for extensive studies of the human prion diseases (Collinge *et al.* 1995*b*). We have successfully transmitted over 20 cases to mice expressing human PrP, including inherited cases that failed to transmit to primates (Collinge *et al.* 1995*a*,*b*), and larger scale studies are in progress to establish the range of transmission characteristics of the human prion diseases and prion titres in peripheral tissues.

Risks of BSE transmission to humans

The issue of whether it is possible for BSE to transit to humans has provoked considerable debate. Clearly we cannot answer the question directly as this would require inoculation of humans with BSE. However, transgenic models may offer a way to address this issue, at least in part. Transmission of prion diseases from one mammalian species to another is often difficult, with only a small proportion of inoculated animals developing disease and then following extremely prolonged incubation periods at first passage—the 'species barrier' (Pattison 1965). The principal determinants of the species barrier are the degree of homology between PrP molecules in the host and inoculum (Prusiner *et al.* 1990) and strain of agent; however, BSE appears to be caused by a single agent strain (Bruce *et al.* 1994). Transgenic mice expressing human PrP, which are competent to produce human PrP^{Sc} and 'human' prions on CJD challenge, offer an opportunity to address the issue of whether bovine prions can induce production of human PrP^{Sc}. To date, results are reassuring. Incubation periods to BSE were unaltered in mice expressing human PrP in addition to mouse PrP, and only mouse PrP^{Sc} appeared to be produced (Collinge *et al.* 1995). A potentially more revealing experiment is to challenge mice expressing only human PrP with BSE (Collinge *et al.* 1995*b*). This experiment is in progress and so far such mice remain well over 420 days post-challenge (mice of this genotype succumb to CJD in around 200 days). However, the end point of this experiment may be 300–400 days away if these mice do not succumb to prion disease but die of old age; it is still too early to draw any firm conclusions and it will be important to measure the fall in incubation period on second passage in mice of this group genotype, as the species barrier is usually quantified in terms of the shortening of incubation period on second and subsequent passage in the same host.

   However, even the presence of a highly effective species barrier between cattle and humans does not exclude the possibility that a few cases of BSE transmission to humans might still occur, given the very large numbers of people that may have been exposed. Clearly, epidemiology cannot reveal whether individual cases have arisen as a result of BSE exposure. There may, however, be an alternative method to achieve this. As mentioned above, BSE appears to be caused by a single prion strain type. This BSE strain is different from over 20 historical or contemporary isolates from sheep or goats with natural scrapie, as determined by study of incubation periods and lesion profiles in mice (Bruce *et al.* 1994). These studies suggest that many of the newly recognized animal prion diseases affecting domestic cats, captive wild cats (puma, cheetah, ocelot), and captive wild ruminants (nyala, gemsbok, eland, Arabian oryx, greater kudu, scimitar-horned oryx) have resulted from transmission of BSE rather than scrapie (Bruce *et al.* 1994), presumably as a result of contaminated feed. The persistence of this characteristic BSE 'signature' on passage through a range of species suggests that it may be possible, by similar strain-typing methods, to determine whether individual CJD cases arose from transmission of BSE. However, it is unknown at present if CJD is caused by one or many different strains of human prion. It will be necessary to determine the full range of human prion strains, some of which may produce similar patterns of pathology in mice to BSE, before the results of such experiments can be interpreted. Transgenic mice expressing only human PrP are susceptible to a range of human prion isolates with short incubation periods (Telling *et al.* 1995; Collinge *et al.* 1995*b*) and studies are in progress to identify and characterize human strains that may cause CJD and to study the transmission characteristics of 'new variant' CJD cases that have been putatively linked to BSE transmission to humans.

References

Alpers, M. (1964). *Kuru: age and duration studies*. Department of Medicine, University of Adelaide.

Alpers, M. P. (1987). Epidemiology and clinical aspects of kuru. In *Prions: novel infectious pathogens causing scrapie and Creutzfeldt–Jakob disease* (ed. S. B. Pruiner and M. P. McKinley), pp. 451–465. Academic Press, San Diego.

Alpers, M. and Rail, L. (1971). Kuru and Creutzfeldt–Jakob disease: clinical and aetiological aspects. *Proceedings of the Australian Association of Neurologists*, **8**, 7–15.

Baker, H. F., Poulter, M., Crow, T. J., Frith, C. D., Lofthouse, R., Ridley, R. M., *et al.* (1991). Amino acid polymorphism in human prion protein and age at death in inherited prion disease. *Lancet*, **337**, 1286.

Bateman, D., Hilton, D., Love, S., Zeidler, M., Beck, J., and Collinge, J. (1995). Sporadic Creutzfeldt–Jakob disease in an 18-year-old in the UK. *Lancet*, **346**, 1155–1156.

Beck, E. and Daniel, P. M. (1987). Neuropathology of transmissible spongiform encephalopathies. In *Prions: novel infectious pathogens causing scrapie and Creutzfeldt–Jakob disease* (ed. S. B. Pruiner and M. P. McKindley), pp. 331–385. Academic Press, San Diego.

Bernoulli, C., Siegfried, J., and Baumgartner, G. (1977). Danger of accidental person-to-person transmission of Creutzfeldt–Jakob disease by surgery. *Lancet*, **i**, 478–479.

Bosque, P. J., Vnencak-Jones, C. L., Johnson, M. D., Whitlock, J. A., and McLean, M. J. (1992). A PrP gene codon 178 base substitution and a 24-bp interstitial deletion in familial Creutzfeldt–Jakob disease. *Neurology*, **42**, 1864–1870.

Britton, T. C., Al-Sarraj, S., Shaw, C., Campbell, T., and Collinge, J. (1995). Sporadic Creutzfeldt–Jakob disease in a 16-year old in the UK. *Lancet*, **346**, 1155.

Brown, P., Rodgers, J. P., Cathala, F., Gibbs, C. J., and Gajdusek, D. C. (1984). Creutzfeldt–Jakob disease of long duration: clinicopathological characteristics, transmissibility, and differential diagnosis. *Annals of Neurology*, **16**, 295–304.

Brown, P., Cathala, F., Raubertas, R. F., Gajdusek, D. C., and Castaigne, P. (1987). The epidemiology of Creutzfeldt–Jakob disease: conclusion of a 15-year investigation in France and review of the world literature. *Neurology*, **37**, 895–904.

Brown, P., Goldfarb, L. G., Brown, W. T., Goldgaber, D., Rubenstein, R., Kascsak, R. J., *et al.* (1991). Clinical and molecular genetic study of a large German kindred with Gerstmann–Sträussler–Scheinker syndrome. *Neurology*, **41**, 375–379.

Brown, P., Galvez, S., Goldfarb, L. G., Neito, A., Cartier, L., Gibbs, C. J. J., *et al.* (1992*a*). Familial Creutzfeldt–Jakob disease in Chile is associated with the codon 200 mutation of the PRNP amyloid precursor gene on chromosome 20. *Journal of Neurological Science*, **112**, 65–67.

Brown, P., Goldfarb, L. G., Kovanen, J., Haltia, M., Cathala, F., Sulima, M., *et al.* (1992*b*). Phenotypic characteristics of familial Creutzfeldt–Jakob disease associated with the codon-178Asn PRNP mutation. *Annals of Neurology*, **31**, 282–285.

Brown, P., Preece, M. A., and Will, R. G. (1992*c*). 'Friendly fire' in medicine: hormones, homografts, and Creutzfeldt–Jakob disease. *Lancet*, **340**, 24–27.

Brown, P., Cervenakova, L., Goldfarb, M. D., McCombie, W. R., Rubenstein, R., Will, R. G., *et al.* (1994*a*). Iatrogenic Creutzfeldt–Jakob disease: an example of the interplay between ancient genes and modern medicine. *Neurology*, **44**, 291–293.

Brown, P., Gibbs, C. J. J., Rodgers Johnson, P., Asher, D. M., Sulima, M. P., Bacote, A., *et al.* (1994*b*). Human spongiform encephalopathy: the National Institutes of Health series of 300 cases of experimentally transmitted disease. *Annals of Neurology*, **35**, 513–529.

Bruce, M., Chree, A., McConnell, I., Foster, J., Pearson, G., and Fraser, H. (1994*c*). Transmission of bovine spongiform encephalopathy and scrapie to mice: strain variation and the species barrier. *Philosophical Transactions of the Royal Society of London (Biology)*, **343**, 405–411.

Bueler, H., Aguzzi, A., Sailer, A., Greiner, R. A., Autenried, P., Aguet, M., *et al.* (1993). Mice devoid of PrP are resistant to scrapie. *Cell*, **73**, 1339–1347.

Bueler, H., Raeber, A., Sailer, A., Fischer, M., Aguzzi, A., and Weissmann, C. (1995). High prion and PrP^{Sc} levels but delayed onset of disease in scrapie-inoculated mice heterozygous for a disrupted PrP gene. *Molecular Medicine*, **1**, 19–30.

Campbell, T. A., Palmer, M. S., Will, R. G., Gibb, W. R. G., Luthert, P., and Collinge, J. (1996). A prion disease with a novel 96-base pair insertional mutation in the prion protein gene. *Neurology*, **46**, 761–766.

Chapman, J., Ben-Israel, J., Goldhammer, Y., and Korczyn, A. D. (1994). The risk of developing Creutzfeldt–Jakob disease in subjects with the PRNP gene codon 200 point mutation. *Neurology*, **44**, 1683–1686.

Chapman, J., Arlazoroff, A., Goldfarb, L. G., Cervenakova, L., Neufeld, M. Y., Werber, E., *et al.* (1996). Fatal insomnia in a case of familial Creutzfeldt–Jakob disease with the codon 200^{Lys} mutation. *Neurology*, **46**, 758–761.

Chazot, G., Brousolle, E., Lapras, C. I., Blattler, T., Aguzzi, A., and Kopp, N. (1996). New variant of Creutzfeldt–Jakob disease in a 26-year-old French man. *Lancet*, **347**, 1181.

Cobb, W. A., Hornabrook, R. W., and Sanders, S. (1973). The EEG of kuru. *Electroencephalography and Clinical Neurophysiology*, **34**, 419–427.

Cochius, J., Human, N., and Esiri, M. (1992). Creutzfeldt–Jakob disease in a recipient of human pituitary derived gonadotrophin: a second case. *Journal of Neurology, Neurosurgery and Psychiatry*, **55**, 1094–1095.

Collinge, J., Harding, A. E., Owen, F., Poulter, M., Lofthouse, R., Boughey, A. M., *et al.* (1989). Diagnosis of Gerstmann–Sträussler syndrome in familial dementia with prion protein gene analysis. *Lancet*, **ii**, 15–17.

Collinge, J., Owen, F., Poulter, M., Leach, M., Crow, T. J., Rossor, M. N., *et al.* (1990). Prion dementia without characteristic pathology. *Lancet*, **336**, 7–9.

Collinge, J., Palmer, M. S., and Dryden, A. J. (1991*a*). Genetic predisposition to iatrogenic Creutzfeldt–Jakob disease. *Lancet*, **337**, 1441–1442.

Collinge, J., Poulter, M., Davis, M. B., Baraitser, M., Owen, F., Crow, T. J. *et al.* (1991*b*). Presymptomatic detection or exclusion of prion protein gene defects in families with inherited prion diseases. *American Journal of Human Genetics*, **49**, 1351–1354.

Collinge, J., Brown, J., Hardy, J., Mullan, M., Rossor, M. N., Baker, H. *et al.* (1992). Inherited prion disease with 144 base pair gene insertion. 2. Clinical and pathological features. *Brain*, **115**, 687–710.

Collinge, J., Palmer, M. S., Campbell, T. A., Sidle, K. C. L., Carroll, D., and Harding, A. E. (1993). Inherited prion disease (PrP lysine 200) in Britain: two case reports. *British Medical Journal*, **306**, 301–302.

Collinge, J., Palmer, M. S., Sidle, K. C. L., Gowland, I., Medori, R., Ironside, J., *et al.* (1995*a*). Transmission of fatal familial insomnia to laboratory animals. *Lancet*, **346**, 569–570.

Collinge, J., Palmer, M. S., Sidle, K. C. L., Hill, A. F., Gowland, I., Meads, J., *et al.* (1995*b*). Unaltered susceptibility to BSE in transgenic mice expressing human prion protein. *Nature*, **378**, 779–783.

Creutzfeldt, H. G. (1920). Über eine eigenartige herdförmige Erkrankung des Zentralnervensystems. *Zeitschrift für die Gesamte Neurologie und Psychiatrie*, **57**, 1–18.

Cuillé, J. and Chelle, P. L. (1936). La maladie dite tremblante du mouton, este-elle inocuable? *Compte rendu de l'Academie des Sciences*, **203**, 1552–1554.

Davies, P. T. G., Jahfar, S., Ferguson, I. T., and Windl, O. (1993). Creutzfeldt–Jakob disease in individual occupationally exposed to BSE. *Lancet*, **342**, 680.

Dlouhy, S. R., Hsiao, K., Farlow, M. R., Foroud, T., Conneally, P. M., Johnson, P., *et al.* (1992). Linkage of the indiana kindred of Gerstmann–Sträussler–Scheinker disease to the prion protein gene. *Nature Genetics*, **1**, 64–67.

Doh ura, K., Tateishi, J., Sasaki, H., Kitamoto, T., and Sakaki, Y. (1989). Pro–Leu change at position 102 of prion protein is the most common but not the sole mutation related to Gerstmann–Sträussler syndrome. *Biochemical and Biophysical Research Communications*, **163**, 974–979.

Doh ura, K., Tateishi, J., Kitamoto, T., Sasaki, H., and Sakaki, Y. (1990). Creutzfeldt–Jakob disease patients with congophilic kuru plaques have the missense variant prion protein common to Gerstmann–Sträussler syndrome. *Annals of Neurology*, **27**, 121–126.

Duffy, P., Wolf, J., and Collins, G. (1974). Possible person-to-person transmission of Creutzfeldt–Jakob disease. *New England Journal of Medicine*, **290**, 692.

Esmonde, T. F. G., Will, R. G., Slattery, J. M., Knight, R., Harries-Jones, R., De Silva, R., *et al.* (1993). Creutzfeldt–Jakob disease and blood transfusion. *Lancet*, **341**, 205–207.

Farlow, M. R., Yee, R. D., Dlouhy, S. R., Conneally, P. M., Azzarelli, B., and Ghetti, B. (1989). Gerstmann–Sträussler–Scheinker disease. I. Extending the clinical spectrum. *Neurology*, **39**, 1446–1452.

Furukawa, H., Kitamoto, T., Tanaka, Y., and Tateishi, J. (1995). New variant prion protein in a Japanese family with Gerstmann–Sträussler syndrome. *Brain Research and Molecular Brain Research*, **30**, 385–388.

Gajdusek, D. C. (1990). Subacute spongiform encephalopathies: transmissible cerebral amyloidoses caused by unconventional viruses. In *Virology* (ed. B. N. Fields and D. M. Knipe), pp. 2289–2324. Raven Press, New York.

Gajdusek, D. C. and Zigas, V. (1957). *New England Journal of Medicine*, **257**, 974–978.

Gajdusek, D. C. and Zigas, V. (1958). *Klinische Wochenschrift*, **36**, 445–459.

Gajdusek, D. C., Gibbs, C. J. J., and Alpers, M. P. (1966). Experimental transmission of a kuru-like syndrome to chimpanzees. *Nature*, **209**, 794–796.

Gasset, M., Baldwin, M. A., Fletterick, R. J., and Prusiner, S. B. (1993). Perturbation of the secondary structure of the scrapie prion protein under conditions that alter infectivity. *Proceedings of the National Academy of Sciences of the USA*, **90**, 1–5.

Gerstmann, J. (1928). Über ein noch nicht beschriebenes Reflexphänomen bei einer Erkrankung des zerebellaren Systems. *Wiener Medizinische Wochenschrift*, **78**, 906–908.

Gerstmann, J., Sträussler, E., and Scheinker, I. (1936). Über eine eigenartige hereditärfamiliäre Erkrankung des Zentralnervensystems. Zugleich ein Beitrag zur frag des vorzeitigen lakalen Alterns. *Zeischrift für Neurologie*, **154**, 736–762.

Ghetti, B., Tagliavini, F., Masters, C. L., Beyreuther, K., Giaccone, G., Verga, L., *et al.* (1989). Gerstmann–Sträussler–Scheinker disease. II. Neurofibrillary tangles and plaques with PrP-amyloid coexist in an affected family. *Neurology*, **39**, 1453–1461.

Gibbs, C. J., Gajdusek, D. C., Asher, D. M., Alphers, M. P., Beck, E., Daniel, P. M., *et al.* (1968). Creutzfeldt–Jakob disease (spongiform encephalopathy): transmission to the chimpanzee. *Science*, **161**, 388–389.

Goldfarb, L. G., Korczyn, A. D., Brown, P., Chapman, J., and Gajdusek, D. C. (1990*a*). Mutation in codon 200 of scrapie amyloid precursor gene linked to Creutzfeldt–Jakob disease in Sephardic Jews of Libyan and non-Libyan origin. *Lancet*, **336**, 637–638.

Goldfarb, L. G., Mitrova, E., Brown, P., Toh, B. K., and Gajdusek, D. C. (1990*b*). Mutation in codon 200 of scrapie amyloid protein gene in two clusters of Creutzfeldt–Jakob disease in Slovakia. *Lancet*, **336**, 514–515.

Goldfarb, L. G., Brown, P., McCombie, W. R., Goldgaber, D., Swergold, G. D., Wills, P. R., *et al.* (1991*a*). Transmissible familial Creutzfeldt–Jakob disease associated with five, seven, and eight extra octapeptide coding repeats in the PRNP gene. *Proceedings of the National Academy of Sciences of the USA*, **88**, 10926–10930.

Goldfarb, L. G., Brown, P., Mitrova, E., Cervenakova, L., Goldin, L., Korczyn, A. D., *et al.* (1991*b*). Creutzfeldt–Jakob disease associated with the PRNP codon 200Lys mutation: an analysis of 45 families. *European Journal of Epidemiology*, **7**, 477–486.

Goldfarb, L. G., Haltia, M., Brown, P., Nieto, A., Kovanen, J., McCombie, W. R., *et al.* (1991*c*). New mutation in scrapie amyloid precursor gene (at codon 178) in Finnish Creutzfeldt–Jakob kindred. *Lancet*, **337**, 425.

Goldfarb, L. G., Brown, P., Haltia, M., Cathala, F., McCombie, W. R., Kovanen, J., *et al.* (1992*a*). Creutzfeldt–Jakob disease cosegregates with the codon 178-Asn PRNP mutation in families of European origin. *Annals of Neurology*, **31**, 274–281.

Goldfarb, L. G., Petersen, R. B., Tabaton, M., Brown, P., LeBlanc, A. C., Montagna, P., *et al.* (1992*b*). Fatal familial insomnia and familial Creutzfeldt–Jakob disease: disease phenotype determined by a DNA polymorphism. *Science*, **258**, 806–808.

Goldfarb, L. G., Brown, P., Little, B. W., Cervenakova, L., Kenney, K., Gibbs, C. J. J., *et al.* (1993). A new (two-repeat) octapeptide coding insert mutation in Creutzfeldt–Jakob disease. *Neurology*, **43**, 2392–2394.

Gomori, A. J., Partnow, M. J., Horoupian, D. S., and Hirano, A. (1973). The ataxic form of Creutzfeldt–Jakob disease. *Archives of Neurology*, **29**, 318–323.

Gore, S. M. (1995). More than happenstance: Creutzfeldt–Jakob disease in farmers and young adults. *British Medical Journal*, **311**, 1416–1418.

Guiroy, D. C., Marsh, R. F., Yanagihara, R., and Gajdusek, D. C. (1993). Immunolocalization of scrapie amyloid in non-congophilic, non-birefringent deposits in golden Syrian hamsters with experimental transmissible mink encephalopathy. *Neuroscience Letters*, **155**, 112–115.

Hadlow, W. J. (1959). Scrapie and kuru. *Lancet*, **ii**, 289–290.

Hainfellner, J. A., Brantner-Inthaler, S., Cervenáková, L., Brown, P., Kitamoto, T., Tateishi, J., *et al.* (1995). The original Gerstmann–Sträussler–Scheinker family of Austria: Divergent clinicopathological phenotypes but constant PrP genotype. *Brain Pathology*, **5**, 201–211.

Hornabrook, R. W. (1968). Kuru—a subacute cerebellar degeneration. The natural history and clinical features. *Brain*, **91**, 53–74.

Hsiao, K., Baker, H. F., Crow, T. J., Poulter, M., Owen, F., Terwilliger, J. D., *et al.* (1989). Linkage of a prion protein missense variant to Gerstmann–Sträussler syndrome. *Nature*, **338**, 342–345.

Hsiao, K. K., Scott, M., Foster, D., Groth, D. F., DeArmond, S. J., and Prusiner, S. B. (1990). Spontaneous neurodegeneration in transgenic mice with mutant prion protein. *Science*, **250**, 1587–1590.

Hsiao, K., Meiner, Z., Kahana, E., Cass, C., Kahana, I., Avrahami, D., *et al.* (1991*a*). Mutation of the prion protein in Libyan Jews with Creutzfeldt–Jakob disease. *New England Journal of Medicine*, **324**, 1091–1097.

Hsiao, K. K., Cass, C., Schellenberg, G. D., Bird, T., Devine, G. E., Wisniewski, H., *et al.* (1991*b*). A prion protein variant in a family with the telencephalic form of Gerstmann–Sträussler–Scheinker syndrome. *Neurology*, **41**, 681–684.

Hsiao, K., Dlouhy, S. R., Farlow, M. R., Cass, C., Da Costa, M., Conneally, P. M., *et al.* (1992*a*). Mutant prion proteins in Gerstmann–Sträussler–Scheinker disease with neurofibrillary tangles. *Nature Genetics*, **1**, 68–71.

Hsiao, K. K., Groth, D., Scott, M., Yang, S. L., Serban, A., Rapp, D., *et al.* (1992*b*). Genetic and transgenetic studies of prion proteins in Gerstmann–Sträussler–Scheinker disease. In *Prion disease of humans and animals* (ed. S. B. Prusiner, J. Collinge, J. Powell, and B. Anderton), pp. 120–128. Ellis Horwood, London.

Hsiao, K. K., Groth, D., Scott, M., Yang, S., Serban, H., Rapp D., *et al.* (1994). Serial transmission in rodents of neurodegenaration from transgenic mice expressing mutant prion protein. *Proceedings of the National Academy of Sciences of the USA*, **91**, 9126–9130.

Jakob, A. (1921*a*). Über eigenartige Erkrankungen des Zentralnervensystems mit bemerkenswertem anatomischen Befund. *Zeitschrift für die Gesamte Neurologie und Psychiatrie*, **64**, 147–228.

Jakob, A. (1921*b*). Über eigenartige Erkrankungen des Zentralnervensystems mit bemerkenswertem anatomischen Befund (spastische Pseudosclerose-Encephalo-myelopathie mit disseminierten Degenerationsherden). *Deutsche Zeitschrift für Nervenheilkunde*, **20**, 132–146.

Jakob, A. (1921*c*). Über eine der multiplen Sklerose klinisch nahestehende Erkrankung des Zentralnervensystems (spastische Pseudosklerose) mit bemerkenswertem anatomischen Befund. *Medizinische Klinik*, **13**, 372–376.

Kitamoto, T., Iizuka, R., and Tateishi, J. (1993*a*). An amber mutation of prion protein in Gerstmann–Sträussler syndrome with mutant prp plaques. *Biochemical Biophysical Research Communications*, **192**, 525–531.

Kitamoto, T., Ohta, M., Dohura, K., Hitoshi, S., Terao, Y., and Tateishi, J. (1993*b*). Novel missense variants of prion protein in Creutzfeldt–Jakob disease or Gerstmann–Sträussler syndrome. *Biochemical and Biophysical Research Communications*, **191**, 709–714.

Klatzo, I., Gajdusek, D. C., and Zigas, V. (1959). Pathology of kuru. *Laboratory Investigations*, **8**, 799–847.

Klitzman, R. L., Alpers, M. P., and Gajdusek, D. C. (1984). *Neuroepidemiology*, **3**, 3–20.

Korczyn, A. D., Chapman, J., Goldfarb, L. G., Brown, P., and Gajdusek, D. C. (1991). A mutation in the prion protein gene in Creutzfeldt–Jakob disease in Jewish patients of Libyan, Greek, and Tunisian origin. *Annals of the New York Academy of Science*, **640**, 171–176.

Krasemann, S., Zerr, I., Weber, T., Poser, S., Kretzschmar, H., Hunsmann, G., *et al.* (1995). Prion disease associated with a novel nine octapeptide repeat insertion in the *PRNP* gene. *Molecular Brain Research*, **34**, 173–176.

Kretzschmar, H. A., Stowring, L. E., Westaway, D., Stubblebine, W. H., Prusiner, S. B., and Dearmond, S. J. (1986). Molecular cloning of a human prion protein cDNA. *DNA*, **5**, 315–24.

Kretzschmar, H. A., Honold, G., Seitelberger, F., Feucht, M., Wessely, P., Mehraein, P., *et al.* (1991). Prion protein mutation in family first reported by Gerstmann, Sträussler, and Scheinker. *Lancet*, **337**, 1160.

Kretzschmar, H. A., Kufer, P., Riethmuller, G., DeArmond, S. J., Prusiner, S. B., and Schiffer, D. (1992). Prion protein mutation at codon 102 in an Italian family with Gerstmann–Sträussler–Scheinker syndrome. *Neurology*, **42**, 809–810.

Laplanche, J. L., Chatelain, J., Launay, J. M., Gazengel, C., and Vidaud, M. (1990). Deletion in prion protein gene in a Moroccan family. *Nucleic Acids Research*, **18**, 22.

Laplanche, J. L., Chatelain, J., Thomas, S., Launay, J. M., Gaultier, C., and Derouesne, C. (1992). Uncommon phenotype of a codon 178 mutation of the human PrP gene. *Annals of Neurology*, **31**, 345.

Laplanche, J.-L., Delasnerie-Lauprêtre, N., Brandel, J. P., Chatelain, J., Beaudry, P., Alpérovitch, A., *et al.* (1994). Molecular genetics of prion diseases in France. French Research Group on Epidemiology of Human Spongiform Encephalopathies. *Neurology*, **44**, 2347–2351.

Laplanche, J. L., Delasnerie Laupretre, N., Brandel, J. P., Dussaucy, M., Chatelain, J., and Launay, J. M. (1995). Two novel insertions in the prion protein gene in patients with late-onset dementia. *Human Molecular Genetics*, **4**, 1109–1111.

Lugaresi, E., Medori, R., Baruzzi, P. M., Cortelli, P., Lugaresi, A., Tinuper, P., *et al.* (1986). Fatal familial insomnia and dysautonomia, with selective degeneration of thalamic nuclei. *New England Journal of Medicine*, **315**, 997–1003.

Masters, C. L., Gajdusek, D. C., and Gibbs, C. J. J. (1981). Creutzfeldt–Jakob disease virus isolations from the Gerstmann–Sträussler syndrome with an analysis of the various forms of amyloid plaque deposition in the virus-induced spongiform encephalopathies. *Brain*, **104**, 559–588.

Mastrianni, J. A., Iannicola, C., Myers, R., and Prusiner, S. B. (1995). Identification of a new mutation of the prion protein gene at codon 208 in a patient with Creutzfeldt–Jakob disease. *Neurology*, **45** (Suppl. 4), A201.

Masullo, C., Pocchiari, M., Macchi, G., Alema, G., Piazza, G., and Panzera, M. A. (1989). Transmission of Creutzfeldt–Jakob disease by dural cadaveric graft. *Journal of Neurology*, **71**, 954–955.

McGowan, J. P. (1922). Scrapie in sheep. *Scottish Journal of Agriculture*, **5**, 365–375.

Medori, R., Montagna, P., Tritschler, H. J., LeBlanc, A., Cortelli, P., Tinuper, P., *et al.* (1992*a*). Fatal familial insomnia: a second kindred with mutation of prion protein gene at codon 178. *Neurology*, **42**, 669–670.

Medori, R., Tritschler, H. J., LeBlanc, A., Villare, F., Manetto, V., Chen, H. Y., *et al.* (1992*b*). Fatal familial insomnia, a prion disease with a mutation at codon 178 of the prion protein gene. *New England Journal of Medicine*, **326**, 444–449.

Meyer, A., Leigh, D., and Bagg, C. E. (1954). A rare presenile dementia associated with cortical blindness (Heidenhain's syndrome). *Journal of Neurology, Neurosurgery and Psychiatry*, **17**, 129–133.

Miyashita, K., Inuzuka, T., Kondo, H., Saito, Y., Fujita, N., Matsubara, N., *et al.* (1991). Creutzfeldt–Jakob disease in a patient with a cadaveric dural graft. *Neurology*, **41**, 940–941.

Monari, L., Chen, S. G., Brown, P., Parchi, P., Petersen, R. B., Mikol, J., *et al.* (1994). Fatal familial insomnia and familial Creutzfeldt–Jakob disease: Different prion proteins determined by a DNA polymorphism. *Proceedings of the National Academy of Sciences of the USA*, **91**, 2839–2842.

Neufeld, M. Y., Josiphov, J., and Korczyn, A. D. (1992). Demyelinating peripheral neuropathy in Creutzfeldt–Jakob disease. *Muscle and Nerve*, **15**, 1234–1239.

Nicholl, D., Windl, O., De Silva, R., Sawcer, S., Dempster, M., Ironside, J. W., *et al.* (1995). Inherited Creutzfeldt–Jakob disease in a British family associated with a noval 144 base pair insertion of the prion protein gene. *Journal of Neurology, Neurosurgery and Psychiatry*, **58**, 65–69.

Nieto, A., Goldfarb, L. G. Brown, P. McCombie, W. R., Trapp., Trapp, S., Asher, D. M., *et al.* (1991). Codon 178 mutation in ethnically diverse Creutzfeldt–Jakob disease families. *Lancet*, **337**, 622–623.

Nisbet, T., MacDonaldson, I., and Bishara, S. (1989). Creutzfeldt–Jakob disease in a second patient who received a cadaveric dura mater graft. *Journal of the American Medical Association*, **261**, 1118.

Oda, T., Kitamoto, T., Tateishi, J., Mitsuhashi, T., Iwabuchi, K., Haga, C., *et al.* (1995). Prion disease with 144 base pair insertion in a Japanese family line. *Acta Neuropathologica (Berlin)*, **90**, 80–86.

Oesch, B., Westaway, D., Walchli, M., McKinley, M. P., Kent, S. B., Aebersold, R., *et al.* (1985). A cellular gene encodes scrapie PrP 27-30 protein. *Cell*, **40**, 735–746.

Owen, F., Poulter, M., Lofthouse, R., Collinge, J., Crow, T. J., Risby, D., *et al.* (1989). Insertion in prion protein gene in familial Creutzfeldt–Jakob disease. *Lancet*, **1**, 51–52.

Owen, F., Poulter, M., Collinge, J., Leach, M., Lofthouse, R., Crow, T. J., *et al.* (1992). A dementing illness associated with a novel insertion in the prion protein gene. *Molecular Brain Research*, **13**, 155–157.

Palmer, M. S., Dryden, A. J., Hughes, T. J., and Collinge, J. (1991). Homozygous prion protein genotype predisposes to sporadic Creutzfeldt–Jakob disease. *Nature*, **352**, 340–342.

Palmer, M. S., Mahal, S. P., Campbell, T. A., Hill, A. F., Sidle, K. C., Laplanche, J. L., *et al.* (1993). Deletions in the prion protein gene are not associated with CJD. *Human Molecular Genetics*, **2**, 541–544.

Pan, K., Baldwin, M. A., Nguyen, J., Gasset, M., Serban, A., Groth, D., *et al.* (1993). Conversion of α-helices into β-sheets features in the formation of the scrapie prion proteins. *Proceedings of the National Academy of Sciences of the USA*, **90**, 10962–10966.

Pattison, I. H. (1965). Experiments with scrapie with special reference to the nature of the agent and the pathology of the disease. In *Slow, latent and temperate virus infections, NINDB monograph 2* (ed. C. J. Gajdusek, C. J. Gibbs, and M. P. Alpers), pp. 249–257. US Government Printing, Washington DC.

Poulter, M., Baker, H. F., Frith, C. D., Leach, M., Lofthouse, R., Ridley, R. M., *et al.* (1992). Inherited prion disease with 144 base pair gene insertion. I: Genealogical and molecular studies. *Brain*, **115**, 675–685.

Prusiner, S. B., Gajdusek, D. C., and Alpers, M. P. (1982). Kuru with incubation periods exceeding two decades. *Annals of Neurology*, **12**, 1–9.

Prusiner, S. B., Scott, M., Foster, D., Pan, K. M., Groth, D., Mirenda, C., *et al.* (1990). Transgenetic studies implicate interactions between homologous PrP isoforms in scrapie prion replication. *Cell*, **63**, 673–686.

Raben, M. (1958). Treatment of a pituitary dwarf with human growth hormone. *Journal of Clinical Endocrinology and Metabolism*, **18**, 901–903.

Ripoll, L., Laplanche, J.-L., Salzmann, M., Jouvet, A., Planques, B., Dussaucy, M., *et al.* (1993). A new point mutation in the prion protein gene at codon 210 in Creutzfeldt–Jakob disease. *Neurology*, **43**, 1934–1938.

Robakis, N. K., Devine, G. E., Jenkins, E. C., Kascsak, R. J., Brown, W. T., Krawczun, M. S. *et al.* (1986). Localization of a human gene homologous to the PrP gene on the p arm of chromosome 20 and detection of PrP-related antigens in normal human brain. *Biochemical and Biophysical Research Communications*, **140**, 758–765.

Salazar, A. M., Masters, C. L., Gajdusek, D. C., and Gibbs, C. J. J. (1983). Syndromes of amyotrophic lateral sclerosis and dementia: relation to transmissible Creutzfeldt–Jakob disease. *Annals of Neurology*, **14**, 17–26.

Salvatore, M., Genuardi, M., Petraroli, R., Masullo, C., D'Alessandro, M., and Pocchiari, M. (1994). Polymorphisms of the prion protein gene in Italian patients with Creutzfeldt–Jakob disease. *Human Genetics*, **94**, 375–379.

Scrimgeour, E. M., Masters, C. L., Alpers, M. P., Kaven, J., and Gajdusek, D. C. (1983). A clinico-pathological study of a case of kuru. *Journal of Neurological Science*, **59**, 265–275.

Seitelberger, F. (1962). Eigenartige familiäre-hereditare Krankheit des zentralen Nervensystems in einer niederösterriechischen Sippe. *Wiener Klinische Wochenschrift*, **41/42**, 687–691.

Simpson, D. A., Lander, H., and Robson, H. N. (1959). *Australasian Annals of Medicine*, **8**, 8–15.

Smith, P. E. M., Zeidler, M., Ironside, J. W., Estibeiro, P., and Moss, T. H. (1995). Creutzfeldt–Jakob disease in a diary farmer. *Lancet*, **346**, 898.

Speer, M. C., Goldgaber, D., Goldfarb, L. G., Roses, A. D., and Pericak-Vance, M. A. (1991). Support of linkage of Gerstmann–Sträussler–Scheinker syndrome to the prion gene on chromosome 20p12-pter. *Genomics*, **9**, 366–368.

Spielmeyer, W. (1992). Die histopathologische Forschung in der Psychiatrie. *Klinische Wochenschrift*, **2**, 1817–1819.

Tabrizi, S. J., Scaravilli, F., Howard, R. S., Collinge, J., and Rossor, M. N. (1996). Grand Round: Creutzfeldt–Jakob disease in a young woman. Report of a meeting of physicians and scientists, St. Thomas' Hospital, London. *Lancet*, **347**, 945–948.

Tagliavini, F., Prelli, F., Ghiso, J., Bugiani, O., Serban, D., Prusiner, S. B., *et al.* (1991). Amyloid protein of Gerstmann–Sträussler–Scheinker disease (Indiana kindred) is an 11 kd fragment of prion protein with an N-terminal glycine at codon 58. *EMBO Journal*, **10**, 513–519.

Tangliavini, F., Giaccone,G., Prelli, F., Verga, L., Porro, M., Trojanowski, J. Q., *et al.* (1993). A68 is a component of paired helical filaments of Gerstmann–Sträussler–Scheinker disease, Indiana kindred. *Brain Research*, **616**, 325–328.

Tange, R. A., Troost, D., and Limburg, M. (1990). Progressive fatal dementia (Creutzfeldt–Jakob disease) in a patient who received homograft tissue for tympanic membrane closure. *European Archives of Otorhinolaryngology*, **247**, 199–201.

Tateishi, J. (1985). Transmission of Creutzfeldt–Jakob disease from human blood and urine into mice. *Lancet*, **ii**, 8463.

Tateishi, J., Koga, M., and Mori, R. (1981). Experimental transmission of Creutzfeldt–Jakob disease. *Acta Pathologica Japan*, **31**, 943–951.

Tateishi, J., Brown, P., Kitamoto, T., Hoque, Z. M., Roos, R., Wollman, R., *et al.* (1995). First experimental transmission of fatal familial insomnia. *Nature*, **376**, 434–435.

Telling, G. C., Scott, M., Hsiao, K. K., Foster, D., Yang, S., Torchia, M., *et al.* (1994). Transmission of Creutzfeldt–Jakob disease from humans to transgenic mice expressing chimeric human–mouse prion protein. *Proceedings of the National Academy of Sciences of the USA*, **91**, 9936–9940.

Telling, G. C., Scott, M., Mastrianni, J., Gabizon, R., Torchia, M., Cohen, F. E., *et al.* (1995). Prion propagation in mice expressing human and chimeric PrP transgenes implicates the interaction of cellular PrP with another protein. *Cell*, **83**, 79–90.

Thadani, V., Penar, P. L., Partington, J., Kalb, R., Janssen, R., Schonberger, L. B., *et al.* (1988). Creutzfeldt–Jakob disease probably acquired from a cadaveric dura mater graft. Case report. *Journal of Neurosurgery*, **69**, 766–769.

Weber, T., Tumani, H., Holdorff, B., Collinge, J., Palmer, M., Kretzschmar, H. A., *et al.* (1993). Transmission of Creutzfeldt–Jakob disease by handling of dura mater. *Lancet*, **341**, 123–124.

Weissmann, C. (1991). Spongiform encephalopathies. The prion's progress. *Nature*, **349**, 569–571.

Westaway, D., DeArmond, S. J., Cayetano-Canlas, J., Groth, D., Foster, D., Yang, S., *et al.* (1994). Degeneration of skeletal muscle, peripheral nerves and the central nervous system in transgenic mice overexpressing wild-type prion proteins. *Cell*, **76**, 117–129.

Will, R. G. (1993). Epidemiology of Creutzfeldt–Jakob disease. *British Medical Bulletin*, **49**, 960–970.

Will, R. and Matthew, W. (1982). Evidence for case-to-case transmission of Creutzfeldt–Jakob disease. *Journal of Neurology, Neurosurgery and Psychiatry*, **45**, 235–238.

Will, R. G., Ironside, J. W., Zeidler, M., Cousens, S. N., Estibeiro, K., Alperovitch, A., *et al.* (1996). A new variant of Creutzfeldt–Jakob disease in the UK. *Lancet*, **347**, 921–925.

Windl, O., Dempster, M., Estibeiro, J. P., Lathe, R., De Silva, R., Esmonde, T., *et al.* (in press). Genetic basis of Creutzfeldt–Jakob disease in the United Kingdom: a systematic analysis of predisposing mutations and allelic variation in the *PRNP* gene. *Human Genetics*.

Wu, Y., Brown, W. T., Robakis, N. K., Dobkin, C., Devine, G. E., Merz, P. *et al.* (1987). A PvuII RFLP detected in the human prion protein (PrP) gene. *Nucleic Acids Research*, **15**, 3191.

3 Pathology of prion diseases

JAMES W. IRONSIDE AND JEANNE E. BELL

Introduction

The neuropathology of prion diseases in animals and humans shares four characteristic features: spongiform change, neuronal loss, reactive astrocytosis, and amyloid plaque formation. Although these four features are characteristic of human and animal prion diseases, there exists a wide spectrum of neuropathology in both groups of disorders, particularly with regard to the distribution and severity of the lesions (Lantos 1992). Substantial advances in the understanding of the protein chemistry and molecular biology of prion diseases (Prusiner 1991; DeArmond 1993a,b) has prompted renewed interest in the neuropathology of these disorders. The emergence of bovine spongiform encephalopathy (BSE) and other 'novel' prion diseases in animals (see Chapter 1), the recognition of new clinical syndromes in human prion diseases (see Chapter 2) and the outbreak of iatrogenic Creutzfeldt–Jakob disease (CJD) in recipients of human pituitary hormones (Gibbs *et al.* 1985) have also been accompanied by further attempts to understand the pathological processes occurring in the central nervous system (CNS) under such circumstances. The recent recognition that spongiform change is not an exclusive feature of human prion diseases (Hansen *et al.* 1989; Bell and Ironside 1993a) has prompted detailed studies in the comparative pathology of human prion diseases and other neurodegenerative disorders occurring in humans, particularly Alzheimer's disease (DeArmond 1993a). Although the transmissible agents responsible for prion disorders are unique, the similarities between the pathology of human and animal prion diseases and other unrelated neurodegenerative disorders imply the existence of common mechanisms of cell injury and death in the CNS.

Human prion diseases

The first human prion diseases to be recognized were CJD, kuru, and Gerstmann–Sträussler syndrome (GSS). The recent advances in knowledge of the molecular biology of the human prion protein (PrP) gene have allowed recognition and characterization of additional human prion disorders (see Chapter 2). One such disorder, fatal familial insomnia (Medori *et al.* 1992), is of particular interest not only with respect to its clinical and genetic features, but in the spectrum of neuropathological changes described, several cases of which appear not to show evidence of spongiform change (Gambetti *et al.* 1993). Furthermore, recent cases of inherited prion diseases have been reported in which all the classical pathological features of CJD are absent (Collinge *et al.* 1990). The ever-widening range of identified abnormalities in the human PrP gene, and the widening clinical spectrum of human prion diseases have resulted in a corresponding widening of diagnostic criteria for this group of disorders:

- clinical features and history
- electroencephalogram abnormalities
- PrP gene abnormalities
- spongiform change in CNS
- PrP accumulation in CNS
- transmissibility.

In practice, it is convenient to retain the main historical categories for classification of human prion diseases with modifications to include newly recognized entities:

- CJD—sporadic, new variant, iatrogenic, or inherited
- GSS—classical, or variants with neurofibrillary tangles
- fatal familial insomnia (FFI)
- atypical prion dementias
- kuru.

This forms a sound basis for clinicopathological correlations and can be readily modified to accommodate new clinical and molecular genetic data.

Macroscopic pathology

Human prion diseases are uniformly fatal neurodegenerative disorders which pursue a variable clinical course, with survival periods ranging from a few months to several years (Bastian 1991). Most patients die from bronchopneumonia or pulmonary embolism as a result of prolonged immobility, with inanition, generalized muscle wasting, and cachexia being common findings in cases with prolonged survival. As with animal prion diseases, no specific abnormalities are detectable outside the CNS at autopsy. Examination of the brain may not reveal any macroscopic abnormality; cerebral cortical atrophy is a characteristic finding in many cases of CJD, although this varies enormously both from case to case and within the various regions of the cortex in an affected case (Tomlinson 1992). The pattern of cortical atrophy may be related to clinical features of the disease, such as atrophy of the visual cortex in cases with cortical blindness.

Occasionally, the brain weight in CJD is reduced to less than 1000 g (Fig. 3.1): cortical atrophy in such cases is usually accompanied by atrophy of the basal ganglia, thalamus, and hypothalamus (Brown *et al.* 1984; Tomlinson 1992). Selective thalamic atrophy is a characteristic feature of FFI (Gambetti *et al.* 1993), and may be detected on gross examination of the brain. These macroscopic abnormalities are not specific, but may be shared with a wide range of other neuro-

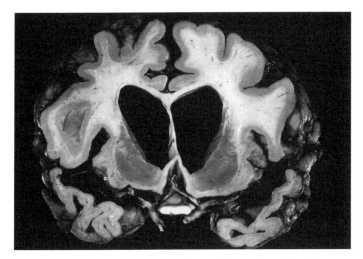

Fig. 3.1 Extreme cerebral atrophy in a case of sporadic CJD involving the cortex and basal ganglia with secondary white matter loss and ventricular dilatation.

degenerative disorders including Alzheimer's disease, Pick's disease, Huntington's disease, and multisystem atrophy. Cerebellar atrophy may be a prominent macroscopic abnormality in some cases of human prion diseases, particularly in kuru and GSS (Tomlinson 1992), and also in iatrogenic CJD occurring in human pituitary hormone recipients (Gibbs *et al.* 1985; Bell and Ironside 1993*a*). In these cases, cerebral cortical atrophy may be absent: a differential diagnosis in such cases would include cerebellar cortical atrophy (Holme's type), olivopontocerebellar atrophy, and other forms of spinocerebellar degeneration, including multisystem atrophy. Hereditary spinocerebellar degeneration is a clinical diagnosis which has been applied clinically to GSS kindreds which have not been studied histologically, emphasizing the need for accurate pathological and genetic studies in such families.

Microscopic pathology

Sporadic CJD

The classical triad of histological abnormalities in human prion diseases is spongiform change, neuronal loss, and reactive astrocytosis (Manuelidis 1985; Lantos 1992). These features are not consistently present throughout the CNS, and vary enormously from case to case and within the CNS in individual cases. Spongiform change consists of a fine vacuolation of the neuropil of the grey matter in which the vacuoles vary in size from around 2 μm to 20 μm (Fig. 3.2a), with larger vacuoles becoming confluent to form irregular cavities (Fig. 3.7a) (Masters and Richardson

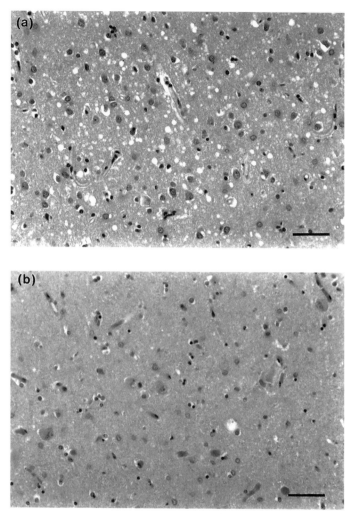

Fig. 3.2 Microvacuolar spongiform change in the cerebral cortex in CJD (a) is accompanied by neuronal loss and reactive gliosis. Haematoxylin and eosin staining. Bar is 50 μm. In FFI (b) neuronal loss and reactive gliosis occur in the absence of spongiform change. Haematoxylin and eosin staining. Bar is 62.5 μm.

1978). Vacuolation of neurones is also occasionally present, although this is usually not a dominant feature. A distinction has been drawn between spongiform change and status spongiosis, where extensive neuronal loss is accompanied by severe reactive gliosis and cavitation of the neuropil, with collapse of the cytoarchitecture (Masters and Gajdusek 1982). Status spongiosis is not confined to human prion diseases, but may occur in other neurodegenerative diseases including Pick's disease and Alzheimer's disease (Bell and Ironside 1993a).

Neuronal loss and reactive astrocytosis tend to be most apparent in the areas of grey matter with spongiform change. As might be expected, neuronal loss is usually most severe in cases with a prolonged clinical history in which there is extensive cortical atrophy with status spongiosis (Tomlinson 1992). Spongiform change of variable severity is usually present in the cerebral cortex (often in layers 2–3), albeit in a patchy distribution. The molecular layer of the cerebellar cortex is usually involved (Fig. 3.3), although confluent vacuolation is unusual at this site (Bell and Ironside 1993*a*). Other neuronal abnormalities may be apparent, including abnormal dendritic patterns, with Purkinje cell torpedoes in the cerebellum (Bastian 1991). Ballooned neurones are occasionally evident in the cerebral cortex; these are most easily visualized on immunocytochemistry for αB crystallin and neurofilament proteins (Nakazota *et al.* 1990; Kato *et al.* 1992). A range of neuronal cytoplasmic inclusions have been described in human prion diseases, including Hirano bodies, neurofibrillary tangles, and small punctate inclusions demonstrable on ubiquitin immunocytochemistry (Ironside *et al.* 1992; Tomlinson 1992). Ubiquitin immunocytochemistry also reveals granular deposition of ubiquinated proteins around areas of spongiform change, which occur in relation to granular deposits of PrP (see below) (Ironside *et al.* 1993*b*). Neuronal nuclear inclusions have also been described; they occur rarely and their precise nature is unknown. Vacuolation of the cerebral white matter is uncommon in CJD (Berciano *et al.* 1990), although a loss of myelinated fibres may be observed as a consequence of neuronal loss and cortical atrophy. Necrotizing lesions in the cerebral white matter have been described in cases of CJD from Japan (Kawata *et al.* 1992); these changes are not characteristic of CJD cases in Western countries and their pathogenesis is uncertain.

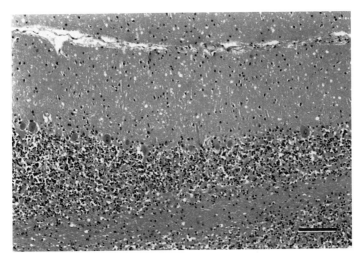

Fig. 3.3 Microvacuolar spongiform change is present in the cerebellar molecular layer in most cases of CJD, accompanied by reactive gliosis and neuronal loss, particularly in the granular layer. Haematoxylin and eosin staining. Bar is 125 μm.

The reactive astrocytosis in human spongiform disease is most apparent in areas with severe spongiform change and neuronal loss. Astrocytic cell processes can be seen to extend around areas of spongiform change (Fig. 3.4) and an extensive network of cell processes can be revealed by immunocytochemistry for glial fibrillary acidic protein around PrP amyloid plaques in both CJD and GSS (Bell and Ironside 1993*a*). Recent studies have demonstrated that a florid microglial reaction occurs in human prion diseases, with marked hyperplasia and hypertrophy of these cells (Fig. 3.5). Microglial cells expressing class II major histocompatibility complex (MHC) are widespread throughout areas of spongiform change and, like the reactive astrocytes, microglial cell processes can be seen to extend around spongiform vacuoles (Ironside *et al.* 1993*a*). Microglial cells are also closely associated with PrP plaques and there is an accumulating body of evidence to suggest that microglia may be involved in the processing of amyloid precursor proteins into amyloid fibrils, in a manner analogous to the β/A4 amyloid plaques which are the major extracellular lesions in the cerebral cortex in Alzheimer's disease (Frackowiak *et al.* 1992).

PrP amyloid plaques have been described in a minority of cases of sporadic CJD, but occur at increased frequencies in kuru (in up to 70% of cases), familial CJD, and, most strikingly, in GSS (Bastian 1991). Historical descriptions of plaque incidence and morphology require revision as PrP immunocytochemistry now provides a sensitive and specific method of plaque detection (Hashimoto *et al.* 1992; Bell and Ironside 1993*a*). Classical plaque morphology in human prion diseases comprises the compact or kuru plaque and larger multicentric plaques which are usually confined to GSS cases (Bastian 1991). The compact plaque in

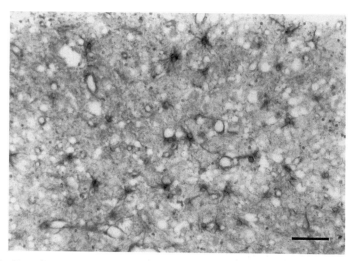

Fig. 3.4   Reactive astrocytosis in the cerebral cortex in CJD, with cell processes extending around spongiform vacuoles. Immunocytochemistry for glial fibrillary acidic protein plus haematoxylin staining. Bar is 50 μm.

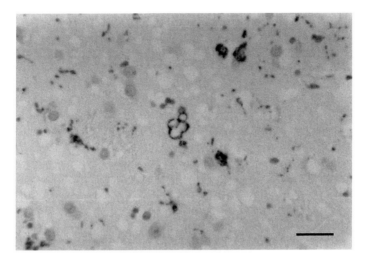

Fig. 3.5 Microglial hypertrophy in the cerebral cortex in CJD, with cell processes extending around spongiform vacuoles (centre). Immunocytochemistry for CD 68 plus haematoxylin staining. Bar is 50 μm.

CJD and kuru consists of a uniform dense core surrounded by a pale halo of radiating fibrils (Fig. 3.6). These are most often seen in the cerebellum, usually in the granular layer or adjacent to Purkinje cells, but PrP immunocytochemistry has revealed a wider distribution in the cerebellum, including the molecular layer of the cortex and the subcortical white matter (Bell and Ironside 1993*a*). Similar

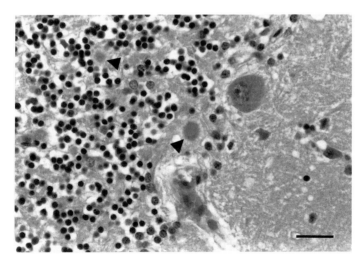

Fig. 3.6 Kuru-type plaques in CJD consist of a homogeneous core surrounded by a halo of radiating fibrils (arrowheads). Haematoxylin and eosin staining. Bar is 25 μm.

plaques may also occur in the cerebrum; cerebral plaques do not appear to occur in human prion diseases in the absence of cerebellar plaques. The large multicentric plaques found in GSS show a striking range of morphological similarities to Alzheimer β/A4 plaques, with a dense plaque core surrounded by a peripheral area in which neuritic processes, astrocytic processes, and microglial cells may be identified. These plaques are usually present in the molecular layer of the cerebellum, but PrP immunocytochemistry has revealed a wider distribution in the cerebellum and cerebrum than historical descriptions suggest (Bell and Ironside 1993*a*).

CJD occurs most frequently in elderly individuals, in which the CNS may show other age-related changes including neuronal loss and cerebral cortical atrophy, 'senile' β/A4 plaques, neurofibrillary tangles, and occasional Lewy bodies in the pigmented nuclei of the thalamus and brainstem (Bell and Ironside 1993*a*). It is important to recognize these abnormalities on histological examination; their significance should be interpreted in light of published data concerning the frequency of these abnormalities in apparently normal elderly individuals and a broad general experience of the examination of the CNS in both normal and demented elderly individuals.

A new variant of CJD in UK and France

A new variant of CJD was recently identified by the CJD Surveillance Unit in UK (Will *et al.* 1996), followed by a report of a similar case in France (Chazot *et al.* 1996). The patients in these reports differed from typical cases of sporadic CJD in terms of the relatively young age at disease onset (average 26.3 years), the prolonged duration of illness (average 14 months) and the clinical features, in which presentation with psychiatric symptoms or dysaesthesiae was common, followed by cerebellar signs and symptoms, with myoclonus or chorea occuring late in the illness. Dementia was not evident until the final stages of the illness, when it was often accompanied by cortical blindness and akinetic mutism. None of these patients showed changes in the electroencephalogram which were characteristic of sporadic CJD, and all were methionine homozygotes at codon 129 with no pathogenic mutations in the PRNP gene.

The neuropathological features in these cases were remarkably similar, and presented a spectrum of changes which were highly unusual for sporadic CJD. Although spongiform change was present in all cases in the cerebral cortex, the most striking abnormality was the presence of multiple kuru-type PrP plaques, many of which were surrounded by a halo of spongiform change (Fig. 3.7b). Similar plaques were present in other regions of the cerebrum and cerebellum. Spongiform change was most evident in the basal ganglia and thalamus, with severe thalamic astrocytosis.

Immunocytochemistry showed widespread accumulation of PrP in the brain, particularly in the cerebellar cortex and occipital cortex. The relationship of these cases to sporadic CJD in older patients is unclear; further studies are required to

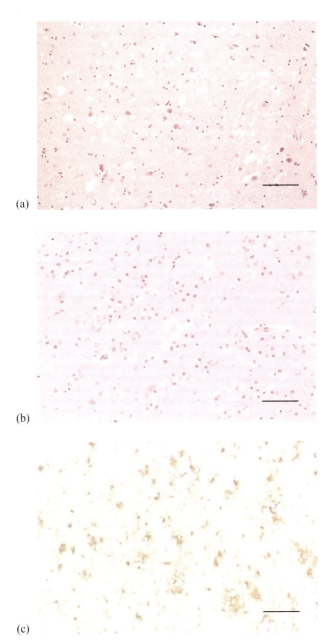

(a)

(b)

(c)

Fig. 3.7 (a) Confluent spongiform change in the cerebral cortex in sporadic CJD with a background of microvacuolar spongiform change, accompanied by neuronal loss and reactive gliosis. Neuronal vacuolation is not present. Haematoxylin and eosin staining. Bar is 75 μm; (b) In the new variant of CJD the cerebral vortex contains kuru-type PrP amyloid plaques, surrounded by spongiform change (*centre*). Haematoxylin and eosin staining. Bar is 75 μm; (c) Deposits of PrP in and around areas of confluent spongiform change in the cortex in sporadic CJD, showing the vacuolar pattern of deposition. PrP immunocytochemistry with haematoxylin staining. Bar is 50 μm;

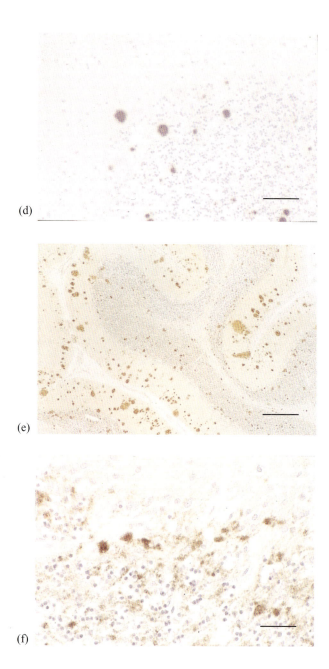

(d) Immunolocalization of PrP (plaque pattern) in the granular layer of the cerebellum in sporadic CJD. Note that the Purkinje cells and molecular layer are unstained. PrP immunocytochemistry with haematoxylin staining. Bar is 50 μm; (e) Cerebellum in GSS shows large irregular PrP-positive plaques in the molecular layer. PrP immunocytochemistry with haematoxylin staining. Bar is 125 μm; (f) PrP positivity in the granular layer in the cerebellum of a growth hormone treated case of CJD. PrP immunocytochemistry plus haematoxylin staining. Bar is 50 μm.

characterize this unusual phenotype and investigate the possibility that these cases are causally related to exposure to the BSE agent via the human foodchain.

Kuru

This variety of human prion disease has become now virtually extinct since the abolition of cannibalism and other related practices in the Fore tribe in New Guinea (Alpers 1987). The predominant clinical manifestations of kuru were related to cerebellar dysfunction (Gajdusek and Vigas 1957), and it is not surprising to find that cerebellar atrophy was a prominent macroscopic abnormality in such cases. The most striking histological abnormality in kuru was the presence of amyloid plaques, which occurred in approximately 70% of cases, particularly in the cerebellum (Klatzo *et al.* 1959). Although most of these kuru plaques were of the compact morphological variety, a range of plaque morphologies was recorded (Neumann *et al.* 1965). PrP immunocytochemistry has confirmed that these plaques are composed of prion protein (Hashimoto *et al.* 1992) and electron microscopy has shown a similar ultrastructural appearance to other PrP plaques occurring in GSS and both sporadic and familial CJD (Field *et al.* 1969). It has been suggested that the formation of PrP plaques in kuru was most widespread in cases with a prolonged clinical history (Alpers 1987); no other factors which might influence PrP plaque formation have yet been identified in this disorder, particularly in relation to PrP genotype.

The earliest published observations on the pathology of this disorder did not indicate that spongiform change was a prominent feature (Klatzo *et al.* 1959), but subsequent studies showed a variable distribution of spongiform change in the cerebral cortex, basal ganglia, thalamus, and cerebellum (Neumann *et al.* 1964). Spongiform change was a prominent finding in experimental transmissions of kuru to chimpanzees (Gajdusek *et al.* 1966); this observation prompted the first experimental transmissions of CJD to primates (Gibbs *et al.* 1968), followed by a similar experiment on GSS (Masters *et al.* 1981).

GSS

The early description of GSS emphasized the large numbers of amyloid plaques in the brain (Gerstmann *et al.* 1936). The most characteristic plaque structure in GSS is the multicentric plaque (Boellaard and Schlote 1980). These plaques are most numerous in the cerebellum, involving predominantly the molecular and granular layers, but also being present in smaller numbers in the cerebellar white matter, the cerebral cortex, and basal ganglia. A variety of plaque morphologies have subsequently been described in this disorder, some of which overlap with those occurring in kuru and sporadic CJD (Boellaard *et al.* 1993); the plaques in GSS are also composed of PrP (Hashimoto *et al.* 1992). Cerebellar involvement in GSS is usually severe, with neuronal loss and reactive gliosis in addition to the presence of PrP plaques. The severity of cerebellar involvement is reflected in the macroscopic abnormalities in GSS, in which cerebellar atrophy predominates.

Spongiform change has been described elsewhere in the CNS, particularly in the superficial cerebral cortex (Hudson *et al.* 1983), but this is by no means a constant feature. In the Indiana GSS kindred neurofibrillary tangles are present in large numbers within the cerebral cortex (Ghetti *et al.* 1993). In this disorder, a mutation exists at codon 198 in the PrP gene, whereas most families with 'classic' GSS have a leucine substitution at codon 102 (Hsiao *et al.* 1989). In these classic cases, neurofibrillary tangle formation is not usually evident. Other PrP gene mutations have been reported in families with GSS, one of which (arginine substitution at codon 217) is associated with cerebral cortical neurofibrillary tangles (Anano *et al.* 1992). It is possible that in the past such cases were misdiagnosed as familial Alzheimer's disease, before molecular genetic studies and PrP immunocytochemistry were available to confirm the nature of the underlying genetic disorder and the precise identity of the amyloid plaques in the CNS (de Courten-Myers and Mandybur 1987; Hart and Gordon 1990).

Iatrogenic CJD

In cases of iatrogenic CJD, the main pathological features described above can all be recognized, although the distribution of the lesions varies from case to case (Bastian 1991; Lantos 1992). However, in cases associated with human pituitary hormone therapy, cerebellar involvement is particularly marked and these cases exhibit gross cerebellar atrophy at autopsy with extensive neuronal loss, widespread spongiform change, and PrP amyloid plaque formation. Immunocytochemical studies have also demonstrated a more widespread distribution of PrP in a diffuse pattern within the cerebellar granular layer in many of these cases (Bell and Ironside 1993*a*).

Fatal familial insomnia and 'prion dementias'

Fatal familial insomnia is an interesting example of an inherited human prion disease with characteristic genetic abnormality at codon 178 in the PrP gene (Medori *et al.* 1992). The clinical features of this disorder are distinctive, and the pathology is correspondingly striking, with severe thalamic gliosis being the predominant abnormality (Fig. 3.2b). Spongiform change has not been reported in all individuals with this disorder, and PrP amyloid plaques are absent. A range of other coexisting neuropathological abnormalities have been reported in this disorder, including atrophy with neuronal loss and gliosis in the olivopontocerebellar system (Gambetti *et al.* 1993).

Another type of pathology has been revealed by immunocytochemical studies for PrP in inherited prion diseases. In one large kindred with a 144 base pair insert in the PrP gene a range of pathological abnormalities have been described in affected demented individuals, ranging from classical CJD to cases without any characteristic pathological abnormalities (Collinge *et al.* 1990). These findings emphasize the variability of the neuropathology in human prion diseases, even in families with an identical genetic mutation. Other factors are presumably involved in the evolution of the neuropathology in these cases, and further research is required to elucidate the other mechanisms involved in the pathogenesis of the structural changes in the brain. The term 'prion dementia' has been coined for cases in such families where routine neuropathological examination of the brain has yielded little in the way of features which are characteristic for human prion diseases (Collinge *et al.* 1990). Immunocytochemistry for PrP however has revealed abnormal deposits of the protein in the brain, particularly in the molecular layer of the cerebellar cortex (Lantos *et al.* 1992). These findings are discussed below, and appear to be unrelated to spongiform change or PrP amyloid plaque formation.

Features shared with other neurodegenerative diseases

Detailed neuropathological studies on human prion diseases have revealed a spectrum of abnormalities which overlap to a considerable extent with other human neurodegenerative disorders, particular Alzheimer's disease. Alzheimer's disease and CJD can occur simultaneously (Powers *et al.* 1991), but this is a very rare event and there is no evidence to support a specific association between these disorders. It is now accepted that spongiform change can occur in a range of other neurodegenerative disorders (Table 3.1), although in such cases the distribution of the abnormality is usually limited to characteristic sites within the brain and appears to be represented by microvacuolation within the neuropil rather than the more extensive confluent form of spongiform change usually present in CJD (Bell and Ironside 1993*a*). The implications of this finding are significant in two ways: first, the pathogenesis of spongiform change is not confined to human prion diseases but is common to other unrelated disorders; second, spongiform change cannot be regarded as pathognomonic for human prion diseases. This should be borne in mind when cortical biopsy is contemplated as an investigation on suspected cases of

Table 3.1 Other conditions involving spongiform change or vacuolation in the CNS in humans

Spongiform change	Alzheimer's disease
	Diffuse Lewy body disease
	Dementia of frontal lobe type (associated with motor neurone disease)
	Pick's disease
Vacuolation of grey and white matter	Status spongiosis
	Cerebral oedema
	Metabolic encephalopathies
	Neuronal storage disorders
	Canavan's disease
	Tissue fixation and processing artefacts

human prion disease, since spongiform change *per se* is not necessarily a specific diagnostic feature for this group of diseases. Other conditions which may be misinterpreted as spongiform change are listed in Table 3.1.

A comparison of the features of prion diseases and Alzheimer's disease is given in Table 3.2. Recently, authors have emphasized the regional progression of Alzheimer's disease in the human brain, which resembles the evolution of disease in murine scrapie following focal inoculation of brain homogenates into the CNS (DeArmond 1993a). Neurofibrillary tangles are a characteristic feature of Alzheimer's disease (Probst *et al.* 1991), and can occur in human prion diseases, particularly in the GSS Indiana kindred (Ghetti *et al.* 1989). Neuritic plaques of the β/A4 type are characteristic of Alzheimer's disease (Probst *et al.* 1991) and yet plaques of similar morphology can occur in human prion disease, being composed of PrP rather than the β/A4 protein. Recent investigations into the Indiana GSS kindred have revealed that deposition of the β/A4 protein can also occur in some cases of human prion disease within PrP plaques, usually at the periphery of the lesion, indicating a similar mechanism for plaque formation in these distinct disorders (Bugiani *et al.* 1993). Other plaque components including neuritic processes, microglial cells, and astrocytic processes have been reported in both PrP and β/A4 plaques; microglial cells are implicated as being of major importance in the evolution of amyloid deposition occurring in both lesions. In contrast to human prion diseases, Alzheimer's disease has been found to be non-transmissable to other species. However, an interesting recent study has shown accumulations of β/A4 protein in the brains of elderly primates following intracerebral inoculation with Alzheimer brain homogenate (Baker *et al.* 1993). Further studies on this phenomenon are required, however, to determine its significance.

Table 3.2   Alzheimer's disease and human prion disease

Similarities
- Most cases occur as sporadic disorders.
- Familial forms occur in both disorders, usually as autosomal dominant conditions with specific genetic mutations.
- Neuronal loss and reactive gliosis occur in the CNS in both disorders.
- Amyloid plaques (β/A4 protein or PrP) are formed in the CNS, with associated neuritic and glial components.
- The precursor of the amyloidogenic protein in both diseases is a normal cell membrane glycoprotein which is also involved in inclusion body myositis.

Differences
- Neurofibrillary tangles are common in Alzheimer's disease but rare in prion diseases.
- No clear evidence that Alzheimer's disease is transmissible (although β/A4 protein deposition may be induced by inoculation of Alzheimer brain homogenate into the CNS of aged primates); CJD, kuru, and GSS can be transmitted to primates and other species.

PrP in skeletal muscle disease

Recent studies have demonstrated that PrP and β/A4 protein deposition are not confined to the CNS but may also be associated with a necrotizing myopathy, inclusion body myositis (Askanas *et al.* 1992, 1993). This is a relatively common age-related muscle disorder associated with filamentous structures within muscle fibres accompanied by muscle fibre degeneration and inflammatory changes. The fibres characteristically contain rimmed vacuoles and amyloid-like filaments that react with antisera to both the β/A4 protein and PrP. This finding is of particular interest in relation to the recent report of a severe generalized skeletal muscle disorder in transgenic mice that express high levels of hamster, mouse, or sheep PrP (Westaway *et al.* 1994). On histological examination this has been found to be a necrotizing myopathy with accumulation of the transgene-associated PrP within the muscle fibres.

Ultrastructural studies in human prion diseases

Detailed ultrastructural studies of human prion diseases are considerably hampered by problems associated with post-mortem autolysis and poor ultrastructural preservation. Fewer cortical biopsies are now performed in suspected cases of human prion disease, and hence opportunities to study in detail the ultrastructural changes associated with this group of disorders are now less readily available. However, previous observers have reported ultrastructural findings relating to spongiform change, which appears to result from dilatation within the nerve cell dendrites and may relate to swelling of the endoplasmic reticulum or Golgi apparatus (Bastian 1991). The precise nature of the spongiform vacuoles in human prion diseases is unknown, as is their mechanism of evolution. Other ultrastructural changes relate to abnormalities in neuronal dendritic processes, and astrocytic changes relating to hyperplasia in reactive astrocytes (Tomlinson *et al.* 1992).

Ultrastructural studies of PrP plaques have suggested that microglial cell processes are intimately associated with the core region of the plaque, and this has been recently confirmed by immunocytochemistry at light microscopic level and confocal scanning laser microscopy (Turner *et al.* 1993). An apparently unique neuronal abnormality, the tubulovesicular body, has been reported in well-preserved biopsies from cases of CJD and in experimental prion disorders (Liberski *et al.* 1990, 1992). The precise nature of this abnormality is uncertain, although some workers have claimed it is related to a postulated infectious agent responsible for this group of disorders. Further studies are required to clarify the precise nature and significance of this unusual finding.

Immunocytochemistry

These descriptions of the classical histopathological findings in human prion diseases highlight the variability between cases of the distribution and severity of lesions, particularly of spongiform change. Why this variability should exist is poorly understood, but pathological studies were given a new impetus when it was recognized that human cases, like the animal prion diseases, are characterized by the accumulation in brain tissue of the disease-related protein, PrP^{CJD} (Bockman *et al.* 1985). It has become clear that PrP^{CJD} is a perverted and insoluble form of a naturally occurring cell surface protein PrP^C which is expressed in many tissues of the body including brain tissue, particularly, on neuronal membranes. The presence of PrP^{CJD} has been demonstrated in brain tissue of prion disease cases by the process of immunoblotting as well as in extracts of brain tissue by Western blotting (Tateishi and Kitamoto 1993). It is clearly of interest to attempt more precise localization of PrP^{CJD} at the cellular level by immunocytochemical investigation, since it might be expected that the disease-related protein would have some topographical relationship with pathology findings. One potential pitfall in this approach is that PrP^{CJD} is so closely related to the normal cellular form of PrP that the antibodies currently available do not clearly separate one form from the other. In spite of this difficulty which is explored in more detail below, quite a number of immunocytochemical surveys have now been published which purport to show the localization of PrP^{CJD} in prion disease cases (Kitamoto and Tateishi 1988; Piccardo *et al.* 1990; Guiroy *et al.* 1991*b*; Powers *et al.* 1991; Hashimoto *et al.* 1992; Lantos *et al.* 1992; Bell and Ironside 1993*a*; Bugiani *et al.* 1993; Hayward *et al.* 1994). Sufficient consensus exists between reports of both human and animal (McBride *et al.* 1988) studies for the results to have credibility.

The UK National CJD Surveillance Unit in Edinburgh has provided the opportunity of applying immunocytochemical techniques to more than 120 cases of human prion disease (Bell and Ironside 1993*a*). These include current cases awaiting diagnosis, archival cases referred from the UK and from abroad, and cases of dementia in which pathological examination has not previously yielded a definitive diagnosis. We have employed a range of antibodies (Table 3.3) and a variety of pre-treatments to enhance the positivity of what is believed to be disease-related PrP^{CJD}, and to reduce background staining and the likelihood of detection of PrP^C. These pre-treatments are based on the experience of other laboratories and published methods (reviewed in Bell and Ironside 1993*a*) (Table 3.4). There are important safety issues in preparation, sectioning, and staining of multiple blocks of brain tissue which remain infective after formalin fixation (Bell and Ironside 1993*a,b*). In brief, Brown *et al.* (1990) have shown that brain tissue from human prion disease cases is effectively decontaminated by immersion of tissue blocks for 60 minutes in 96% formic acid, after formalin fixation and before processing. Serendipitously, this procedure also enhances immunostaining for many features of interest in tissue sections and is particularly valuable in the pre-treatment of sections stained for the presence of PrP^{CJD} (Kitamoto *et al.* 1987). In most immunocytochemical studies which have investigated the localization of PrP^{CJD}, formic acid has been used as a pre-treatment and the absence of staining in control sections obtained from non-spongiform dementias has been taken as evidence for the specificity of the reaction.

Table 3.3 PrP antibodies

Antibody	Clonality	Antigen	Source	Dilution
ME7	Polyclonal	Scrapie fibrils	Dr J. Hope	1 in 500, 30 min
IB4	Polyclonal		Edinburgh	1 in 500, 30 min
IB3	Polyclonal			1 in 1000, overnight
IA8	Polyclonal			1 in 1800, overnight (with pre-treatment)
RO73	Polyclonal	Hamster prion	Dr S. Prusiner	1 in 400, 30 min
611	Monoclonal		California	1 in 2000, overnight (with pre-treatment)
1755	Polyclonal	Synthetic peptide (partial sequence sheep SAF protein)	Dr H. Diringer Berlin	1 in 1500, overnight (with pre-treatment)
SP30	Polyclonal	Synthetic peptide (partial sequence sheep PrP)	Prof. B. Anderton London	1 in 1500, overnight
SP40	Polyclonal			1 in 1500, overnight
3F4	Monoclonal	Synthetic peptide (residues 108–111 of human PrP^C)	Dr Kascsak New York	1 in 1500, overnight
PrP Nott.	Polyclonal	Synthetic peptide (Diringer sequence)	Prof. R. J. Mayer	1 in 1000, overnight
KG9	Monoclonal	Recombinant (bovine PrP)	Dr C. Birkett (Compton)	1 in 2000, overnight

Table 3.4 Possible pre-treatment schedules for PrP^{CJD} immunocytochemistry

- 80–100% formic acid, 5–60 min.
- 4 M guanidine thiocyanate 2 h.
- Proteinase K 10 μg/ml, 15 min, 37°C.
- Pepsin 10%, 30 min, 37°C.
- Hydrolytic autoclaving, 2.5 mM HCl, 10 min, 121°C.
- Hydrated autoclaving, distilled water, 10 min, 120°C.
- 30% formic acid, 1 min in microwave oven.
- 96% formic acid 60 min followed by 4 M guanidine thiocyanate, 2 h, 4°C.

For further details, see Bell and Ironside 1993a.

The method for PrP^{CJD} immunocytochemistry currently in use in the National CJD Surveillance Unit (see Appendix) has evolved over a number of years and has been modified by our experience in using a variety of different antibodies (Table 3.3). It seems that different antibodies require slight variations in the pre-staining protocol in order to achieve optimal results. Although there are some differences in the features demonstrated by different antibodies, in general the staining patterns are reproducible. In any particular case of human prion disease, the application of different antibodies and different pre-treatment demonstrates the same basic pattern of PrP positivity but the topography and form of PrP-positive features do vary from case to case. Manipulations of the pre-treatments, in particular the application of autoclave pre-treatment (Kitamoto *et al.* 1992*a,b*), serves to enhance the positivity, and consistently brings out features which are not well shown with other pre-treatments. Background staining is also reduced by autoclave pre-treatment as compared with other methods.

To clarify the full spectrum of PrP immunolocalization in human prion disease cases, small blocks of tissue from frontal, parietal, temporal, and occipital cerebral cortex have been investigated, together with basal ganglia, thalamus, hypothalamus, brainstem, and cerebellum. Spinal cord, pituitary, and pituitary stalk have also been examined when available. It is necessary to examine this rather large number of blocks in each case because it has become clear that immunolocalization of PrP is as variable in prion disease cases as is the pattern of standard pathology. Nevertheless certain generalities about the pattern of PrP positivity become evident from studying a large number of cases. PrP immunostaining patterns appear to be of two main types; these are in the form of perivacuolar deposits and defined plaques (Bell and Ironside 1993*a*). In the presence of severe spongiform change in neocortical grey matter, irregular strongly positive deposits of PrP are present within coalescing vacuoles and around the periphery of these lesions (Fig. 3.7c). This form of PrP staining in spongiform cortex we have called the vacuolar pattern of PrP deposition. In those cases characterized by small discrete vacuoles scattered diffusely in the cortical neuropil, much less PrP positivity is seen in the cortex which may indeed appear to be negative unless the most stringent pre-treatments are employed. The second distinctive pattern of PrP positivity is that associated with plaque formation in prion disease case (Fig. 3.7d). Plaques may or may not be visible in routinely stained sections and in sections stained to demonstrate the presence of amyloid. However the application of PrP antibodies, particularly following autoclave pretreatment, may reveal plaques in greater numbers than otherwise apparent and in wider distribution around the brain (Kitamoto and Tateishi 1988; Piccardo *et al.* 1990; Guiroy *et al.* 1991*b*; Powers *et al.* 1991; Hashimoto *et al.* 1992; Lantos *et al.* 1992; Bell and Ironside 1993*a*; Bugiani *et al.* 1993; Hayward *et al.* 1994). Most frequently the sites of plaque accumulation include the granular layer and, to a lesser extent, the central white matter and molecular layers of the cerebellum (Fig. 3.7d). Well defined plaques are also sometimes seen in the basal ganglia, thalami, brainstem, and cerebral cortex. The density of PrP staining in prion plaques may not be uniform within and between plaques, and the classic well defined 'kuru' plaques often have pale centres. Sometimes the plaques are arranged in linear arrays particularly along the Purkinje cell layer (Fig. 3.8) and within granular layer of the cerebellum. Cerebellar deposits, particularly in the form of large, confluent, and rather irregularly shaped PrP-positive plaques, are most conspicuous in cases of GSS (Fig. 3.7e). Purkinje cells appear negative in PrP-stained preparations in all cases of prion disease (Fig. 3.8).

More subtle forms of positivity for PrP are seen in many cases. Close examination of the deep grey matter of the brain, and of the brain stem, shows that many fibre tracts appear positive, apparently within neuronal processes (Fig. 3.9). Some neurones appear to be outlined by granular PrP-positive deposits (Fig. 3.10) suggestive of synaptic accumulations at the surface of the perikaryon, and in some instances intra-neuronal staining appears to be present. Similar punctate perineuronal PrP deposits have been described by Kitamoto *et al.* (1992*a*) in cases of CJD subjected to autoclave pre-treatments, and co-localization with synaptophysin was suggested. Punctate granular staining of astrocyte cytoplasm is also sometimes observed, similar to that reported in animals (Diedrich *et al.* 1991) particularly in those cases which show marked cortical and basal ganglionic gliosis (Bell and Ironside 1993*a*). Concurrent investigation using antibodies to cell-specific products may be useful in an attempt to identify the cells and structures which are PrP positive. In this way antibodies to glial fibrillary acidic protein, synaptophysin, and neurofilament, as well as microglial markers, (Ironside *et al.* 1993*a*) are of value in close serial sections or in double immunofluorescent preparations.

Considerable variation in PrP immunostaining is seen in the human prion diseases. In some cases, particularly in archival material which may have been fixed for long periods, there may be some difficulty in demonstrating PrP positivity in many areas of the brain despite the presence of classical spongiform changes.

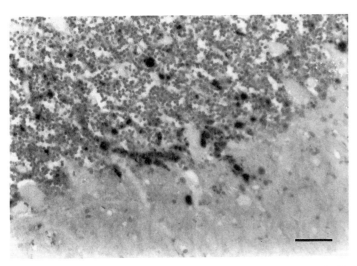

Fig. 3.8 Linear arrays of small plaque-like deposits of PrP in and close to the Purkinje cell layer of the cerebellum in sporadic CJD. Note that the Purkinje cells themselves are PrP negative. PrP immunocytochemistry plus haematoxylin staining. Bar is 50 μm.

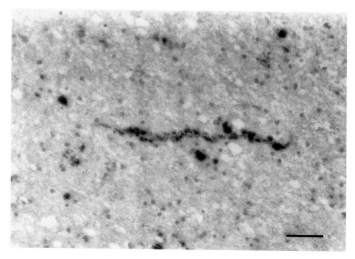

Fig. 3.9 Fibre tracts show focal PrP positivity in the basal ganglia in some cases of CJD. Slight spongiform change is also apparent. PrP immunocytochemistry plus haematoxylin staining. Bar is 50 μm.

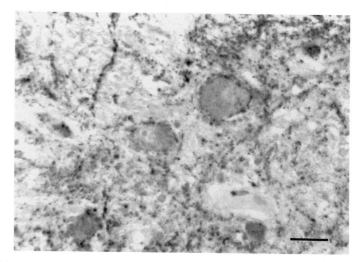

Fig. 3.10 Three neurones in this brainstem nucleus are outlined by small granular PrP-positive deposits apparently at or on the neuronal membrane although neuronal cytoplasm and nuclei are negative. PrP immunocytochemistry plus haematoxylin staining. Bar is 22 μm.

Factors such as post-mortem delay or duration of formalin fixation may influence the results of immunostaining studies quite apart from the variable protein load in the particular tissue under examination. Whether there is a reliable correlation in any particular section between the density of PrP immunopositivity and the quantity of PrP present is open to question. It is clear, however, that significant deposits of PrP^{CJD}, as demonstrated by immunocytochemical techniques, may be present in parts of the brain which do not show obvious spongiform change. This includes the granular layer of the cerebellum which is not spongiform, although it may show atrophy and neuronal depletion. Conversely parts of the cortex which do show spongiform change, especially of the non-confluent variety, are sometimes virtually negative for PrP^{CJD}. This is frequently seen in the molecular layer of the cerebellum and, often, in the cerebral cortex as well. These points highlight the dangers inherent in the examination of a single sample of brain tissue from a particular case, either at biopsy or in autopsy examination. The practice of biopsy in suspected prion dementia cases should be discouraged (Metters 1992) despite the pressing urgency of making a definitive diagnosis in particular cases.

Regional distribution of plaques and spongiform change

The variability of topographic distribution of classical pathology and PrP immunopositivity is not just of diagnostic significance but also of scientific interest. A full understanding of spongiform encephalopathies and prion dementias must take account of this apparent focal distribution and provide an adequate explanation for the variation in pattern. The pathological changes are neither global nor obviously in functionally related parts of the brain and they vary from case to case. In classic sporadic CJD at least part of the neocortical ribbon shows some spongiform change and this frequently involves the occipital calcarine cortex or the inferior temporal gyrus (though often sparing the cornu ammonis proper) and the parietal cortex. When spongiform change is diffuse and characterized by multi-loculated confluent vacuoles, the diagnosis is easy to establish. However, the spongiform change is often more subtle (Manuelidis 1985; Bastian 1991; Lantos 1992) and represented only by sparse microcystic cavities in the neuropil. Potential sources of confusion are listed in Table 3.1 and in these cases PrP immunostaining may be of help, although negative results do not rule out the diagnosis of prion disease. Marked spongiform change may also be present in the basal ganglia, with or without cortical spongiform change. The presence of well defined plaques, demonstrated by the presence of amyloid or of PrP positivity, may or may not be a significant accompanying feature of spongiform change in classical sporadic CJD. Plaques may be numerous in the cerebellum or may be very sparse indeed (Kitamoto and Tateishi 1988; Tateishi *et al.* 1992). Their presence correlates well with the degree of cerebellar atrophy, particularly in the vermis, but does not necessarily related to the presence or absence of severe spongiform change elsewhere in the brain. Cases of sporadic CJD that present clinically with a preponderance of cerebellar signs and symptoms may show more spongiform change in the molecular layer of the cerebellum than in the cerebral cortex. PrP-positive plaques are often a prominent feature in the cerebellum in such cases (Masters and Gajdusek 1982; Jones *et al.* 1985) (Fig. 3.7d).

Although the pattern of pathology, distribution of spongiform change, and of plaques, are so variable in sporadic cases of CJD, some more particular patterns of pathology are evident within the even rarer cases of inherited prion diseases (Goldfarb *et al.* 1990*a,b*; Nieto *et al.* 1991). GSS cases show more accentuated immunopathological changes in the cerebellum in that PrP^{CJD} appears to be more widespread in GSS than in CJD (Bugiani *et al.* 1993; Bell and Ironside 1993*a*) (Fig. 3.7d and e). Cases with PrP base pair inserts may show cerebellar PrP deposits in the absence of the usual pathology features of human prion diseases (Gambetti *et al.* 1993).

In fatal familial insomnia the main burden of pathology appears to be in the thalamus which may show spongiform change but more often displays prominent gliosis without sponge, and certainly contains deposits of PrP positivity (Manetto *et al.* 1992; Gambetti *et al.* 1993). In those cases of atypical dementia in which mutations of the PrP gene have been found, evidence of PrP deposition, together with spongiform change and other changes, are often topographically quite limited but are found to be present focally when a thorough and wide ranging investigation of the neuropathology is undertaken. Pathology changes are most noticeable in the basal ganglia and in the cerebellum in atypical cases examined in our laboratory.

It is of interest that the iatrogenic cases, particularly those acquiring CJD following administration of pituitary-derived hormones (Tintner *et al.* 1986; Weller *et al.* 1986), show rather characteristically a cerebellar pattern of disease with cerebellar atrophy, molecular layer spongiform change, and PrP positivity which is diffuse rather than in plaque form, particularly in the granular layer (Fig. 3.7f). Neocortical spongiform change, and concomitant PrP positivity, may be very circumscribed in the iatrogenic cases.

To return again to the question of reliability of PrP immunostaining, the emerging consensus from studies employing different protocols and different antibodies generates some confidence that the PrP visualized in this way is disease related (Bell and Ironside 1993*a*). The absence of staining in non-demented, age-matched controls does suggest that there is little or no cross-staining of the normal cellular form of PrP. Whether this form of PrP is present in insufficient quantity, or has been removed by pre-staining protocols in these preparations, is not known. Although it is time-consuming and inconvenient to employ complex pre-treatment schedules, it is clear that the range of PrP-positive features within diseased brains is being extended, particularly by studies with the newer monoclonal antibodies. This suggests that some disease-related PrP deposits are harder to detect than others, even in the same case. Sensitivity of immunocytochemical detection is clearly an important issue in this context.

It seems that PrP immunocytochemistry is becoming a useful tool to increase our understanding of basic disease processes in the brains of patients affected by human prion diseases. A thorough understanding of the distribution of lesions, and of the load of disease-related PrP, might provide clues as to how the disease process is initiated and transmitted throughout the CNS. As the patterns of PrP distribution become better understood, it will be important to incorporate these findings into clinicopathological correlations.

Clinicopathological correlations

Sporadic CJD

Classic cases of CJD have traditionally been divided into subacute, intermediate, and amyotrophic cases (Masters and Gajdusek 1982). In the amyotrophic cases a dementing process is accompanied by muscle atrophy and weakness and there is some doubt as to whether this form represents a true subset of CJD. The subacute and intermediate cases form a spectrum of progressive dementia in which the time to death varies from six months to two years (Manuelidis 1985). Myoclonus is a characteristic symptom in a high proportion of cases and most have a highly abnormal and typical form of electroencephalogram, characterized by spike formation. The variability of pathology findings in classic CJD cases means that some areas of the neocortical grey matter may appear virtually normal, emphasizing the risks of inadequate focal examination of cases, particularly at biopsy. The more extensive cases of neocortical spongiform change are clearly correlated with profound dementia and akinetic mutism which may characterize the terminal stages of the disease (Masters and Richardson 1978; Will 1991*b*). Although the final detail of neurological signs and symptoms may be difficult to determine in mute, immobile, and demented patients, it is clear that some cases show cortical blindness and this condition results from pathological changes in the calcarine cortex. Visual pathways may also be involved although this is less clear in the human cases than in corresponding studies in scrapie. Some patients with sporadic CJD present first with a cerebellar syndrome and while the initial symptom of ataxia may be rapidly overtaken by a dementing process, it is evident from pathological examination of the brain that such cases do show cerebellar atrophy, cerebellar spongiform change, and sometimes profuse PrP-positive cerebellar plaques. If dementia is not a prominent feature such cerebellar cases may be diagnosed as paraneoplastic syndrome (Will and Matthews 1984; Mizutani and Shiraki 1985).

Careful correlations between clinical signs and symptoms and classical pathological features such as spongiform change and gliosis have been performed in human cases in the past (Mizutani and Shiraki 1985). The added dimension of PrP^{CJD} immunolocalization may throw further light on clinicopathological correlation, particularly because of the intimate relationship between PrP^{CJD} and the infective agent, even if these two are not identical. Although PrP^{CJD} plaques are not seen in all CJD cases, there is some evidence that their presence correlates with longer clinical duration (Kitamoto and Tateishi 1988).

The importance of detailed clinicopathological correlation is heightened when considering new CJD cases in the wake of the bovine spongiform encephalopathy epidemic (Wells *et al.* 1992). The recent identification of a new variant of CJD in 10 young patients in UK and one in France (Will *et al.* 1996; Chazot *et al.* 1996) has led the suggestion that these cases may be causally linked to BSE, possibly as a result of exposure to bovine brain or spinal cord tissue in the food chain in the 1980s. Further studies, including experimental strain typing experiments, are required to investigate this hypothesis.

Inherited human prion diseases

Before the genetic pathology of the PrP gene was explored, it was evident from familial cases of CJD, and from GSS cases, that the clinical picture was somewhat different from classical sporadic CJD (Collinge *et al.* 1989; Brown *et al.* 1991). The onset is usually at a slightly younger age and the duration of the disease is longer. First presentation is often related to cerebellar signs and symptoms, and from pathological examination of these cases, it is clear that the cerebellum is usually heavily involved. Whether the more significant degree of cerebellar pathology in such cases relates to the greater clinical duration is not fully understood but seems probable. It may be that putative spread of the infective agent through the CNS of familial cases occurs at a slower rate than in sporadic cases, highlighting the fact that this process is not understood at present. Within individual families there is sometimes a rather wide range of clinical and pathological findings. Familial cases have all to date been shown to have an identifiable PrP gene abnormality (see Chapter 2), as detailed above but the pathology changes are often far from uniform in individuals with the same PrP genotype. However, particular PrP mutations do determine the clinical manifestations and disease duration to a large extent (Kitamoto *et al.* 1992*b*; DeArmond 1993*b*). The mechanisms involved in this variation remain poorly understood. Recent descriptions of atypical dementias characterized by gene mutations, and which lack classical spongiform change (Collinge *et al.* 1990), only add to the perplexities of pathogenesis. If the accumulation of PrP^{CJD} is not always followed by spongiform change, it may be that the two are not closely related and that the latter is not causally linked to the former.

Iatrogenic cases

Iatrogenic cases of spongiform encephalopathy include cases of CJD in comparatively young patients who have been treated for short stature or for infertility with cadaver-derived pituitary hormones (Weller *et al.* 1986; Collinge *et al.* 1991; Will 1991*a*; Brown *et al.* 1992). Iatrogenic CJD has also followed neurosurgical procedures, corneal grafting, and dura mater grafting (Duffy *et al.* 1974). In such cases the likely incubation period from introduction of the agent to the development of clinically manifested disease can be estimated with some degree of accuracy, whereas the timing of initiation of events and commencement of the latent period in sporadic CJD is completely unknown. It is of interest that iatrogenically induced cases display presymptomatic periods which vary according to the site of inoculation. Those treated with peripheral injections of extract such as contaminated pituitary preparations, have a longer incubation period than those inoculated centrally, as in neurosurgical procedures (Brown *et al.* 1992). While cases which follow neurosurgical or grafting procedures tend to develop classical CJD with neocortical spongiform change, the more characteristic picture in patients treated with pituitary-derived hormones is that of a cerebellar pattern of disease. Before this iatrogenic form of CJD was clearly recognized and received sufficient publicity, some of these patients were thought to have a primary cerebellar degeneration or paraneoplastic syndrome and others were thought to have recurrence of the cerebellar tumour which had led to treatment with pituitary hormones in the first place.

It is of interest to speculate how the infective agent reaches the CNS from a peripheral point of injection. Haematogenous transport remains a possibility. Recent studies on the spinal cord in cases of iatrogenic CJD in growth hormone recipients in the UK have demonstrated PrP^{CJD} accumulation in the spinal cord by immunocytochemistry, particularly in the substantia gelatinosa, suggesting entry of the transmissible agent into the CNS by sensory axons. A similar pattern of accumulation has also been identified in a subset of patients with sporadic CJD; the pathogenetic implications of this finding are at present unclear and require further investigation.

Comparison with animal prion diseases

Naturally occurring animal prion diseases

As in the human prion diseases, neuropathology is characterized by spongiform change, neuronal loss, reactive astrocytosis, and PrP amyloid plaque formation (Fraser 1993). The spongiform change corresponds closely to that in human disease although neuronal vacuolation is usually a more pronounced feature, with large single or multiple vacuoles distending the neuronal cell bodies. As in the human diseases, there is a considerable variation in the distribution, incidence, and relative severity of these abnormalities in different sites within the CNS, particularly in scrapie (Fraser 1993). Vacuolation of neuronal perikarya has also been described as an incidental finding in the brain of sheep, cattle, and goats; it is also noted that vacuolation of CNS can occur in a wide range of viral infections, metabolic disorders, and toxic states which can affect the grey and white matter and should not be confused with the spongiform change characteristic of animal prion diseases (Wells *et al.* 1992, Fraser 1993). Detailed descriptions of the pathological features of the animal prion diseases are given in Chapter 4.

Experimental scrapie

A wide range of animals have been used as hosts in experimental transmission studies of scrapie, but the mouse and hamster have been most extensively studied, particularly in relation to scrapie strain variation (Kim *et al.* 1990; Scott 1993).

Several distinct scrapie strains have been isolated by serially passaging scrapie or BSE from sheep, goat, and cattle sources in mice (Bruce 1993). The identification of scrapie strains relates to observations and measurements of the disease characteristics in the mouse host, including the incubation period, clinical features, the severity and distribution of the neuropathological lesions in the CNS, transmission characteristics from the mouse brain, and susceptibility to inactivation. Of these, one of the major differences between scrapie strains is the variation in incubation period between initial infection and clinical disease in genetically identical hosts. In mice, the *Sinc* (scrapie incubation) gene also influences the incubation periods of experimental scrapie and it is now thought that this gene encodes PrP, with two distinct alleles being identified which consistently differ in predicted protein sequence by two amino acids (Westaway *et al.* 1987). Scrapie strains also show reproducible differences in the nature, location, and severity of neuropathology in the mouse brain, relating to spongiform change, amyloid plaque formation, and neuronal loss (Scott 1993). These features have been studied by developing lesion profiles for the various scrapie strains, which imply the ability of the agent to replicate in different neuronal populations, indicating a variation in neuronal susceptibility to the disease (Bruce 1993; De Armond 1993*a,b*).

Experimental transmissions with two strains of the scrapie agent chosen for different incubation periods has demonstrated a 'blocking' effect where a strain with a relatively long incubation period delays or prevents the transmission of a strain with a shorter incubation period when injected subsequently (Bruce 1993). Scrapie strains are stable within identical individual host species, but may differ significantly in their properties on passage to mice with a different *Sinc* genotype. Strain variation has been identified in naturally occurring prion diseases in sheep and goats. In contrast, transmissions of BSE from cattle, kudu, and nyala to mice all show similar transmission characteristics. BSE transmission from cattle to sheep, goats, and pigs and subsequent passage from these secondary hosts into mice show similar transmission characteristics, indicating that the BSE agent is unchanged when passaged through a range of species and that the donor species has little influence on the disease characteristics on transmission to mice. The uniformity of transmission results with different sources of the BSE agent suggests that a single strain may be responsible for this epidemic, in keeping with the uniformity of the pathology described in cattle with BSE (Bruce 1993).

These findings have considerable potential implications for human spongiform encephalopathies, particularly in light of the postulated effect of BSE on the incidence of human prion diseases. CJD and related disorders have been transmitted experimentally to a variety of animals, including mice, and although there is evidence of some variation in the pathological characteristics of the transmitted human agents, accurate strain typing has not yet been performed (Mori *et al.* 1989). If BSE does have a major effect on human prion diseases, then strain typing of BSE-related human CJD might be expected to show uniform characteristics in experimental mice, similar to those seen for BSE in cattle and other similar disorders occurring in kudu and nyala.

The significance for human prion disease of the pathological variation in scrapie strains is as yet uncertain. Certain similarities exist between the distribution and nature of the neuropathology in some scrapie strains and the neuropathological features reported in sporadic human prion diseases. However, a variety of other host character-istics have to be taken into consideration when assessing these similarities and it is not possible to draw any firm conclusions from the information available at present.

Transgenic animal models of prion diseases

A variety of transgenic animal models now exist for the study of prion diseases; these include mice containing the human PrP gene with the characteristic GSS mutation at codon 102. These mice develop a spontaneous neurodegenerative disor-der characterized by the histological features of the human disease, including amyloid plaque formation (Hsiao *et al.* 1990; DeArmond 1993*b*). Transgenic mice have also been developed which express both hamster and mouse PrP. Careful studies on these animals have demonstrated that infectious scrapie prions (PrP^{Sc}) bind selectively to homologous cellular prion protein (PrP^C), which are then con-verted into PrP^{Sc} molecules (Prusiner *et al.* 1990). When different experimental scrapie strains were introduced into these transgenic mice, the distribution of the neuropathology was unique for each prion isolate. This variable pattern of neu-ropathology implies differing susceptibility of neuronal subgroups in the CNS to different scrapie prion strains; this finding has obvious relevance for human disease as well as animal prion disorders. The development of these animal models allows unique insights into the pathogenesis of prion diseases, particularly with regard to the evolution of the characteristic neuropathological features.

Conclusion

The recognition of the broadening clinical spectrum of prion diseases in humans and animals has been matched by advances in the understanding of the molecular genetics of prion diseases. These developments have in turn been accompanied by more detailed studies of the pathological mechanisms and structural changes occur-ring within the CNS. Modern investigative techniques, particularly PrP immunocy-tochemistry, have revealed a far wider range of abnormalities in the CNS than was recognized in earlier descriptions of the neuropathology of prion diseases. In human prion diseases, these findings are of value in the differential diagnosis of neurodegenerative disease. Studies of animal models of prion disease, particularly the murine scrapie model and more recently transgenic animal studies, have allowed a more detailed investigation into the relationship between molecular genetic abnormalities and neuropathology than hitherto possible. The enormous potential of the transgenic animal models for prion diseases will also allow detailed studies on the evolution of the structural changes in the CNS and their relationship with the deposition of PrP and other host proteins. The considerable overlap in the pathological features between human prion diseases and Alzheimer's disease indicates the existence of common disease mechanisms resulting in neuronal damage and death in these two unrelated disorders; further work is required to pursue this intriguing comparison. PrP and β/A4 protein also seem to be involved in skeletal muscle disorders, particularly inclusion body myositis; this involvement may also be studied in transgenic animal models for prion disease. In animal prion diseases, the emergence of BSE has demonstrated a stereotyped neuropathology in affected animals which implies a single strain effect with respect to the causative agent, and emphasizes a close relationship between prion agents and neuropathology which may yield further clues in future investigations into the pathogenesis of the CNS damage in these unique disorders.

References

Alpers, M. (1989). Epidemiology and clinical aspects of kuru. In *Prions: novel infectious agents causing scrapie and Creutzfeldt–Jakob disease*, (ed. S. B. Prusiner and M. P. McKinley), pp. 451–467. Academic Press, San Diego.

Anano, N., Yagishita, S., Yokoi, S., Itoh, Y., Kinoshita, J., Mizutani, T., *et al.* (1992). Gerstmann–Sträussler syndrome–variant type: amyloid plaques and Alzheimer's neurofibrillary tangles in cerebral cortex. *Acta Neuropathologica*, **84**, 15–23.

Askanas, V., King, E. W., and Alverez, R. B. (1992). Light and electron microscopic localisation of β-amyloid protein in muscle biopsies of patients with inclusion-body myositis. *American Journal of Pathology*, **141**, 31–36.

Askanas, V., Bilak, M., Engel, W. K., Alvarez, R. B., Tome, F., and Leclerc, A. (1993). Prion protein is abnormally accumulated in inclusion-body myositis. *NeuroReport*, **5**, 25–28.

Baker, H. F., Ridley, R. M., Duchen, L. W., Crow, T. J., and Bruton, C. J. (1993). Evidence for the experimental transmission of cerebral β-amyloidosis to primates. *International Journal of Experimental Pathology*, **74**, 441–454.

Bastian, F. O. (ed.) (1991). *Creutzfeldt–Jakob disease and other transmissible human spongiform encephalopathies*. Mosby Year Book, St Louis.

Bell, J. E. and Ironside, J. W. (1993a). Neuropathology of spongiform encephalopathies in humans. *British Medical Bulletin*, **49**, 738–777.

Bell, J. E. and Ironside, J. W. (1993b). How to tackle a possible Creutzfeldt–Jakob disease necropsy. *Journal of Clinical Pathology*, **46**, 193–197.

Berciano, J., Berciano, M. T., Polo, J. M., Figols, J., Ciudad, J., and Lafarga, M. (1990). Creutzfeldt–Jakob disease with severe involvement of cerebral white matter and cerebellum. *Virchows Archiv A Pathology Anatomy*, **417**, 533–538.

Bockman, J. M., Kingsbury, D. I., McKinley, M. P., Bendheim, P. E., and Prusiner, S. B. (1985). Creutzfeldt–Jakob disease prion proteins in human brains. *New England Journal of Medicine*, **312**, 73–78.

Boellaard, J. W. and Schlote, W. (1980). Subakutte spongiforme Encephalopathie mit multiformer Plaquebildung. *Acta Neuropathologica*, **49**, 205–212.

Boellaard, J. W., Doerr-Schott, J., and Schlote, W. (1993). Mini plaques and shapeless cerebral amyloid deposits in a case of Gerstmann–Sträussler–Scheinker's syndrome. *Acta Neuropathologica*, **86**, 532–535,

Brown, P., Goldfarb, L. G., Brown, W. T., Goldgaber, D., Rubenstein, R., Kascsak, R. J., *et al.* (1991). Clinical and molecular genetic study of a large German kindred with Gerstmann–Straussler–Scheinker syndrome. *Neurology*, **41**, 375–379.

Brown, P., Rodgers-Johnson, P., Cathala, F., Gibbs, C. J., and Gajdusek, D. C. (1984). Creutzfeldt–Jakob disease of long duration: clinicopathological characteristics, transmissibility and differential diagnosis. *Annals of Neurology*, **16**, 295–304.

Brown, P., Wolff, A., and Gajdusek, D. C. (1990). A simple and effective method for inactivating virus infectivity in formalin-fixed tissue samples from patients with Creutzfeldt–Jakob disease. *Neurology*, **40**, 887–890.

Brown, P., Preece, M. A., and Will, R. G. (1992). 'Friendly fire' in medicine: hormones, homografts, and Creutzfeldt–Jakob disease. *Lancet*, **340**, 24–27.

Bruce, M. E. (1993). Scrapie strain variation and mutation. *British Medical Bulletin*, **49**, 822–838.

Bugiani, O., Giaccone, G., Verga, L., Pollo, B., Frangione, B., Farlow, M. R., *et al.* (1993). βPP participates in PrP-amyloid plaques of Gerstmann–Sträussler–Scheinker disease, Indiana kindred. *Journal of Neuropathology and Experimental Neurology*, **52**, 66–70.

Chazot, G., Broussole, E., Lapras, C. I., Blattler, T., Aguzzi, A., and Kopp, N. (1996). New variant of Creutzfeldt–Jakob disease in a 26-year-old French man. *Lancet*, **347**, 1181.

Collinge, J., Harding, A. E., Owens, F., Poulter, M., Lofthouse, R., Boughey, A. M., *et al.* (1989). Diagnosis of Gerstmann–Sträussler syndrome in familial dementia with prion protein gene analysis. *Lancet*, **ii**, 15–17.

Collinge, J., Owen, F., Poulter, M., Leach, M., Crow, T. J., Rossor, M. N., *et al.* (1990). Prion dementia without characteristic pathology. *Lancet*, **336**, 7–9.

Collinge, J., Palmer, M. S., and Dryden, A. J. (1991). Genetic predisposition to iatrogenic Creutzfeldt–Jakob disease. *Lancet*, **337**, 1441–1442.

de Courten-Myers, G. and Mandybur, T. I. (1987). Atypical Gerstmann–Sträussler syndrome or familial spinocerebellar ataxia and Alzheimer's disease? *Neurology*, **37**, 269–275.

DeArmond, S. J. (1993*a*). Alzheimer's disease and Creutzfeldt–Jakob disease: overlap of pathogenic mechanisms. *Current Opinion in Neurology*, **6**, 872–881.

DeArmond, S. J. (1993*b*). Overview of the transmissable spongiform encephalopathies: Prion protein disorders. *British Medical Bulletin*, **49**, 725–737.

Diedrich, J. F., Bendheim, P. E., Kim, Y. S., Carp, R. I., and Haase, A. T. (1991). Scrapie-associated prion protein accumulates in astrocytes during scrapie infection. *Proceedings of the National Academy of Science of the USA*, **88**, 375–379.

Duffy, P., Wolf, J., Collins, G., De Voc, A. G., Streeten, B., and Cowen, D. (1974). Possible person to person transmission of Creutzfeldt–Jakob disease. *New England Journal of Medicine*, **290**, 692–693.

Field, E. J., Mathews, J. D., and Raine, C. S. (1969). Electron-microscopic observations on the cerebellar cortex in kuru. *Journal of the Neurological Sciences*, **8**, 209–224.

Frackowiak, J., Wisniewski, H. M., Wegiel, J., Merz, G. S., Iqbal, K., and Wang, K. C. (1992). Ultrastructure of the microglia that phagocytose amyloid and the microglia that produce β-amyloid fibrils. *Acta Neuropathologica*, **84**, 225–233.

Fraser, H. (1993). Diversity in the neuropathology of scrapie-like diseases in animals. *British Medical Bulletin*, **49**, 792–809.

Gajdusek, D. C., and Vigas, V. (1957). Degenerative disease of the central nervous system in New Guinea: the endemic occurrence of 'kuru' in the native population. *New England Journal of Medicine*, **257**, 974–978.

Gajdusek, D. C., Gibbs, C. J., and Alpers, M. P. (1966). Experimental transmission of a kuru-like syndrome in chimpanzees. *Nature*, **209**, 794–796.

Gambetti, P., Peterson, R., Monari, L., Tabaton, M., Autillo-Gambetti, L., Cortelli, P., *et al.* (1993). Fatal familial insomnia and the widening spectrum of prion diseases. *British Medical Bulletin*, **49**, 980–994.

Gerstmann, J., Straussler, E., and Scheinker, I. (1936). Ueber eine eigengartige hereditärfamiliare Erkrankung des Zentralnervensystems, zugleich ein Beitrag zur Frage des vorzeitigen lokalen Alterns. *Zeitzschrift für die gesamte Neurologie und Psychiatrie*, **154**, 736–762.

Ghetti, B., Tagliavina, F., Masters, C. L., Beyreuther, K., Giaccone, G., Verga, L., *et al.* (1989). Gerstmann–Sträussler–Scheinker disease. II. Neurofibrillary tangles and plaques with PrP amyloid coexist in an affected family. *Neurology*, **39**, 1453–1461.

Gibbs, C.J., Gajdusek, D. C., Asher, D. M., Alpers, M. P., Beck, E., Daniel, P. M., *et al.* (1968). Creutzfeldt–Jakob disease (subacute spongiform encephalopathy): transmission to the chimpanzee. *Science*, **161**, 388–389.

Gibbs, C. J., Joy, A., Heffner, R., Franko, M., Miyazaki, M., Asher, D., *et al.* (1985). Clinical and pathological features and laboratory confirmation of Creutzfeldt–Jakob disease in a recipient of pituitary-derived human growth hormone. *New England Journal of Medicine*, **313**, 734–738.

Goldfarb, L. G., Brown, P., Goldgaber, D., Garruto, R. M., Yanaghara, R., Asher, D. M., *et al.* (1990*a*). Identical mutation in unrelated patients with Cruetzfeldt–Jakob disease. *Lancet*, **336**, 174–175.

Goldfarb, L. G., Mitrova, E., Brown, P., Toh, B. H., and Gajdusek, D. C. (1990*b*). Mutations in codon 200 of scrapie amyloid protein gene in two clusters of Creutzfeldt–Jakob disease in Slovakia. *Lancet*, **336**, 514–515.

Goodbrand, I. A., Ironside, J. W., Nicolson, D., and Bell, J. E. (1995). Prion protein accumulation in the spinal cords of patients with sporadic and growth hormone associated Creutzfeldt–Jakob disease. *Neuroscience Letters*, **183**, 127–130.

Guiroy, D. C., Yanagihara, R., and Gajdusek, D. C. (1991*b*). Localisation of amyloidogenic proteins and sulfated glycosaminoglycans in nontransmissible and transmissible cerebral amyloidoses. *Acta Neuropathologica*, **82**, 87–92.

Hansen, L. A., Masliah, E., Terry, R. D., and Mirra, S. S. (1989). A neuropathological subset of Alzheimer's disease with concomitant Lewy body disease and spongiform change. *Acta Neuropathologica*, **78**, 194–201.

Hart, J. and Gordon, B. (1990). Early-onset dementia and extrapyramidal disease: clinicopathological variant of Gerstmann–Sträussler–Scheinker or Alzheimer's disease. *Journal of Neurology, Neurosurgery and Psychiatry*, **53**, 932–939.

Hashimoto, K., Mannen, T., and Nobuyuki, N. (1992). Immunohistochemical study of kuru plaques using antibodies against synthetic prion protein peptides. *Acta Neuropathologica*, **83**, 613–617.

Hayward, P. A. R., Bell, J. E., and Ironside, J. W. (1994). Prion protein immunocytochemistry: The development of reliable protocols for the investigation of Creutzfeldt–Jakob disease. *Neuropathology and Applied Neurobiology*, **20**, 375–383.

Hsiao, K., Baker, H. F., Crow, T. J., Poulter, M., Owen, F., Terwilliger, J. D., *et al.* (1991). Linkage of a prion protein missense variant to Gerstmann–Straussler syndrome. *Nature*, **338**, 342–345.

Hsiao, K. K., Scott, M., Foster, D., Groth, D. F., DeArmond, S. J., and Prusiner, S. B. (1990). Spontaneous neurodegeneration in transgenic mice with mutant prion protein. *Science*, **250**, 1587–1590.

Hudson, A. J., Farrell, M. A., Kalnins, R., and Kaufmann, J. C. E. (1983). Gerstmann–Sträussler–Scheinker disease with coincidental familial onset. *Annals of Neurology*, **14**, 670–678.

Ironside, J. W., Barrie, C., McCardle, L., and Bell, J. E. (1993*a*). Microglial reactions in human spongiform encephaloathies (abstract). *Neuropathology and Applied Neurobiology*, **19**, 57.

Ironside, J. W., McCardle, L., Hayward, P. A. R., and Bell, J. E. (1993*b*). Ubiquitin immunocytochemistry in human spongiform encephalopathies. *Neuropathology and Applied Neurobiology*, **19**, 134–140.

Jones, H. R., Hedley-Whyte, E. T., Freiberg, S. R., and Baker, R. A. (1985). Ataxic Creutzfeldt–Jakob disease: diagnostic techniques and neuropathologic observations in early disease. *Neurology*, **35**, 254–257.

Kato, S., Hiran, A., Umahara, T., Llena, J. F., Herz, F., and Ohama, E. (1992). Ultrastructural and immunohistological studies of ballooned cortical neurons in Creutzfeldt–Jakob disease: expression of aB-crystallin, ubiquitin and stress-response protein 27. *Acta Neuropathologica*, **84**, 443–448.

Kawata, A., Masakazu, S., Oda, M., Hayashi, H., and Tanabe, H. (1992). Creutzfeldt–Jakob disease with congophilic kuru plaques: CT and pathological findings of the cerebral white matter. *Journal of Neurology, Neurosurgery and Psychiatry*, **55**, 849–851.

Kim, Y. S., Carp, R. I., Callahan, S., and Wisniewski, H. M. (1990). Incubation periods and histopathological changes in mice injected stereotaxically in different brain areas with the 87V scrapie strain. *Acta Neuropathologica*, **80**, 388–392.

Kitamoto, T. and Tateishi, J. (1988). Immunohistochemical confirmation of Creutzfeldt–Jakob disease with a long clinical course with amyloid plaque core antibodies. *American Journal of Pathology*, **131**, 435–443.

Kitamoto, T., Ogomori, K., Tateishi, J., and Prusiner, S. B. (1987). Methods in laboratory investigation: formic acid pretreatment enhances immunostaining of cerebral and systemic amyloids. *Laboratory Investigation*, **57**, 230–236.

Kitamoto, T., Shin, R. W., Doh-ura, K., Tomokane, N., Miyazono, M., Muramoto, T., *et al.* (1992*a*). Abnormal isoform of prion protein accumulates in the synaptic structures of the central nervous system in patients with Creutzfeldt–Jakob disease. *American Journal of Pathology*, **140**, 1285–1289.

Kitamoto, T., Doh-ura, K., Muramoto, T., Miyazono, M., and Tateishi, J. (1992*b*). The primary structure of the prion protein influences the distribution of abnormal prion protein in the CNS. *American Journal of Pathology*, **141**, 271–277.

Klatzo, I., Gajdusek, D. C., and Zigas, V. (1959). Pathology of kuru. *Laboratory Investigation*, **8**, 799–847.

Lantos, P. L. (1992). From slow virus to prion: a review of transmissible spongiform encephalopathies. *Histopathology*, **20**, 1–11.

Lantos, P. L., McGill, I. S., Janota, I., Doey, L. J., Collinge, J., Bruce, M. T., *et al.* (1992). Prion protein immunocytochemistry helps to establish the true incidence of prion diseases. *Neuroscience Letters*, **147**, 67–71.

Liberski, P. P., Yanagihara, R., Gibbs, C. J., and Gajdusek, D. C. (1990). Appearance of tubulovesicular structures in experimental Creutzfeldt–Jakob disease and scrapie precedes the onset of clinical disease. *Acta Neuropathologica*, **79**, 349–354.

Liberski, P. P., Budka, H., Sluga, E., Barcikowska, M. and Kwiecinski, H. (1992). Tubulovesicular structures in Creutzfeldt–Jakob disease. *Acta Neuropathologica*, **84**, 238–243.

Manetto, V., Medori, R., Cortelli, P., Montagna, P., Tinuper, P., Baruzzi, A., *et al.* (1992). Fatal familial insomnia: clinical and pathological study of five new cases. *Neurology*, **42**, 312–319.

Manuelidis, E. E. (1985). Creutzfeldt–Jakob disease. *Journal of Neuropathology and Experimental Neurology*, **44**, 1–17.

Masters, C. L. and Gajdusek, D. C. (1982). The spectrum of Creutzfeldt–Jakob disease and the virus-induced spongiform encephalopathies. In *Recent Advances in Neuropathology 2*, (ed. W. T. Smith and J. B. Cavanagh), pp. 139–164. Churchill Livingstone, Edinburgh.

Masters, C. L. and Richardson, E. P. (1978). Subacute spongiform encephalopathy (Creutzfeldt–Jakob disease). The nature and progression of spongiform change. *Brain*, **101**, 333–334.

Masters, C. L., Gajdusek, D. C., and Gibbs, C. J. (1981). Creutzfeldt–Jakob disease: virus isolations from the Gerstmann–Sträussler syndrome. *Brain*, **104**, 559–588.

McBride, P. A., Bruce, M. E., and Fraser, H. (1988). Immunostaining of cerebral amyloid plaques with antisera raised to scrapie-associated fibrils (SAF). *Neuropathology and Applied Neurobiology*, **14**, 325–336.

Medori, R., Tritschler, J. H., LeBlanc, A., Villare, F., Manetto, V., Ghen, H. Y., *et al.* (1992). Fatal familial insomnia, a prion disease with a mutation at codon 178 of the prion protein gene. *New England Journal of Medicine*, **7**, 444–449.

Metters, J. S. (1992). Neuro and ophthalmic surgery procedures in patients with, or suspected to have, or at risk of developing CJD or GSS. *Letter PL(92)CO/4 to Consultants and Health Managers*, Department of Health, London.

Mizutani, T. and Shiraki, H. (ed.) (1985). *Clinicopathological aspects of Creutzfeldt–Jakob disease*. Elsevier, Amsterdam.

Mori, S., Hamada, C., Kumanishi, T., Fukuhara, N., Ichihashi, Y., Ikuta, F., *et al.* (1989). A Creutzfeldt–Jakob disease agent (Echigo-1 strain) recovered from brain tissue showing the 'panencephalopathic type' disease. *Neurology*, **39**, 1337–1342.

Nakazato, Y., Hirato, J., Ishida, Y., Hoshi, S., Hasegawa, M., and Fukuda, T. (1990). Swollen cortical neurons in Creutzfeldt–Jakob disease contain a phosphorylated neurofilament epitope. *Journal of Neuropathology and Experimental Neurology*, **49**, 197–205.

Neumann, M. A., Gajdusek, D. C., and Zigas, V. (1965). Neuropathologic findings in exotic neurologic disorders among natives of the highlands of New Guinea. *Journal of Neuropathology and Experimental Neurology*, **18**, 486–507.

Nieto, A., Goldfarb, L. G., Brown, P., McCombie, W. R., Trapp, S., Asher, D. M., *et al.* (1991). Codon 178 mutation in ethnically diverse Creutzfeldt–Jakob disease families. *Lancet*, **337**, 622–623.

Piccardo, P., Safar, J., Ceroni, M., Gajdusek, D. C., and Gibbs, C. J. (1990). Immunohistochemical localization of prion protein in spongiform encephalopathies and normal brain tissue. *Neurology*, **40**, 518–522.

Powers, J. M., Liu, Y., Hair, L. S., Kascsack, R. J., Lewis, L. D., and Levy, L. A. (1991). Concomitant Creutzfeldt and Alzheimer diseases. *Acta Neuropathologica*, **83**, 95–98.

Probst, A., Langui, D., and Ulrich, J. (1991). Alzheimer's disease. A description of the structural lesions. *Brain Pathology*, **1**, 229–239.

Prusiner, S. B. (1991). Molecular biology of prion diseases. *Science*, **252**, 1515–1522.

Prusiner, S. B., Scott, M., Foster, D., Pan, K. M., Groth, D., Mirenda, C., *et al.* (1990). Transgenetic studies implicate interactions between homologous PrP isoforms in scrapie prion replication. *Cell*, **63**, 73–686.

Scott, J. R. (1993). Scrapie pathogenesis. *British Medical Bulletin*, **49**, 778–791.

Tateishi, J. and Kitamoto, T. (1993). Developments in diagnosis for prion diseases. *British Medical Bulletin*, **49**, 971–979.

Tateishi, J., Kitamoto, T., Doh-ura, K., Boellaard, J. W., and Peiffer, J. (1992). Creutzfeldt–Jakob disease with amyloid angiopathy: diagnosis by immunologic analysis and transmission experiments. *Acta Neuropathologica*, **83**, 559–563.

Tintner, R., Brown, P., Hedley-Whyte, E. T., Rappaport, E. B., Piccardo, C. P., and Gajdusek, D. C. (1986). Neuropathologic verification of Creutzfeldt–Jakob disease in the exhumed American recipient of human pituitary growth hormone. *Neurology*, **36**, 932–936.

Tomlinson, B. E. (1992). Creutzfeldt–Jakob disease. In *Greenfield's neuropathology*, (5th edn) (ed. J. H. Adams and L. W. Duchen), pp. 1366–1375. Edward Arnold, London.

Turner, C., Bell, J. E., and Ironside, J. W. (1993). Localisation of microglia in CNS amyloid plaques: an immunocytochemical and confocal microscopic study. *Journal of Pathology*, **170**, 401.

Weller, R. O., Steart, P. V., and Powell-Jackson, J. D. (1986). Pathology of Creutzfeldt–Jakob disease associated with pituitary-derived human growth hormone administration. *Neuropathology and Applied Neurobiology*, **12**, 117–129.

Wells, G. A. H., Wilesmith, J. W., and McGill, I. S. (1992). Bovine spongiform encephalopathy. *Brain Pathology*, **1**, 69–78.

Westaway, D., Goodman, P. A., Mirenda, C. A., McKinley, M. P., Carlson, G. A., and Prusiner, S. B. (1987). Distinct prion proteins in short and long scrapie incubation period mice. *Cell*, **51**, 651–662.

Westaway, D., DeArmond, S. J., Cayetano-Canlas, J., Groth, D., Foster, D., Yang, S., *et al.* (1994). Degeneration of skeletal muscle, peripheral nerves, and the central nervous system in transgenic mice overexpressing wild-type prion proteins. *Cell*, **76**, 117–129.

Will, R. G. (1991*a*). An overview of Creutzfeldt–Jakob disease associated with the use of human pituitary growth hormone. *Developments in Biological Standardisation*, **75**, 85–86.

Will, R. G. (1991*b*). The spongiform encephalopathies. *Journal of Neurology, Neurosurgery and Psychiatry*, **54**, 761–763.

Wiil, R. G., Ironside, J. W., Zeidler, M., Cousens, S. N., Estebeiro, K., Alperovitch, A. *et al.* (1996). A new variant of Creutzfeldt–Jakob disease in the UK. *Lancet*, **347**, 921–925.

Will, R. G. and Matthews, W. B. (1984). A retrospective study of Creutzfeldt–Jakob disease in England and Wales 1970–79 I: clinical features. *Journal of Neurology, Neurosurgery and Psychiatry*, **47**, 134–140.

Appendix

Protocol for PrP immunocytochemistry

1. Float 5 μm sections on to slides coated with Vectabond.
2. Sections to water.
3. Picric acid 15 min (to remove formalin pigment).
4. Water.
5. Hydrogen peroxide 30 min (to block endogenous peroxide).
6. Water.
7. Autoclave in distilled water 121°C for 10 min.
8. Water.
9. 96% formic acid 5 min.
10. Water.
11. 4 M guanidine thiocyanate 2 h at 4°C.
12. Water followed by Tris buffer.
13. Blocking serum 10 min.
14. Primary PrP antibody: duration depends on specific antibody (Table 3.3)
15. Wash in Tris buffer.

16. Secondary antibody (1:200) for 30 min.
17. Wash in Tris buffer.
18. Avidin biotin for 30 min.
19. Wash in Tris buffer.
20. Visualize with diaminobenzidine.
21. Wash in water.
22. Counterstain lightly with haematoxylin.
23. Dehydrate, clear, and mount sections in Pertex.

4 Animal prion diseases

R. BRADLEY

Introduction

Until 1985 there were six subacute, transmissible spongiform encephalopathies or prion diseases: three in humans (Creutzfeldt–Jakob disease (CJD), Gerstmann–Sträussler syndrome (GSS), and kuru), and three in animals (scrapie of sheep and goats, transmissible mink encephalopathy (TME) and chronic wasting disease (CWD) of some wild Cervidae (deer) species in North America. Since 1985, another 12 species have had spongiform encephalopathy confirmed (Table 4.1). There is epidemiological evidence to suggest that 11 of the 12 'new' diseases are related to the

Table 4.1 Naturally occurring transmissible spongiform encephalopathies reported since 1985

Host	Disease	First report	Reported distribution
Nyala	SE	1987	England
Cattle	Bovine SE	1987	Great Britain, Republic of Ireland, Oman*, Falkland Islands*, Denmark*, Switzerland, France, Italy*, Portugal*, Canada*, Germany*
Gemsbok[+]	SE	1988	England
Arabian oryx[+]	SE	1989	England
Greater kudu	SE	1989	England
Eland[+]	SE	1989	England
Cat	Feline SE	1990	British Isles
Moufflon[+]	Scrapie	1992	England
Puma[+]	Feline SE	1992	England
Cheetah[+]	Feline SE	1992	Australia*, Great Britain, Republic of Ireland*
Scimitar horned oryx[+]	SE	1993	England
Ocelot[+]	Feline SE	1994	Scotland

SE, spongiform encephalopathy.
[+]Transmission not attempted;
*Presumptively exposed in Great Britain.

advent of bovine spongiform encephalopathy (BSE). Experimental transmission to mice, and sometimes other species, has been proved in four of these. The final species, moufflon (a primitive wild sheep) was probably infected with scrapie.

The purpose of this chapter is to describe briefly the clinical features, pathology, epidemiology, and control of the animal prion diseases. However, some features are common to all of them, so to avoid repetition some of the general features will be discussed separately.

General features

Scrapie is the oldest subacute transmissible spongiform encephalopathy and the clinical signs were well known to sheep farmers and described in the literature of the 18th century, for example by Leopoldt (1759). Epidemics and declines in the incidence of scrapie were reported in sheep in Great Britain and mainland Europe, notably in Germany and the Danube valley, during the late 18th century and in the 19th century. Besnoit and Morel (1898) were the first to describe characteristic vacuoles in the perikaryon (cell body of a nerve cell) of ventral horn cells of the spinal cord in sheep with scrapie. This was the prelude to defining the pathology, common to all of the diseases of the group, as a spongiform encephalopathy in which the other subsequently reported important features were:

● the occurrence of vacuolation in neurites (processes of nerve cells) in grey matter neuropil;
● loss of neurones;
● astrocytosis (increase of supporting cells called astrocytes);
● sometimes, occurrence of amyloid plaques.

On 6 July 1934, Cuillé and Chelle from the veterinary school in Toulouse, France, inoculated a ewe with spinal cord from an affected sheep and, after an incubation period of 15 months, scrapie resulted. This did not occur in a control sheep (Cuillé and Chelle 1936). This was the first report of experimental transmission of scrapie. Transmission is the single most important criterion that enables the scrapie group of diseases to be distinguished from other non-transmissible spongiform encephalopathies, such as hepatic encephalopathy of humans and animals.

Cuillé and Chelle (1939) were also the first to transmit scrapie experimentally to goats. Later Chelle (1942) reported natural scrapie in the species. Goats, which appear to be uniformly susceptible to scrapie, were subsequently used to study the disease under laboratory conditions. However, this was expensive and cumbersome. These problems were alleviated when Chandler (1961) reported transmitting scrapie to mice, thus providing a relatively cheap model system for studying the experimental disease. A vast expansion of the research into this enigmatic disease and the agent causing it then took place. This led to an understanding of the pathogenesis of the experimental disease (Dickinson and Outram 1979; Kimberlin 1979, 1986; Kimberlin and Walker 1988, 1989*a,b*).

Pathogenesis

When experimental scrapie in rodents is compared with conventional virus diseases, an obvious difference is the remarkable uniformity of the pathogenesis and clock-like precision of the length of the incubation period. This remains provided a small number of variables are kept constant, such as the agent strain, infectivity titre, amount inoculated and the route of administration, and importantly the consistency of the host genotype.

Following experimental infection of mice by non-neural, peripheral routes pathogenesis essentially involves the lymphoreticular system before the central nervous system (CNS) (Kimberlin and Walker 1988). Other organs are, for the most part, either not involved (for example, muscle) or only transiently so (for example, blood) and even then only at low titres following experimental challenge. Following replication in fixed cells of the lymphoreticular system – possibly follicular dendritic cells (Fraser and Brown 1994; O'Rourke *et al.* 1994) – infection spreads via visceral autonomic nerves to the thoracic spinal cord. It then moves rostrally to the brain and caudally to the lumbosacral spinal cord via nerve tracts, at the rate of 1 mm per day. When certain clinical target areas are reached and sufficient agent replication and functional damage have occurred, disease ensues (Kimberlin and Walker 1988). These and other studies in Suffolk sheep (Hadlow *et al.* 1982) and goats (Hadlow *et al.* 1980) with natural scrapie, in mink with experimental TME (Hadlow *et al.* 1987*a*), and in experimental murine scrapie show that some tissues remain free of detectable infectivity throughout the incubation period. Also, the infectivity titre in terminal clinical cases is highest in the CNS, and next highest in the lymphoreticular system. Most other tissues have low or minimal levels of infectivity which is detectable only in the clinical phase of disease or late in the incubation period. Such data provide basic guidance and enable judgements to be made on the risk to humans of exposure to tissues and organs from food animals infected with scrapie-like agents which might be human pathogens.

Efficiency of routes of transmission

One other important feature of scrapie-like infections has been investigated using mice and hamsters. (The hamster has been a useful experimental animal to study experimental scrapie as some models—for example, using scrapie strain 263K— have incubation periods of under 100 days, which is shorter than in mice infected with any murine scrapie strains.) The relative efficiencies of infection by different routes, as measured by titration of standard brain inocula (Kimberlin and Walker 1988) show that the oral route of infection is about 100 000 times less efficient than inoculation directly into the brain within a species. It is little different across a species barrier (Kimberlin and Walker 1988, 1989*b*; Kimberlin 1994). Other routes are intermediate, in the order from most to least efficient: intravenous > intraperitoneal > sub-cutaneous. This also has important implications for disease control for consumers of animal products (naturally well protected by the low efficiency of transmission by mouth) and recipients of biological products from animals administered by the oral, or the more efficient parenteral routes. Both these potential problems have been addressed in the measures adopted for BSE control. In this context it is important to mention another factor: the species barrier.

The species barrier

From the collective studies of experimental and natural disease it seems there are natural restraints which resist the transmission of spongiform encephalopathy from one species to another under natural conditions. One is the strain of agent. The other is the variation in the *PrP* genotype between the donor and recipient species. In humans exposed to infected animal tissues little can be done to influence these factors, so the only protective measure that is practical and effective is to reduce exposure to tissues that might carry agents which might potentially be a danger. This is the basis of the measures adopted to control BSE. In animals, lowering exposure is still an important way of reducing the risk of between-animal transmission, but recent advances in molecular genetics raise the possibility of control by selectively breeding animals with incubation periods which exceed the commercial lifespan. For example, scrapie could be controlled in sheep by selection of *PrP* genotypes resistant to experimental and natural challenge with scrapie agent (in other words, animals with a long incubation period). Such methods, using simple blood tests, are now gaining favour and so far seem to be a qualified success. In cattle this is not an option because polymorphisms detected in the *PrP* gene do not appear to confer resistance and all cattle seem, like mink, to be uniformly susceptible to the disease.

Strains of agent and Sinc *gene*

Another important discovery was the role of a major gene called *Sinc* (for *s*crapie *inc*ubation period) that affects the incubation period in mice (Dickinson *et al.* 1968). Dickinson and co-workers developed in-bred strains of mice which respond differently to two major strains of murine scrapie (Dickinson and Fraser 1979). *Sinc* has two alleles: *s7* for short incubation, and *p7* for long incubation. One group of scrapie strains typified by strain ME7 have short incubations in homozygous *s7* mice, and longer incubations in homozygous *p7* mice. Another group of strains, typified by the 22A strain, have the opposite properties. Individual members of each strain group can be distinguished by the distribution and severity of the spongiform change (the lesion profile, Fraser 1979) within certain anatomical locations in the brain. It is thus possible to type and compare isolates obtained from natural incidents of disease in different species, or the same species from different geographical locations or over time periods, provided of course those strains transmit to mice. Some strains of natural scrapie and TME do not transmit to mice, but all isolates from brains of cattle so far tested do.

Some 20 different strains of scrapie agent have been determined by serial passage in mice. However, the biological characteristics of the BSE agent differ from those strains of scrapie isolated on first passage in mice from historical or contemporary incidents of natural sheep scrapie (Bruce *et al.* 1994). Furthermore, the biological characteristics of the agent isolated at first passage in mice from the brains of three unrelated cats, a greater kudu, a nyala with natural spongiform encephalopathy, and a sheep, goat, and pig with spongiform encephalopathy resulting from experimental transmission from brain tissue from cows with confirmed BSE, are remarkably similar to those of the BSE agent, in their incubation period and lesion profile. On present evidence, therefore, the biological properties of the BSE agent are retained on natural or experimental transmission to other species, despite the fact that the *PrP* gene shows considerable sequence differences between these species. The *PrP* gene (*Prnp*) and *Sinc* are tightly linked genetically and are probably the same. *Sinc* is also referred to as *Prn-i*. The *Prnp* alleles seen in short and long incubation time mice are designated *Prnp*ᵃ and *Prnp*ᵇ and encode proteins which differ by two amino acids at residues 108 (leucine–phenylalanine) and 189 (threonine–valine) (Westaway *et al.* 1987).

Another important finding from these studies is that the incubation periods in two inbred mouse strains with the same *Sinc* genotype *s7* (RIII and C57 black) were very different when they were inoculated with the same dose of BSE-infected cow brain. This contrasts with transmissions from natural cases of scrapie where differences in incubation periods in the two mouse strains were not large. Also, with isolates from BSE cases the difference in incubation period was substantially reduced on subsequent mouse-to-mouse passage in either mouse strain. This could reflect so far undiscovered differences in sequences of the *PrP* gene between the two strains, or some unknown regulation of the *PrP* gene, or the effect of another gene at a different locus (Bruce *et al.* 1994).

Confirmation of disease

Diagnosis and confirmation of the diseased state can be made by several methods including PrP^Sc detection as follows:

1. Presence of clinical signs leads to a suspicion of disease and a clinical diagnosis.

2. Presence of characteristic, bilaterally symmetrical, microscopic lesions of spongiform change in grey matter neuropil of the brain leads to confirmation of spongiform encephalopathy. If this is also supplemented by the immunohistochemical demonstration of PrP^Sc in areas with vacuolation or demonstration of PrP^Sc-positive plaques (if they exist), this lends additional weight to the diagnosis of prion disease. These examinations are done on formalin-fixed tissues.

3. Using detergent extracts of unfixed, fresh, or frozen brain or cervical spinal cord grey matter (including that accidentally mutilated or affected by autolytic change) two other methods of prion disease diagnosis are available. These rely upon the

detection of either PrP^{Sc} by immunoblotting (western blotting) or of disease-specific aggregated fibrils by electron microscopy (EM). The latter are shown following treatment with proteinase K, electron-dense staining and examination by EM. These fibrils are usually referred to as scrapie-associated fibrils (Merz *et al.* 1981, 1984). Detailed protocols for diagnosis or confirmation of BSE and scrapie in member states by these methods have been adopted by the European Commission (1994).

Scrapie

Scrapie (for reviews see Kimberlin 1981; Detwiler 1992) affects most breeds of sheep. It has a widespread distribution but has been successfully eradicated from Australia, where it was established only locally and briefly following importation (Bull and Murnane 1958), from New Zealand, and from some locations and flocks in Iceland. Some countries of south America and Europe are probably also free of the disease. Scrapie in moufflon (*Ovis musimon*) has been recorded only in Great Britain (Wood *et al.* 1992a). Goat scrapie is much rarer than sheep scrapie but probably has a similar distribution. Scrapie affects adult sheep of any age but the modal age of occurrence is 42 months. Cases are very rare in sheep under one year old.

Epidemiology and genetics

It is commonly accepted that scrapie is an infectious and contagious disease and importing countries wishing to protect their native scrapie-free flocks from infection base their controls on this view. However, Parry (1983) was convinced the disease was hereditary. This notion was based on many years of meticulous research on sheep farms. Although his views are not widely supported now, it is clear that the genes *Sip* and *PrP* are particularly important in sheep, in that they control the incubation period of the disease and, under some conditions, particular alleles can determine whether or not clinical disease will result during the sheep's lifetime. Even though we do not know for certain that *Sip* and *PrP* are congruent there is evidence that they are linked and could be the same (Hunter *et al.* 1989, 1991; Goldmann *et al.* 1991a). One problem however is that there are more alleles of the *PrP* gene than of *Sip*. Studies reported by Foster and Hunter (1991) and Hunter *et al.* (1991) show that these genes control susceptibility to both experimental and natural scrapie respectively.

As has been mentioned earlier, the expression of clinical disease is a result of the interaction of the infectious agent with the host *PrP* genotype. Once it is recognized that there are variables on both sides of this equation (there are various strains of agent and polymorphisms in the coding region of the *PrP* gene sequence), then one has to consider the possibilities for various outcomes when various combinations of agent strain and host genotype interact. Goldmann *et al.* (1994) investigated such possibilities experimentally, by challenging Cheviot sheep with BSE agent, SSBP/1 (A group) scrapie, and scrapie isolate CH1641 (C group strain). CH1641 differs from SSBP/1 and other A group strains in that the alleles of *Sip* act in the opposite way, namely with incubation being shorter in *pA* homozygotes than in *sA* homozygotes (Foster and Dickinson 1988). Goldmann *et al.* (1991*a*) had previously shown that there was an apparently simple association between one polymorphic form of the *PrP* gene (namely the allele with valine at codon 136 instead of alanine) and SSBP/1, in that the former allele conferred an increased susceptibility to disease in Cheviot sheep. The study reported by Goldmann *et al.* (1994) showed, in contrast, a much lower disease incidence following infection of SSBP/1-susceptible sheep with either BSE or CH1641 agents, showing a more complex host genetic control when the strain of agent is changed. These two agent strains induce disease in Cheviot sheep that are homozygous for glutamine at codon 171. The low incidence of disease following challenge with BSE or CH1641 can be attributed to the allele with arginine at codon 171, rather than glutamine. The arginine allele confers a four-to six-fold prolongation of the healthy state, which means that disease does not occur in the average normal lifespan. The codon 136 dimorphism (valine versus alanine) has a minor modulating effect on incubation period in heterozygous sheep inoculated with BSE, the valine allele lengthening the period. Homozygosity at this site may also have an influence. Whereas the arginine 171 allele delays, it does not prevent the onset of disease following challenge with SSBP/1. The 136 dimorphism with this strain has the major effect on disease susceptibility and the 171 codon modulates the incubation period. Caution must be exercised in applying the results of experimental studies in particular breeds of sheep to the field situation, not least because some breeds such as the Manech and Préalpes (Laplanche *et al.* 1993), and Suffolks (Westaway *et al.* 1994) do not exhibit polymorphisms at codon 136 of the *PrP* gene, and Lacaunes very rarely do (Laplanche *et al.* 1993). It is concluded that the functional effects of the two domains of the *PrP* gene (codons 136 and 171) alternate, depending on the isolate of the infecting agent.

It cannot be inferred from these studies that the BSE agent and CH1641 scrapie strain are the same. That they are different is clear, because the BSE agent consistently transmits from brain material to mice, whereas CH1641 does not.

The complete strain typing of isolates from field cases of scrapie or BSE can take up to 10 years. However, the relative dominance of valine 136 over arginine 171 or vice versa, for disease incidence, provides a useful practical method to distinguish A group and C group strains present in a flock. This has importance for disease control because it is now possible to select sheep for low susceptibility to scrapie A strains by selecting those carrying the alanine 136 allele. However, such sheep would be susceptible to C strains. It is therefore important to know, not only the *PrP* genotypes, but also the type of strains present in affected sheep in the flock or, if scrapie does not exist, the strain group most likely to be encountered if the risk of scrapie introduction was to be prevented or reduced.

BSE has been experimentally transmitted to sheep and goats including by the oral route (Foster *et al.* 1993). The risk of BSE infection to sheep in this context must be considered, though there is no evidence at present that transmission has occurred in the field. This is because few sheep were fed concentrate rations containing ruminant protein. In July 1988 a ban on feeding ruminant protein to ruminants was brought in in Great Britain and now it is prevented by the ban on feeding mammalian protein to ruminant animals throughout the EU (Commission Decision 94/381/EC 1994).

Scrapie has not been shown to develop in genetically susceptible sheep without exposure to infection. Scrapie tends to become endemic once introduced into a flock or country, and sheep are the only known reservoir of infection. The infection is maintained and disseminated by maternal and, more importantly, horizontal transmission. The precise means of spread is not certain but Pattison *et al.* (1972, 1974) showed that placenta from Swaledale ewes with scrapie was infective for both sheep and goats by feeding, thus establishing a source and route of infection that was plausible for natural transmission of disease and could explain why scrapie is difficult to eradicate and so easily becomes endemic. There are numerous instances reported where scrapie has been introduced into countries, regions or flocks by movement of apparently normal sheep incubating the disease (Brash 1952; Bull and Murnane 1958; Hourrigan *et al.* 1979).

The question of whether or not sheep (or goats) can be clinically silent carriers of scrapie infection is unanswered. Such a mechanism could explain the sudden and unexpected appearance of scrapie in a previously clinically free flock, if a mutant and more pathogenic strain became selected. Sometimes scrapie can appear in a flock following the introduction of a scrapie-free ram, with susceptibility alleles, which may alter the subsequent genetic susceptibility of offspring kept for breeding to the prevailing strains of agent.

Other than placenta, there is no detectable infectivity in body fluids, secretions, and excretions (including urine, faeces, milk, blood, and saliva) (Hadlow *et al.* 1982). Tissues other than those of the central nervous or lymphoreticular systems from subclinically affected animals are much less likely transmit disease (and may be incapable of doing so) by the inefficient oral route because infectivity titres are so low. Under natural conditions exposure would not occur and now, in member states of the EU, the mammalian protein feed ban prevents access to infectivity via meat and bone meal and feed. Many, but not all, sheep with scrapie exhibit severe pruritus and rub to relieve it, causing skin ulceration. However, skin has not shown infectivity (Stamp *et al.* 1959), and nor has semen or a range of male and female reproductive tissues (Hadlow *et al.* 1982). The same is true in goats (Hadlow *et al.* 1980). One study (Foster *et al.* 1992) has however shown that offspring with susceptible *PrP* genotypes derived from dams experimentally infected with SSBP/1 and their unwashed embryos, transferred and gestated in scrapie-free *pApA* surrogate dams can develop scrapie, suggesting that some form of vertical (maternal) transmission can occur by this route. A second study in the USA however, showed no such transmission when embryos were washed three times before transfer (Foote *et al.* 1986; Bradley 1994*a*). There is also some evidence that sheep may become infected via contaminated pasture (Greig 1940), buildings, or equipment. The natural resistance of the scrapie agent to physical and chemical disinfection would aid such indirect transmission. Presumably the source of contamination would be placenta.

Clinical signs

Onset of scrapie is insidious and likely only to be recognized in the earliest stage by an experienced shepherd. The early signs are behavioural, and sheep may lead or trail a driven flock and respond unusually to the sheep dog. The dominant sign in the fully developed disease is pruritus. This is relieved by rubbing against objects (causing damage to and loss of the fleece (Fig. 4.1) and sometimes skin ulceration), or by biting or chewing the feet, for example. Horned breeds of goats use their horns with great precision to relieve irritation on the back and other parts. In sheep, if the lower back is rubbed a satisfying nibbling response results. Pruritus is not invariable. For example, it is not a feature of historical rida (Icelandic scrapie). Teeth grinding, tremor (locally or generally), and abnormal low head and ear carriage can also be seen. Ataxia is a common finding exhibited as gait incoordination, hypermetria, trotting, or 'bunny hopping'. Some sheep show hypersensitivity to sound, movement, or touching. Rumination may be reduced, but feeding is not, and condition is usually only lost in the pre-terminal phase of clinical disease. Water metabolism may be upset and is exhibited by frequent drinking and voiding small quantities of urine

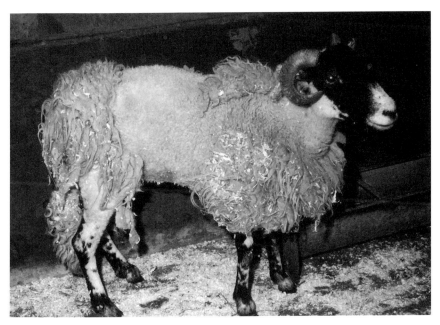

Fig. 4.1 Sheep with advanced scrapie showing poor condition and loss of fleece. (Courtesy of Mr G. A. H. Wells and Mr S. A. C. Hawkins. Crown copyright.)

repeatedly. Not all sheep show all the signs, which are progressive, lasting usually a few weeks or months. However, scrapie lesions can be found in sheep found dead without premonitory signs (Clark 1991; Clark and Moar 1992; Clark *et al.* 1994). In the UK since the advent of BSE, there has been no reported change in the age of onset, clinical signs, duration of disease, or neuropathology. There is some evidence for an increase in incidence of scrapie in sheep but this cannot be attributed to the occurrence of BSE. Scrapie was made a notifiable disease in member states of the EU on 1 January 1993. Wood *et al.* (1992*b*) reported case histories of scrapie in 20 goats in which common signs were hyperaesthesia, ataxia, and pruritus.

Pathology

The classical features of spongiform encephalopathy occur in sheep and goats with scrapie. In contrast to some transmissible spongiform encephalopathies, vacuolation in the cytoplasm of neurones is conspicuous and a pathognomic feature. The vacuoles are empty in paraffin sections stained with haematoxylin and eosin. They are particularly evident in neurones of the mid brain, pons, medulla, and ventral and lateral horns of the spinal cord. Proliferation of astrocytes is also a conspicuous feature (Parry 1983). The other features of spongiform encephalopathies are also present, notably vacuolation of grey matter neuropil, neuronal cell loss (sometimes, but hard to prove without morphometric analysis), and amyloidosis (seen in just over half of 20 natural scrapie cases; Gilmour *et al.* 1985). Wood *et al.* (personal communication) have recently completed a report on the neuropathology of natural sheep scrapie in brains submitted to the Central Veterinary Laboratory, Weybridge, UK, over more than a decade. They reported lesions in the cerebral cortex in some cases and were able to distinguish certain patterns of disease between different breeds. A report has been prepared for publication. In goats, lesions were seen in the brainstem, cerebellum, diencephalon, corpus striatum, and in the neopallium or cerebral cortex. Amyloid deposits were seen in three of 20 goats (Wood and Done 1992). In sheep, scrapie-associated fibrils (Stack *et al.* 1991) and PrP^{Sc} can be detected in detergent extracts of brain. Studies in the USA (Race *et al.* 1992), Japan (Ikegami *et al.* 1991), and the UK (Mohri *et al.* 1992) have shown that immunoblotting methods applied to spleen or lymph node biopsies may sometimes be successful in detecting experimentally or naturally scrapie-affected animals. This is not yet sufficiently well developed for use under farm conditions and in any case does not detect infection. PrP^{Sc} can also be detected in tissue sections of brain from affected sheep by immunocytochemistry. Scrapie-associated fibrils have been detected in goats with scrapie (Perrin *et al.* 1991).

Diagnosis

Scrapie can be readily recognized once signs have developed adequately, enabling a clinical diagnosis to be made. Confirmation is by one or other of the methods described in the protocols (European Commission 1994).

Control

Prevention of infection via feed in the member states of the EU is by the ban on feeding mammalian protein to ruminant animals (Commission Decision 94/381/EC 1994). Some other countries have taken similar precautions. All countries have regulations controlling the importation of sheep and goats in regard to scrapie. The lack of a diagnostic test which can be used on the live animal hinders control and certification of scrapie freedom. It will be undoubtedly easier to establish flock freedom rather than country freedom, but even this demands extensive monitoring, maintenance of impeccable breeding records, accurate and complete identification of all animals, and strict veterinary control, including extensive post-mortem examinations looking for evidence of scrapie.

Once scrapie has occurred, and if it is not possible or justifiable to slaughter out, disinfect and rest the farm, then there are three alternatives (Kimberlin 1981). The first is to cull blood-line relatives of affected sheep – that is, the affected case and all male and female antecedents and male and female progeny. The second is to cull only in the female line including female antecedents and all female progeny intended for breeding. The third option, which is now being developed, is the selection of breeding animals which have a low susceptibility to the scrapie strains likely to be encountered in the flock. This demands, like the other methods, certain additional measures:

(1) individual identification of all animals and records of matings;
(2) purchase of new breeding animals of known *PrP* genotype from scrapie-free sources, preferably of an age at which scrapie is unlikely to occur;
(3) collection and safe disposal of placenta;
(4) avoidance of the use of lambing pens;
(5) use of different lambing areas in subsequent years and effective disinfection of buildings and equipment.

If breeding and identification records do not exist it will take at least three years before effective culling can begin.

Transmissible mink encephalopathy

Mink farming and husbandry

Mink (*Mustela vison*) are members of the carnivorous family Mustelidae, which comprises about 25 genera and includes weasels and ferrets. Captive mink kept in cages are aggressive animals, prone to fighting and biting each other and cannibalizing the dead. They are farmed for their lustrous fur mainly in North America, and central and northern Europe. In the northern hemisphere females are bred in March and whelp in May. Kits are weaned by July, caged separately to prevent fur damage, and, following the autumnal moult, are pelted in November and December when pigment has migrated fully into the hair shafts.

Mink lack a caecum, and have a small stomach and short digestive tract, necessitating small, frequent, digestible meals high in fat (about 20%) and protein (25–35%, depending upon their physiological state). Such a demand is met usually by feed of fish, poultry, or animal origin. Dry pelleted feeds are available but traditionally mink are fed 'wet' using animal offals mixed with cooked cereal. Feed is the major cost of any mink enterprise and centrally prepared wet feed is cheaper than the dry version. Feed can contain sheep or cattle offals or material derived from them. Feed is placed on the top of cages which mink climb to consume. Mink are naturally clean animals, defecating at a single site.

Mink ranchers are now aware that a number of diseases (some of which are vaccinated against) can be transmitted via feed, and these include tuberculosis, Aujeszky's disease, anthrax, botulism, tularaemia, brucellosis, clostridial infections, aleutian disease, and of course TME. Strict control of feed sources restricts their occurrence.

Occurrence of TME

TME is a rare disease occurring only in farmed mink, which are a dead-end host. It is invariably fatal and mortality is usually very high, approaching 100 per cent of adults on an affected farm. Hartsough and Burger (1965) first reported TME, although it had been recognized on mink ranches in Wisconsin and Minnesota since 1947. Outbreaks have since been reported in: Idaho (in 1963); Wisconsin (including at Hayward and Stetsonville in 1985); Ontario, Canada; Finland; Germany; and Russia. It has never been recorded in the UK.

Clinical signs

The onset of disease is insidious and detectable in its earliest phase only by those experienced in mink husbandry. The primary changes are behavioural. There is increased aggressiveness, hyperexcitability, and hyperaesthesia. Affected mink make frenzied attacks on objects moved along the cage side, show exaggerated responses to touch and sound, and become careless in defecating. They become reluctant to climb to the cage roof to consume feed, so intake is reduced and condition lost. Ataxia of the hind limbs progressively develops resulting in lateral falling. The initial hyperexcitability declines and mink become stuporous with a low head carriage. The tail may be uncharacteristically carried over the back like that of a squirrel but this is not seen in experimentally inoculated animals. Inconstant signs include tremor and circling but terminal blindness is common. Finally locomotion becomes impossible, with hind limbs being held flexed against the body. Compulsive biting and self-mutilation occur and this may result in haemorrhage (Fig. 4.2) which can be fatal. Mink will tenaciously bite on to a pencil and can thus suspend themselves vertically and even fall asleep in this position. Death in a debilitated state is preceded by a state of deep somnolence. Dead mink may have their jaws tightly clamped to the wire mesh of the cage. The clinical course is usually a

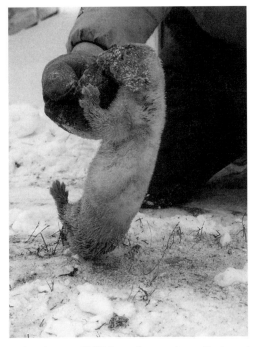

Fig. 4.2 Experimental end-stage TME in an intraperitoneally inoculated, violet, female (Chediak–Higashi syndrome) mink. The mink is suspended by biting on to the gloved hand and the coat is soiled with faeces and blood resulting from self-mutilation. (Courtesy of Professor R. F. Marsh.)

few weeks but can be very short or longer. For a review of the clinical and other aspects of TME see Marsh and Hadlow 1992.

Pathology

In North American mink with TME, the characteristic features of spongiform encephalopathy are present, with bilaterally symmetrical grey matter spongiform change and astrogliosis being the dominant lesions. The spongiform lesions are more evident rostrally than caudally and are most severe in the cerebral cortex, especially in the gyri of the frontal lobes, the amygdaloid nucleus, corpus striatum, and thalamus. The lesions in the mid and hind brain are less severe and more variable. The cerebellum and spinal cord are usually spared (Marsh and Hadlow 1992).

Pathogenesis

There is little doubt that the source of TME infection is feed infected with the causal agent, but mink may not become infected simply by eating it. Experimentally, TME can be transmitted by intradermal inoculation (Marsh and Hanson 1979) and subcutaneous inoculation (Hadlow *et al.* 1987*a*). Under natural circumstances infection may be initiated via wounds caused by fighting between litter mates at feeding time. Such wounds result in penetration of the skin by teeth contaminated with infected feed. Another infection source may be cannibalism of lactating dams by offspring (Burger and Hartsough 1965).

The pathogenesis of experimental TME has been studied in 26 mink challenged subcutaneously with mink-passaged TME from the Idaho outbreak (Hadlow *et al.* 1987*a*). Mink were singly killed sequentially, at intervals of one to four weeks up to 28 weeks post-inoculation, by which time no clinical signs had been observed, and at intervals thereafter when they had. The infectivity titre in a range of neural and non-neural tissues (including lymph nodes, spleen, thymus, liver, intestine, and bone marrow) was estimated by intracerebral bioassay in susceptible mink, thus eliminating any barrier effect from the use of a different host species and maximizing the detection of infectivity. This study showed extremely little replication of the agent during the pre-clinical stage of infection and that which was detected was largely limited to lymph nodes draining the site of inoculation. Infectivity was first detected in the CNS at 20 weeks after inoculation and mild clinical disease appeared at 32 weeks. Early spongiform change was detected in the sigmoid gyrus of the frontal cortex at 28 weeks. Once detected in brain and spinal cord, infectivity appeared in many extra-neural sites, but at much lower titres than in the CNS. Other routes than subcutaneous experimental challenge gave similar results (Marsh *et al.* 1969*a*). It was concluded that mink are not natural hosts for the TME agent.

Diagnosis

Suspicion of disease is based on the distinctive and progressive clinical signs and confirmation is by one or other of the post-mortem methods described in European Commission (1994).

Epidemiology

The origin of infection is infected feed. The minimum incubation period following feed exposure is seven months and the maximum one year (Marsh and Hadlow 1992). The only known reservoirs of animal transmissible spongiform encephalopathy infection, in countries affected with TME, are sheep or goats infected with scrapie. It has been presumed that infected sheep tissues or material derived from them (such as insufficiently decontaminated meat and bone meal) and fed to mink are the most likely source. However, scrapie has never been successfully transmitted to mink by the oral route, although it will transmit when parenteral routes are used, but after prolonged incubations (11–12 months (Hanson *et al.* 1971), or 16–24 months (Marsh and Hanson 1979)) which are no longer than those usually observed in the natural disease. Despite these reports, sheep cannot be eliminated as a source of TME infection since there are many strains of scrapie agent and it may be that TME will only result when challenge is made with a so far untested and specific strain.

BSE has been experimentally transmitted to mink with mean incubation periods of 12 months after intracerebral inoculation and 15 months after feeding but neither the clinical signs (which are quite unlike natural TME) nor the neuropathology (lesion distribution) were identical with natural North American TME (Robinson *et al.* 1994).

Anecdotal evidence from the Stetsonville outbreak of TME indicated that large amounts of products from fallen or sick cattle were fed and that no sheep material was fed at all (Marsh *et al.* 1991). Cattle material was also fed in the Ontario outbreak (Hadlow and Karstad 1968).

Bridges *et al.* (1991) cast some doubt upon whether one can eliminate scrapie-infected sheep as a source of TME even in the Stetsonville outbreak. However, Marsh *et al.* (1991) successfully passaged TME through cattle and back to mink (by feeding and by intracerebral inoculation) with clinical signs and neuropathology in the mink similar to that in the natural disease. The authors concluded that the results suggested the presence of previously unrecognized scrapie-like infection in cattle in the USA. However, a risk analysis has cast doubt on this view, not least because no BSE-like disease has been observed in USA cattle despite clinical and pathological surveillance for the disease.

There is no evidence for maternal transmission of natural, North American TME. Indeed, kits retained for breeding and derived from affected but non-cannibalized dams have not developed TME in three USA outbreaks despite observation over several years (R. F. Marsh, personal communication). However, one Russian report (Chikhov *et al.* 1983) suggests that experimental Russian TME may be maternally transmitted and reduce reproductive performance. Positive transmission was based on detection of spongiform lesions in the brain. Current views would insist that detection of scrapie-associated fibrils or PrP^{Sc} should be accomplished before maternal transmission is confirmed. Even if it was, it may reflect different strains of agent, different mink *Prp* genotypes, and a different pathogenesis in this particular experimental disease.

Experimental transmission of TME to other species and TME strains

TME has been experimentally transmitted to raccoons and skunks (Eckroade *et al.* 1973) and to the European ferret, pine marten, beech marten, Syrian and Chinese hamster, rhesus monkey, stumptail macaque, squirrel monkey, sheep, goat, and cattle (Barlow 1972; Marsh and Hadlow 1992), but not to cats or chickens (Marsh *et al.* 1969*b*). Attempts to transmit TME to mice usually fail (Taylor *et al.* 1986) though Barlow and Rennie (1970) claim success. Interestingly experimental transmission of the Idaho strain of TME to 20 Cheviot sheep and 19 dairy goats resulted in a scrapie-like disease in five sheep and nine goats (Hadlow *et al.* 1987*b*). Lesions occurred in the cerebral cortex but bioassay of tissues in pastel mink showed no detectable infectivity in lymphoid tissues or intestine except for a trace in the proximal colon of one goat.

Two strains (hyper and drowsy) of TME agent, which have distinctive biological properties after transmission in hamsters, produce disease-specific PrP^{Sc} with different physicochemical properties (Bessen and Marsh 1992; Marsh and Bessen 1994), showing that the existence of distinct strains of agent with different biological properties is not just the prerogative of the scrapie agent.

Control and prevention of TME

The precise origin of TME is unknown, whether from sheep, goats, or other species whose tissues may be fed to mink before or after processing. Control of the disease depends therefore on the exclusion from the diet of potentially infected, high-titred offals derived from species affected by transmissible spongiform encephalopathies. For practical purposes this means that central nervous and lymphoreticular system tissues from sheep, goats, and cattle should not be fed unless they are processed by a system that would reduce scrapie and BSE infectivity to a negligible level. When an outbreak of TME occurs it is usually such a dramatic affair that the only action that can be taken is to destroy humanely all affected mink and any offspring that have cannibalized affected dams and to safely destroy the cages and other equipment before restocking with disease- and infection-free animals.

Chronic wasting disease

Species affected and geographical occurrence

CWD is a scrapie-like, naturally occurring transmissible spongiform encephalopathy of deer (family Cervidae) reported only from Colorado and Wyoming in the USA or in zoological parks receiving animals from these locations (Williams and Young 1992). Essentially the disease is restricted to captive animals held in wildlife facilities where experimental nutritional, metabolic, and disease studies are conducted. A few cases have occurred in zoos and there are unpublished reports of a small number of incidents in free-living animals in Colorado and Wyoming which have been confirmed by microscopic examination of the brain (Williams and Young 1992).

The species affected are:

- *Odocoileus hemionus hemionus* — mule deer
- *O. hemionus columbianus* — black-tailed deer
- *O. virginianus* — mule deer × white-tailed deer
- *Cervus elaphus nelsoni* — Rocky Mountain elk.

CWD has not been reported outside North America. It is important to note that spongiform encephalopathy has not occurred in Cervidae in the UK. All the ruminant species in the UK that have been affected by a transmissible spongiform encephalopathy belong to the family Bovidae which includes cattle, sheep, and goats. Experimental transmission of CWD from deer to mink, ferrets, squirrel monkeys, mule deer, and goat has been successful (Williams and Young 1992).

Historical and epidemiology

Williams and Young (1980) first reported CWD which had occurred in captive mule deer in a wildlife facility in Colorado over a 12-year period from 1967. The disease affects only adults, the youngest case being 18 months old and the oldest nine years, but most cases occur in three- to four-year-old animals. In the period 1974–1979, 53 of 67 mule deer and one black-tailed deer had succumbed. Clearly this degree of morbidity and mortality (the disease is invariably fatal) had a serious economic effect and seriously interfered with the wildlife research programme and the options for disposing of surplus animals.

Since 1974 about 90% of deer in the facility have been offspring of trapped, pregnant, wild deer, separated from the dam 1–5 days after birth, and reared artificially on an animal-protein-free diet (other than bovine or ovine milk or products derived therefrom). The dams were returned to the wild. The remainder of the herd was supplemented by a few young adult deer trapped in the wild, orphan fawns captured in the wild, or by offspring from resident does bred in captivity. One black-tailed deer originated from Oregon. CWD has occurred in representative animals from all these sources and suggests no familial or genetic association. There is no evidence that CWD has a feed origin, at least since 1974 when records were available.

Williams and Young (1982) also reported CWD in six Rocky Mountain elk in the same facilities as housed deer in Colorado and Wyoming. The disease followed the first occurrence in mule deer by two years, and, assuming a similar incubation period for the disease in each species, it has been assumed that CWD was naturally transmitted from deer to elk. Elk had fence-line contact with clinically normal and CWD-affected deer and were occasionally maintained in pens previously holding such deer. Elk that contracted CWD were largely caught wild in Wyoming, either as adults or orphans, but some were born to resident dams or born in a zoological park and reared in the facility. CWD has developed in deer or elk in locations previously free of the disease but following movement of animals from affected premises.

How the disease is transmitted is not known but maternal and horizontal transmission must be considered, the latter particularly if one assumes between-species transmission. A number of other species susceptible to transmissible spongiform encephalopathies (cattle, sheep, moufflon, and goats) or not known to be susceptible (bighorn sheep, bighorn × moufflon, pronghorn, moose, white-tailed deer, black back antelope, and mountain goat) have been in direct or indirect contact with CWD cases but none has succumbed. So the origin and maintenance of disease in these facilities remains an enigma no different from that of scrapie itself.

Clinical signs

Some of the clinical signs of CWD in deer and elk are shared, others are distinct. The common signs are weight loss (Fig. 4.3) emaciation, certain behavioural changes, teeth grinding, and excessive salivation (Fig. 4.4). The distinctive feature of CWD in deer is polyuria resulting from polydypsia which is far more common in deer (affecting 77% of cases) than in elk (10%). There is difficulty in swallowing, oesophageal dilation, and regurgitation of rumen contents in deer, but not elk. These features are responsible for terminal aspiration pneumonia, which is a common post-mortem finding. Behavioural changes detected by experienced animal attendants may be the first signs of clinical onset and eventually they affect all deer. They include decreased association with pen-mates, change in behavioural response to attendants, low head and ear carriage, a blank facial expression, repetitive walking in fixed patterns, and periods of somnolence. In elk, behavioural signs are similar and include hyperexcitability and hyperaesthesia. Hind limb ataxia is relatively uncommon but slightly more frequent in elk, though overall a clinical diagnosis is easier in deer. Pruritus is not seen in deer or elk.

Pathology

Gross lesions are related to the polydypsia and loss of body condition, especially in deer. Some deer (13%), but no elk, show a dilated oesophagus; aspiration pneumonia can exist in both.

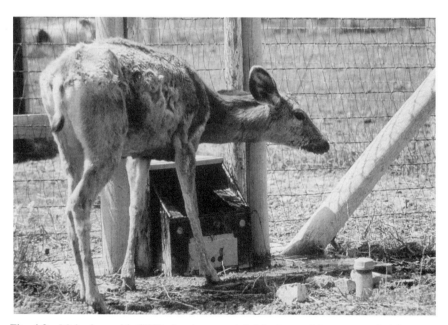

Fig. 4.3 Mule deer with CWD showing emaciated body condition, vacant facial expression, and low head carriage. (Courtesy of Dr E. S. Williams.)

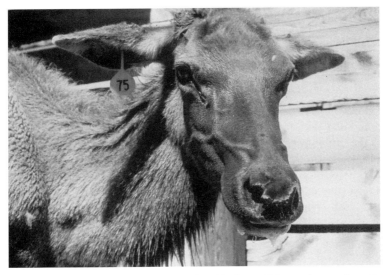

Fig. 4.4   Rocky Mountain elk showing emaciated body condition and excessive salivation. (Courtesy of Dr E. S. Williams.)

A comprehensive light microscopical study of the neuropathology of nine mule deer and six elk has been reported by Williams and Young (1993). All the characteristic signs of spongiform encephalopathy exist in both species, including vacuolation of neurones, neuronal degeneration and loss, astrocytosis, and amyloid plaque formation. There are only minor differences in lesions and their distribution between deer and elk. Lesions in the olfactory tubercle, cortex, hypothalamus, and parasympathetic vagal nucleus of deer are consistent and severe enough to be pathognomic of CWD, but are milder in elk in these locations. By contrast, there were more severe lesions in the thalamus of elk in which there were also some white matter lesions. Amyloid plaques, which also react positively for PrP^{PSc} (Guiroy *et al.* 1991*a,b*), occur in deer but are only seen in elk by the latter method. The severity and distribution of lesions is apparently unaffected by the duration of the clinical signs. Overall the lesion distribution in CWD more closely resembles that in BSE and scrapie than TME. The ultra-structural pathology in captive mule deer also resembles that in other transmissible spongiform encephalopathies.

Fibrils morphologically similar to scrapie-associated fibrils from hamsters with scrapie have been demonstrated in detergent extracts of brains from Rocky Mountain elk (Guiroy *et al.* 1993). Similar extracts showed protein bands with relative molecular masses of 26–30 kDa which reacted positively to anti-PrP^{Sc} serum by western blotting. Immuno-dot blots were also positive.

Diagnosis

Clinical signs are more readily observed in deer than in elk but in the early stages only by experienced stock attendants. Unlike TME, CWD is a sporadic disease but the cumulative mortality over a two-year period may reach 90%. Clinical suspicion must be followed by pathological confirmation by one of the recognized methods (European Commission 1994).

Prevention and control

Eradication of CWD from captive facilities has been attempted more than once (Williams and Young 1992) but failed, even when all deer and elk were killed and buried, the soil turned, and structures and pastures repeatedly sprayed with hypochlorite, and followed by a 12-month period during which no cervids were kept. The reasons for the failure are unknown but could include remaining contamination of pasture or buildings, carrier animals of other domestic or wild species, or re-introduction from the wild. At present there seems to be no useful control method other than humane slaughter and safe destruction of affected animals and an embargo on the movement of animals from affected facilities to other facilities or the wild.

Bovine spongiform encephalopathy

History

Sarradet (1883) reported a case of a scrapie-like disease in an eight-year-old Gasconne cow. The signs were indeed very similar to those of scrapie of sheep, a disease well known by practitioners in France. However, no pathological confirmation is available since spongiform lesions were not described until 1898. Since no other reports have been found since, it is tempting to suggest that an error in diagnosis had been made. An alternative explanation might be the rare occurrence of a familial, hereditary type of BSE due to a pathogenic mutation in the *PrP* gene. There is no way of knowing now, but such cases would be, as in humans, very rare indeed, and would almost certainly escape detection by the standard systems of surveillance pertaining until the emergence of BSE.

The first two BSE cases were confirmed in November 1986 at the Central Veterinary Laboratory, Weybridge, UK. Brains had been submitted for diagnosis from two cows exhibiting unusual and progressive neurological signs by veterinary investigation officers in southern England. The lesions were scrapie-like and, as a result, practitioners were requested to voluntarily report suspect cases showing similar clinical signs. Increasing numbers of suspect animals were reported, expanding the pathological experience of the disease, and in 1987 epidemiological studies were started. It was later confirmed that BSE was indeed a new disease with the first clinical case probably occurring in April 1985 (Wilesmith *et al.* 1988). The Ministry of Agriculture Fisheries and Food and Department of Health set up an independent working party on BSE to determine the implications of the disease in relation to both animal health and any possible human health hazards, and to advise on any necessary measures. Professor Sir Richard Southwood, who chaired the working party, reported in February 1989 and various interim and final recommendations were adopted.

Epidemiology

BSE, and the equivalent disease in captive wild Bovidae, had an origin in meat and bone meal. This was derived from waste animal tissues, including those from ruminants, by rendering, and incorporated into proprietary concentrate rations or protein supplements fed to cattle (Wilesmith *et al.* 1988). A ban on the feeding of ruminant protein to ruminant animals in Great Britain was put in place from 18 July 1988. From 8 August 1988 cattle clinically suspected to have BSE were compulsorily slaughtered and destroyed so no part could enter any food chain. Non-ruminant species however, could be fed potentially infected tissues from cattle incubating the disease, usually in the form of meat and bone meal, until 15 September 1990. From that date a ban was imposed in the UK on the feeding of specified bovine offals, or protein material derived from them, to any species of animal and bird. The specified bovine offals comprise brain, spinal cord, tonsil, thymus, spleen, and intestine. However, no spongiform encephalopathy has ever developed in any pig or poultry anywhere in the world even when fed such material.

Effective exposure of cattle, especially dairy cattle and notably dairy calves, commenced suddenly in 1981–82. This increase in exposure has been associated with the reduction in use of hydrocarbon solvent extraction of fat during the rendering process that produces meat and bone meal (Wilesmith *et al.* 1991). This change presumably permitted an increased amount of infectivity to escape inactivation and was sufficient to produce disease at a detectable incidence. All breeds of cattle and both sexes appear to be equally susceptible.

The epidemiological features are consistent with a source from sheep scrapie, but an origin from a cattle-adapted strain of scrapie cannot be excluded (Wilesmith *et al.* 1988). The epidemic was amplified by the recycling of infected cattle tissue resulting in a marked increase in incidence from mid-1989 (Wilesmith 1994).

To January 1995 there have been over 141 000 cases of confirmed BSE in Great Britain. The rate of acquisition of new cases has shown a significant and progressive decline; for example 36.4% fewer cases were reported in the period July to December 1994 than in the same period in 1993. The decline in incidence of affected herds (Fig. 4.5) preceded the decline in incidence of cases (Fig. 4.6). Earlier, as the epidemic was developing, the increase in annual incidence was by new herds becoming infected, rather than by more cattle developing disease in herds already affected.

There has been a consistently low within-herd incidence of BSE throughout the epidemic, always below 3%, slightly rising during the epidemic and now declining. Furthermore, by 12 January 1995, 72% of all herds affected by BSE had had only four cases or less and 37% had had only one case. There are two possible reasons for this low incidence. The first would be that disease occurs in an uncommon susceptible type of animal governed by a specific *PrP* gene sequence. Though two

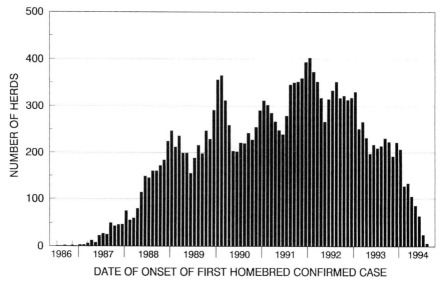

Fig. 4.5 Epidemic curve of BSE herds with homebred cases in the UK between 1986 and October 1994.

polymorphisms of the coding region of the bovine *PrP* gene have been determined (Hunter *et al.* 1994), one results in no change in the coded amino acid. The other codes for either five or six copies of an octapeptide repeat sequence so that three possible genotypes could exist (5/5; 5/6; 6/6). None of these has shown a specific association with BSE occurrence (Goldmann *et al.* 1991*b*; Hunter *et al.* 1994). The uniform susceptibility of different breeds to natural and experimental BSE excludes genetic variation in cattle as a major factor in the occurrence of BSE (Kimberlin and Wilesmith 1994).

The more plausible reason for the low incidence of BSE is that the average exposure to infection in feed has been at a low level. Kimberlin and Wilesmith (1994) calculated, albeit with certain assumptions, that the average contamination of an infected batch of feed might have been as low as 14 oral LD_{50} per tonne. One assumption they made was that infectivity was uniformly distributed. However, it is more likely that infectivity exists in 'packets' and the incidence in any exposed cohort would depend on the frequency of occurrence of these packets.

At 18 November 1994 the confirmed incidence in dairy herds was 52.5% and in suckler herd 14.1%. The reason for the lower incidence in the latter is that beef calves are suckled and usually receive no meat and bone meal or compounded feed. Those cases that do occur are mostly derived from the dairy herd where they would have been exposed. Over 90% of BSE cases in dairy herds occur in Holstein Friesian cows, but this simply reflects the numerical size of the breed. The modal age of occurrence before the decline in incidence in younger cattle, resulting from the feed ban was 60 months, which probably reflects the modal incubation period.

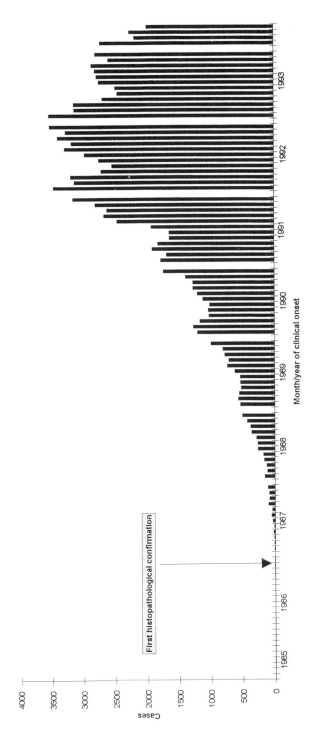

Fig. 4.6 Confirmed cases of BSE by month and year of clinical onset.

No infectivity has been detected in reproductive tissues or placenta of clinically affected cattle. The most appealing evidence for the absence of significant maternal transmission is that the observed incidence of BSE in the offspring of confirmed cases is no greater than would be expected if feed were the only source of infection (Bradley and Wilesmith 1993; MAFF 1994). However, even if maternal transmission did occur at 100% incidence (and there is certainly no evidence for that) the epidemic could not be maintained under British farming practices, as the necessary 1:1 contact rate could not be sustained. The conclusion from these and epidemiological studies is that there is no evidence to support maternal transmission though neither can it be ruled out (Bradley 1994*b*; MAAF 1994).

As a result of the control measures introduced in July 1988 (feed ban) and September 1990 (specified bovine offals ban), new infections via feed are now extremely unlikely. Although the former ban was immediately very effective (Hoinville 1994) it was not completely so because contaminated feed prepared before July 1988 was still in the feed supply chain. Gradually however, this was eliminated, along with possible cross-contamination by feed which may legitimately have contained ruminant protein containing derivatives of specified bovine offals destined for pig or poultry feeding and prepared using the same premises and equipment. This could theoretically have continued until the ban was introduced to protect animals and birds in September 1990. By 12 January 1995 there had been over 15 000 cases of BSE in animals born after the 1988 feed ban. None were born in 1992 or later, 797 were in cattle born in 1990 and only eight in cattle born in 1991. Both the number of suspect cases and confirmed cases (on average 85% of suspects are confirmed) have progressively declined. The decline was first noted, as expected, in cattle two to three years old in 1991 (Wilesmith and Ryan 1992) and has been sustained so the incidence is now zero (MAFF 1994). In successive years a decline has occurred in each age class in turn up to and including cattle five to six years old, and the earlier declines have been maintained. It is expected this process will continue until BSE is eliminated.

BSE has occurred only in animals imported from the UK in the Sultanate of Oman, the Falkland Islands, Canada, Denmark, Germany, and Italy. Some or all of the cases reported in the Republic of Ireland, France, Switzerland, and Portugal have occurred in native-born cattle. The number of cases outside the UK is much lower than the number in the UK but there is evidence that, even for these, meat and bone meal is the origin.

The experimental host range for BSE has been investigated. Successful transmission following parenteral challenge has occurred in cattle, sheep, goats, pigs (Dawson *et al.* 1990), mice, marmosets, and mink. Oral transmission was successful in sheep, goats, mice, and mink but not pigs. Hamsters and chickens were challenged but no disease resulted (Bradley 1994*b*). A wide range of tissues (over 40) from clinically affected, confirmed cases of BSE have shown no detectable infectivity by bioassay in susceptible mice, and this includes muscle (meat), milk, semen, and a range of lymphoreticular tissues (Bradley 1994*b*). Infectivity has however been consistently detected in brain from affected cases at titres similar to those occurring in natural sheep scrapie (Kimberlin 1994). The infectivity titre in peripheral nerve and extraneural tissues of cattle with clinical BSE is at least 1000 times lower than in the comparable tissues from sheep with clinical scrapie. Thus infectivity in extraneural cattle tissues shows a degree of similarity to that in mink with TME (see TME section) and argues similarly that cattle are an unnatural host for the BSE agent and that, with no obvious means of cattle-to-cattle transmission, the species is a dead-end host for BSE.

A study of determine the temporal and spatial development of infectivity and pathology following oral exposure of calves at four months of age to a single, large (100 g) dose of affected cattle brain homogenate is in progress. Results so far available show that at 10 and 14 months of age (six and 10 months after dosing), infectivity is detectable in the distal ileum (Wells *et al.* 1994*a*). This is among the first tissues in which infectivity is found in Suffolk sheep with natural scrapie (Hadlow *et al.* 1982) and is explained by the fact that the intestine at these sites contains Peyer's patches of lymphoreticular tissue in which presumably the agent replicates.

Clinical signs

The neurological signs of BSE are:

(1) changes in mental status exhibited as apprehension, frenzy, and nervousness of doorways;

(2) changes in sensation, notably hyperaesthesia to touch and sound (Kimberlin 1992; Wells *et al.* 1987);

(3) abnormalities of posture (Fig. 4.7) and movement, particularly low head carriage, hind limb ataxia, tremors, and falling.

Of these the signs most frequently recorded are apprehension, hyperaesthesia, and ataxia (Wilesmith *et al.* 1992).

General signs include loss of condition (Fig. 4.7) and milk yield. Rumination is reduced (Austin and Simmons 1993).

The duration of clinical signs varies from seven days to 14 months, but is typically one to two months. There is considerable variation in the presence and severity of clinical signs and, given a quiet environment, they can temporarily subside. Latent signs may become manifest by stress, such as that caused by transport. Signs are progressive and end in recumbency and death, though now, with statutory intervention following notification, most affected animals are killed relatively early in the clinical course. In the UK, after removal of the brain for confirmation of disease, all parts of the carcase are normally incinerated.

Pathology

Lesions are restricted to the CNS and resemble those in scrapie. They include microcystic cavitation of grey matter neuropil (spongiosis or spongiform change),

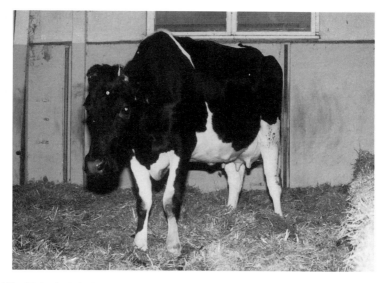

Fig. 4.7 Holstein Friesian cow BSE showing a vacant stare, low head carriage, and a wide-based hind limb stance. (Courtesy of Mr G. A. H. Wells and Mr S. A. C. Hawkins. Crown copyright.)

single or multiple vacuolation of neuronal perikarya (Wilesmith and Wells 1991), astrocytosis represented by astrocyte hypertrophy (Wells *et al.* 1991), neuronal cell loss particularly in the vestibular complex (Jeffrey *et al.* 1992; Jeffrey and Halliday 1994), and the presence of PrP^{Sc} adjacent to, and associated with, areas of vacuolation in grey matter neuropil and on the surface of neurones (Wells *et al.* 1994*b*). In contrast to scrapie, in BSE a greater diagnostic importance is ascribed to the neuropil vacuolation than neuronal vacuolation. The lesions of BSE have been consistent throughout the epidemic, supporting the view that only one major agent strain is involved (Bruce *et al.* 1994). This consistency of lesion permits statutory diagnosis on a single section of medulla at the obex (Wells *et al.* 1989). Suitable brain stem material can be collected via the foramen magnum, thus improving safety and reducing costs. The differential diagnoses of BSE include focal white matter vacuolation in the substantia nigra, cerebral listeriosis, polio-encephalomalacia, and a range of other familiar or previously unrecorded lesions (McGill and Wells 1993).

The ultrastructural pathology of the brain in BSE mimics that in other naturally occurring transmissible spongiform encephalopathies, though Liberski *et al.* (1992) reported finding membrane-bound neuronal inclusions composed of 10 nm diameter tubules in axon terminals.

BSE brains contain PrP^{Sc} and scrapie-associated fibrils (Hope *et al.* 1988; Wells *et al.* 1994*c*). Of particular importance is the excellence of the correlation between examination for fibrils and histopathology of well-fixed brains (Wells *et al.* 1994*c*). The correlations were poor when brains were autolysed but a study by Scott *et al.*

(1992), revealed that fibril detection was of excellent diagnostic value when autolysis rendered brains unsuitable for histopathology.

Diagnosis

Clinical diagnosis of disease to an accuracy of around 85% overall (over 90% of cases in four- to five-year-olds are subsequently confirmed) is possible by simple examination, particularly if conducted over a period. Confirmation of disease post-mortem by one of the established methods is essential (European Commission 1994).

Control

Control of BSE is beyond the scope of this paper, but further details can be found in the publications of Bradley and Wilesmith (1993), Bradley (1994*b*), MAFF (1994), and Taylor (1994).

Controls are best perceived as having objectives to protect both human health and animal health. Some of the measures were stimulated following advice from the Southwood working party and its successor the Spongiform Encephalopathy Advisory Committee.

The major measures for the protection of public health in the UK are:

(1) the compulsory slaughter and complete destruction of cattle clinically suspected to have BSE (August 1988);

(2) the specified bovine offals ban for human consumption (November 1989), extended to include thymus and intestine from cattle of all ages in November 1994 to eliminate any minuscule risks.

There are additional guidelines to control any risks from cattle tissues used during the manufacture of, or in, pharmaceutical products.

The major measures for the protection of animal health (MAFF 1994) include:

(1) the compulsory notification of suspect cases, restriction of their movement, and, if parturient, isolation in approved premises until 72 hours after calving, safe disposal of the placenta and other products and disinfection of the premises (June 1988);

(2) the ban on feeding ruminant animals ruminant derived protein (July 1988) now supplemented by Commission Decision 94/381/EC 1994 which specifies mammalian protein must not be fed, unless it is possible to exclude any ruminant-derived material;

(3) the ban on feeding animals and birds specified bovine offals or products therefrom (September 1990, November 1994).

The European Commission, World Health Organization, Office International des Epizooties, and other governments or agencies have also adopted similar guidelines or recommendations to reduce risks from trading in cattle or cattle products.

Spongiform encephalopathy in captive wild ruminants

History

A single case of spongiform encephalopathy (SE) in a captive nyala (*Tragelaphus angasi*) was identified in a 30-month-old female in 1986 before the first brains from cows affected with BSE were submitted for diagnosis in the UK Central Veterinary Laboratory at Weybridge. This was the herald of the BSE epidemic but did not arouse interest despite publication in the Report of the Chief Veterinary Officer for that year (Anon 1987). A case report was subsequently published (Jeffrey and Wells 1988).

During the next six years a total of 14 further cases of SE had been recognized in five new species as follows:

- gemsbok (*Oryx gazelle*) (one case)

- Arabian oryx (*Oryx leucoryx*) (one case)

- greater kudu (*Tragelaphus strepsiceros*) (six cases)

- eland (*Taurotragus oryx*) (five cases)

- scimitar-horned oryx (*Oryx dammah*) (one case).

All these animals belong to the family Bovidae within the order Artiodactyla. In December 1989 member organizations of the Federation of Zoological Gardens of Great Britain and Ireland had 2675 individuals of 62 species of Artiodactyla recorded in these collections (Kirkwood and Cunningham 1994*a*). This is an underestimate of the totals as non-member representatives are not included. Thus a much larger population of related species is at risk (assuming a common exposure, see below) than has succumbed.

Epidemiology

The epidemiology of spongiform encephalopathy in captive wild ruminants has been comprehensively reviewed and reported (Kirkwood and Cunningham 1994*a,b*). Spongiform encephalopathy in these species is temporally and geographically coincident with the occurrence of BSE suggesting an association with the latter disease. This notion is supported by two other pieces of evidence. First, these (and other Artiodactyla) have been exposed to proprietary feeds or protein supplements of containing ruminant-derived protein believed to be the source of the BSE epidemic (see section on BSE). Secondly brain tissue from the nyala and one greater kudu inoculated into mice showed the same biological characteristics as seven isolates from BSE cases (Bruce *et al.* 1994). These data strongly suggest not only a common origin of infection, but also a common major strain being responsible for BSE, and SE in captive wild ruminants.

The feeding of ruminant-derived protein was not conclusively proved or disproved for the nyala, but was more certain in the gemsbok, Arabian oryx, the first affected kudu, and eland. Four kudu, three eland, and the scimitar-horned oryx were born after the ban on feeding ruminant protein to ruminant animals. However, by December 1994 over 14 000 cases of BSE had been confirmed in cattle born after the ban and, despite the ban, feed seems still to have been the most likely source. Feed cannot therefore be ruled out as the source for all the captive wild ruminant cases.

The strongest case for an origin other than by feed can be made in the kudu, which were all from one collection. Five cases have occurred in eight animals born since 1987 (Kirkwood *et al.* 1994) but although the first may have been derived from infected feed, subsequent cases may have resulted from animal-to-animal transmission. The second case was the offspring of the first suggesting at least the possibility of maternal transmission. The dam of four confirmed cases remains alive so if case-to-case transmission occurs perhaps horizontal transmission occurs, as in scrapie, particularly as one case occurred in an introduced animal 27 months after transfer (Kirkwood *et al.* 1994). The high incidence of disease in the small herd suggests that greater kudu are particularly susceptible to the agent. This is supported by the comparatively short incubation period (minimum 19 months).

A source of infection for some eland could be contamination of their enclosure by fluids dripping from vehicles carrying split bovine heads for lions and tigers (which did not succumb to spongiform encephalopathy). Interestingly two cats that scavenged in the meat room where feed for lions and tigers were prepared succumbed to feline spongiform encephalopathy (FSE) (see section on FSE).

Clinical signs

The duration of clinical signs has ranged from one to 56 days in kudu, eight to 21 days in eland, 21 days in the nyala, seven days in the gemsbok, 22 days in the Arabian oryx, and 18 days in the scimitar-horned oryx (Kirkwood and Cunningham 1994*a*).

Nyala

Hind limb ataxia was followed by episodes of abnormal head posture, persistent licking, and nibbling of the tail base and rump leading to ulceration. There was frequent micturition (Jeffrey and Wells 1988).

Gemsbok

There was a sudden onset of frequent episodic collapse but the condition of the animal was good (Kirkwood and Cunningham 1994*a*).

Eland

Collectively, there was weight loss, drooling, muscle tremor, and dullness. Hypermetria, head pressing, clear nasal discharge, and standing alone were inconstant features (Fleetwood and Furley 1990; Kirkwood and Cunningham 1994*a*).

Arabian oryx

Weight loss and muscle tremors were followed by ataxia, somnolence, and depression (Kirkwood *et al.* 1990, Kirkwood and Cunningham 1994*a*).

Greater kudu

Two animals showed no clinical signs. These had been culled for management reasons but brains examined post-mortem showed spongiform encephalopathy (Cunningham *et al.* 1993). Not all kudu showed all the signs but head tilt was consistently observed. Other prominent signs included weight loss, muscle tremor, lip licking, nose twitching, depression, ataxia, and hypermetria (Kirkwood and Cunningham 1994*a,b*; Kirkwood *et al.* 1990, 1992).

Scimitar-horned oryx

This animal had a nasal discharge, a cough, and weight loss, and later collapsed.

Genetics

The coding regions of the *PrP* gene of the Arabian oryx and greater kudu have been sequenced and compared with the corresponding sheep and cattle sequences (Poidinger *et al.* 1993). The Oryx gene showed only one amino acid different from that of sheep. The kudu gene showed four amino acid differences from that of cattle which gene it resembled more closely. There are too little data to evaluate what influence in the *PrP* gene sequence in these species has on the susceptibility to spongiform encephalopathy.

Pathology

In general, spongiform encephalopathy of captive wild Bovidae resembles BSE most closely. In the nyala, for example, neuropil vacuolation involved principally the brain stem grey matter and was most severe and frequent in the medulla, particularly affecting the dorsal nucleus of the vagus nerve and the nucleus of spinal tract of the trigeminal nerve. Lesions diminished abruptly rostrally and caudally, though mild neuropil vacuolation occurred as far rostral as the hippocampus. Some white matter vacuolation was also seen in the mid-brain and brainstem and cytoplasmic, neuronal vacuolation was seen prominently in the dorsal vagal nucleus. Neither astrocytosis nor amyloid was detected (Jeffrey and Wells 1988). The lesions in greater kudu (Kirkwood *et al.* 1990, 1992), Arabian oryx (Kirkwood *et al.* 1990), and eland (Fleetwood and Furley 1990) were not significantly different, though brainstem lesions in the oryx were less severe than in kudu.

Examination for either scrapie-associated fibrils or PrP^{Sc}, or both, has been conducted in one eland, several kudu, and the scimitar-horned oryx, all with positive results (Kirkwood and Cunningham 1994*a,b*).

Diagnosis

Clinical suspicion of unexplained, progressive, neurological disease should be investigated post-mortem by microscopic examination of the brain coupled with one or other of the diagnostic methods for PrP^{Sc} (European Commission 1994).

Control

All ruminant species, including captive wild Bovidae, in the member states of the EU are protected by the ban on feeding mammalian protein to ruminant animals (Commission Decision 94/381/EC 1994). If feed is the only source of transmissible spongiform encephalopathy infection this ban should be sufficient to protect all ruminant species from new infections via feed. It remains to be seen if there is proven maternal or horizontal transmission in any affected species (especially greater kudu), or if a carrier state occurs. Until then control on movement of affected species from affected collections is vital. All zoos in the UK and Ireland are aware of the clinical signs and pathology of the diseases. Carcases from affected groups should not enter any feed chain, and they are best incinerated (Cunningham 1991).

Feline spongiform encephalopathy

History

Wyatt *et al.* (1990) were the first to report feline spongiform encephalopathy (FSE) in a domestic cat more than three years after the first case of BSE had been confirmed. The cat, a five-year-old, neutered Siamese (*Felis cattus*) had been referred to the Bristol Veterinary School exhibiting progressive ataxia and neuro-logical signs. Following treatment, to which there was no response, the cat was euthanased and microscopic examination of the brain confirmed the presence of spongiform encephalopathy typical of a scrapie-like disease.

A review of reports or tissue sections from cats with neurological disease held in archive in UK veterinary schools from 1975 revealed none that satisfied a patholog-ical diagnosis of spongiform encephalopathy and so, like BSE earlier, FSE was adjudged to be a new disease. However, experimentally induced FSE resulting from inoculation of human brain suspensions from patients with CJD was first accomplished in May 1972 (Amyx *et al.* 1983). These authors reported transmis-sion in 34% of attempts. The cat has been used as an experimental animal to study transmissible spongiform encephalopathies in the USA (Amyx *et al.* 1983; Gourmelon *et al.* 1987) and Slovakia (Mitrova and Mayer 1977).

The clinical signs of experimental CJD in cats and natural FSE are broadly similar (Amyx *et al.* 1983; Pearson *et al.* 1993). However, sleep abnormalities were more frequently reported in the experimental disease and this aspect has been studied (Gourmelon *et al.* 1987) in cats inoculated with animal-passaged CJD agent. In these cats, only discrete to minimal spongiosis was found microscopically so this experimental disease differed markedly from the lesions typical of transmissible spongiform encephalopathies.

FSE has also been reported in three species of captive wild Felidae, a puma (*Felis concolor*) (Willoughby *et al.* 1992), four cheetahs (*Acinonyx jubatus*) (Kirkwood and Cunningham 1994*a,b*), and an ocelot (*Felis pardalis*).

Occurrence of FSE in domestic cats and captive wild Felidae

FSE has occurred in cats in all regions of Great Britain, in Northern Ireland, and some smaller offshore islands, with one case in an indigenous cat in Norway. To 31 December 1994, 61 cases had been reported from the UK.

With the exception of two of the four cheetah (Peet 1992), all the wild cat species developed disease in Great Britain. Two cheetah, one exported to Australia and one to the Republic of Ireland, were presumably exposed to infection in Great Britain before export.

Clinical signs

Domestic cats

Clinical signs in five English cats have been described in detail by Wyatt *et al.* (1991) with single reports in Scottish cats from Leggett *et al.* (1990) and Synge and Waters (1991). All cats had progressive neurological disease involving locomotor disturbances, abnormal behaviour, and altered sensory responses. Pearson *et al.* (1993) report that the mean age of occurrence in 24 cats was six years (range two to 10), with most cases occurring in neutered cats of both sexes from widely geographically separated locations.

Behavioural signs of timidity or aggression preceded invariable and progressive locomotor dysfunction, hind limb ataxia, and/or an ability to judge distances accurately. Ataxia in advanced cases affected also the forelimbs, often with a rapid, crouching, hypermetric gait. Hyperaesthesia and altered grooming (usually decreased, and resulting in an unkempt coat) were common signs. Hypersalivation, polyphagia, polydypsia, and abnormal head posture occurred at a lower frequency. The duration of the clinical period of disease was typically two to three months.

Captive wild Felidae

In these species ataxia is a consistent feature and the clinical signs progress typically over a three to eight week period. The puma was apprehensive, had difficulty in balancing and showed a fine, whole-body tremor (Willoughby *et al.* 1992). Cheetah exhibited, in addition to progressive ataxia, variable signs including hyperaesthesia, weight loss, falling, and muscle spasms.

Pathology

The neuropathology of FSE in all species shows the cardinal signs of a scrapie-like transmissible spongiform encephalopathy, but the lesions are more florid than in

BSE of cattle, and are more prominent in the cerebral cortex, corpus striatum, medial geniculate body, and thalamus. There are usually severe vacuolar changes accompanied by an intense astrocytic and microglial reaction (Wells and McGill 1992). In the puma, neuropil vacuolation was most conspicuous in the inferior colliculi and cerebellar cortex (molecular and granular layers). Wallerian degeneration was also reported in the spinal cord with associated gliosis.

Scrapie-associated fibrils and PrP^{Sc} have been detected in detergent extracts of brains from five affected cats (Pearson *et al.* 1992). Fibrils were also detected in the absence of PrP^{Sc} in the brains of two cats, one with neurological signs and meningioma, and one with neurological signs but a brain appearing normal with microscopic examination. These apparent abnormalities are being further investigated. PrP^{Sc} was detected by immunocytochemistry in the medulla and cervical spinal cord of the puma, in association with SE lesions (Willoughby *et al.* 1992).

Epidemiology

The temporal and geographical occurrence of FSE suggests an origin from BSE rather than scrapie. Furthermore, the biological characteristics of the isolates in mice from three unrelated cats reported by Bruce *et al.* (1994) and Fraser *et al.* (1994) are remarkably similar to those of agents isolated from seven cattle with BSE. This strengthens the support for either a common origin, or an origin from infected tissues from cattle with BSE or a product derived therefrom. There are insufficient cases of FSE in domestic cats with adequate histories to analyse, with confidence, the epidemiology. However, it seems probable that, as in BSE, the origin is infected feed. The particular ingredient is not known since cats have a wide range of diets and, being generally free-ranging animals, there is less control of intake than in other domestic species. However, it is pertinent that no case has so far occurred in a cat born after the imposition in September 1990 of a ban on the feeding of specified bovine offals to any species of animal or birds.

The probable origin of infection for the captive wild cats is clearer because all had access to CNS tissue from cattle, including cattle unfit for human consumption, before the offals ban was in place. FSE has not been reported in lions, tigers, or a range of other captive wild Felidae which may have been similarly exposed to cattle CNS.

Diagnosis

Clinical suspicion of disease is aroused by unaccountable changes of behaviour and progressive ataxia, and disease confirmed by one of the methods mentioned in the EC report (European Commission 1994). It should be borne in mind that there have been few examinations of scrapie-associated fibrils and PrP in Felidae and there are some anomalies with fibril detection; therefore interpretation of results should be cautious until examination of sufficient cases and controls has been completed.

Control

Disease can be prevented by implementing an effective ban on specified bovine offals. Infection may also be prevented by ensuring adequate processing of potentially infected bovine tissues before use in cat feed. Such processes must be shown to inactivate the BSE agent so that no detectable infectivity remains, and must be validated by the national veterinary authorities. Carcases from diseased animals confirmed to have spongiform encephalopathy should be safely disposed of, ideally by incineration, and of course must enter no feed chain. The controls assume no other origin than a feed source.

All zoos in the UK and the Republic of Ireland have been alerted to the occurrence of spongiform encephalopathies in captive wild species and have been informed of the clinical signs and pathological findings (Cunningham 1991). Zoo authorities are aware of the potential risks in exporting animals of affected species to other zoos or returning them to the wild.

References

Amyx, H. L., Gibbs, C. J., Jr, and Gajdusek, D. C. (1983). Experimental Creutzfeldt–Jakob disease in cats. In *Virus non conventionels et affections du système nerveux central* (ed. L. A. Court and F. Cathala), pp. 358–362. Masson, Paris.

Anon (1987). Report of the Chief Veterinary Officer. *Animal Health 1986*, p. 69. HMSO, London.

Austin, A. R. and Simmons, M. M. (1993). Reduced rumination in bovine spongiform encephalopathy and scrapie. *Veterinary Record*, **132**, 324–325.

Barlow, R. M. (1972). Transmissible mink encephalopathy: pathogenesis and nature of the aetiological agent. *Journal of Clinical Pathology*, **25** (Supplement 6), 102–109.

Barlow, R. M. and Rennie, J. C. (1970). Transmission experiments with a scrapie-like encephalopathy of mink. *Journal of Comparative Pathology*, **80**, 75–79.

Besnoit, M. M. and Morel G. (1898). Note sur lésions nerveuses de la tremblante du mouton. *Revue Vétérrinaire T.*, **XXIII(LV)**, 397–400.

Bessen, R. A. and Marsh, R. F. (1992). Biochemical and physical properties of the prion protein from two strains of the transmissible mink encephalopathy agent. *Journal of Virology*, **66**, 2096–2101.

Bradley, R. (1994*a*). Embryo transfer and its potential role in control of scrapie and bovine spongiform encephalopathy (BSE). *Livestock Production Science*, **38**, 51–59.

Bradley, R. (1994*b*). Les encéphalopathies spongiformes animales en Grande Bretagne. *Bulletin Société Vétérinaire Pratique de France*, **78**, 339–366.

Bradley, R. and Wilesmith, J. W. (1993). Epidemiology and control of bovine spongiform encephalopathy (BSE). *British Medical Bulletin*, **49**, 932–959.

Brash, A. G. (1952). Scrapie in imported sheep in New Zealand. *New Zealand Veterinary Journal*, **1**, 27–30.

Bridges, V., Bleem, A., and Walker, K. (1991). Risk of transmissible mink encephalopathy in the US. In *Animal health insight, Fall*, pp. 7–14. USDA:APHIS:VS Animal Health Information, Washington DC.

Bruce, M., Chree, A., McConnell, I., Foster, J., Pearson, G., and Fraser, H. (1994). Transmission of bovine spongiform encephalopathy and scrapie to mice: strain variation and the species barrier. *Philosophical Transactions of the Royal Society of London, Series B*, **343**, 405–411.

Bull, L. B. and Murnane, D. (1958). An outbreak of scrapie in British sheep imported into Victoria. *Australia Veterinary Journal*, **34**, 213–215.

Burger, D. and Hartsough, G. R. (1965). Encephalopathy of mink. II Experimental and natural transmission. *Journal of Infectious Diseases*, **115**, 393–399.

Chandler, R. L. (1961). Encephalopathy in mice produced by inoculation with scrapie brain material. *Lancet*, **i**, 1378–1379.

Chelle, P.-L. (1942). Un cas de tremblante chez la chévre. *Bulletin de l'Academie Vétérinaire de France*, **95**, 294–295.

Chikhov, V. A., Dukur, I. I., and Geller, V. I. (1983). Ministry of Agriculture of the RSFSR. Spread of encephalopathy in mink. All Russian fur-animal science and production group, Afanasiev Institute for research into fur-animal and rabbit production. Cage husbandry of mink, fox, sable, polar fox, nutria and rabbit. In *Collected Scientific Work*, Vol. 29, pp. 241–245.

Clark, A. M. (1991). Diagnosis of scrapie. *Veterinary Record*, **128**, 214.

Clark, A. M. and Moar, J. A. E. (1992). Scrapie: a clinical assessment. *Veterinary Record*, **130**, 377–378.

Clark, A. M., Moar, J. A. E., and Nicholson, J. T. (1994). Diagnosis of scrapie. *Veterinary Record*, **135**, 560.

Commission Decision 94/381/EC. (1994). Concerning certain protection measures with regard to bovine spongiform encephalopathy and the feeding of mammalian-derived protein. *Official Journal of the European Commission*. No. L 172/23, 7 July 1994, Brussels.

Cuillé, J. and Chelle, P.-L. (1936). La maladie dite tremblante du mouton est-elle inoculable? *Comptes Rendus Academie des Sciences*, **203**, 1552–1554.

Cuillé, J. and Chelle, P.-L. (1939). Transmission expérimentale de la tremblante chez la chèvre. *Comptes Rendus Academie des Sciences*, **208**, 1058–1060.

Cunningham, A. A. (1991). Bovine spongiform encephalopathy and British zoos. *Journal of Zoo and Wildlife Medicine*, **22**, 304–308.

Cunningham, A. A., Wells, G. A. H., Scott, A. C., Kirkwood, J. K., and Barnett, J. E. F. (1993). Transmissible spongiform encephalopathy in greater kudu (*Tragelaphus strepsiceros*). *Veterinary Record*, **132**, 68.

Dawson, M., Wells, G. A. H., Parker, B. N. J., and Scott, A. C. (1990). Primary parenteral transmission of bovine spongiform encephalopathy to the pig. *Veterinary Record*, **127**, 338.

Detwiler, L. A. (1992). Scrapie. *Revue Scientifique et Technique, Office International des Epizooties*, **11**, 491–537.

Dickinson, A. G. and Fraser, H. (1979). An assessment of the genetics of scrapie in sheep and mice. In *Slow transmissible diseases of the nervous system* (ed. S. B. Prusiner and W. J. Hadlow), Vol. 2, pp. 367–385. Academic Press, London.

Dickinson, A. G. and Outram, G. W. (1979). The scrapie replication-site hypothesis and its implications for pathogenesis. In *Slow transmissible diseases of the nervous system* (ed. S. B. Prusiner and W. J. Hadlow), Vol. 2, pp. 13–31. Academic Press, London.

Dickinson, A. G., Meikle, V. M. H., and Fraser H. (1968). Identification of a gene which controls the incubation period of some strains of scrapie agent in mice. *Journal of Comparative Pathology*, **78**, 293–299.

Eckroade, R. J., Zu Rhein, G. M., and Hanson, R. P. (1973). Transmissible mink encephalopathy in carnivores: clinical, light and electron microscopic studies in racoons, skunks, and ferrets. *Journal of Wildlife Diseases*, **9**, 229–240.

European Commission. (1994). *Transmissible spongiform encephalopathies. Protocols for the laboratory diagnosis and confirmation of bovine spongiform encephalopathy and scrapie.* A report from the Scientific Veterinary Committee. CEC, Brussels.

Fleetwood, A. J. and Furley, C. W. (1990). Spongiform encephalopathy in an eland. *Veterinary Record*, **126**, 408–409.

Foote, W. C., Call, J. W., Bunch, T. D., and Pitcher, J. R. (1986). Embryo transfer in the control of transmission of scrapie in sheep and goats. *Proceedings of the United States Animal Health Association*, **90**, 413.

Foster, J. D. and Dickinson, A. G. (1988). The unusual properties of CH1641, a sheep-passaged isolate of scrapie. *Veterinary Record*, **123**, 5–8.

Foster, J. D. and Hunter, N. (1991). Partial dominance of the sA allele of the *Sip* gene for controlling experimental scrapie. *Veterinary Record*, **128**, 548–549.

Foster, J. D., McKelvey, W. A. C., Mylne, M. J. A., Williams, A., Hunter, N., Hope, J., *et al.* (1992). Studies on maternal transmission of scrapie in sheep by embryo transfer. *Veterinary Record*, **130**, 341–343.

Foster, J. D., Hope, J., and Fraser, H. (1993). Transmission of bovine spongiform encephalopathy to sheep and goats. *Veterinary Record*, **133**, 339–341.

Fraser, H. (1979). Neuropathology of scrapie: the precision of the lesions and their diversity. In *Slow transmissible diseases of the nervous system* (ed. S. B. Prusiner and W. J. Hadlow), Vol. 2, pp. 387–406. Academic Press, London.

Fraser, H. and Brown, K. (1994). Peripheral pathogenesis of scrapie in normal and immuno-compromised mice. *Animal Technology*, **45**, 21–23.

Fraser, H., Pearson, G. R., McConnell, I., Bruce, M. E., Wyatt, J. M., and Gruffydd-Jones, T. J. (1994). Transmission of feline spongiform encephalopathy to mice. *Veterinary Record*, **134**, 449.

Gilmour, J. S. Bruce, M. E., and MacKellar, A. (1985). Cerebrovascular amyloidosis in scrapie-affected sheep. *Neuropathology and Applied Neurobiology*, **11**, 173–183.

Goldmann, W., Hunter, N., Benson, G., Foster, J. D., and Hope, J. (1991*a*). Different scrapie-associated fibril proteins (PrP) and encoded by lines of sheep selected for different alleles of the *Sip* gene. *Journal of General Virology*, **72**, 2411–2417.

Goldmann, W., Hunter, N., Martin, T., Dawson, M., and Hope, J. (1991*b*). Different forms of the bovine *PrP* gene have five or six copies of a short, G-C-rich element within the protein-coding exon. *Journal of General Virology*, **72**, 201–204.

Goldmann, W., Hunter, N., Smith, G, Foster, J., and Hope, J. (1994). *PrP* genotype and agent effects in scrapie: change in allelic interaction with different isolates of agent in sheep, a natural host of scrapie. *Journal of General Virology*, **75**, 989–995.

Gourmelon, P., Amyx, H. L., Baron, H., Lemercier, G., Court, L., and Gibbs, C. J., Jr (1987). Sleep abnormalities with REM disorder in experimental Creutzfeldt–Jakob disease in cats: a new pathological feature. *Brain Research*, **411**, 391–396.

Greig, J. R. (1940). Observations on the transmission of the disease by mediate contact. *Veterinary Journal*, **96**, 203–206.

Guiroy, D. C., Williams, E. S., Yanagihara, R., and Gajdusek, D. C. (1991*a*). Topographic distribution of scrapie amyloid-immunoreactive plaques in chronic wasting disease in captive mule deer (*Odocoileus hemionus hemionus*). *Acta Neuropathologica*, **81**, 475–481.

Guiroy, D. C., Williams, E. S., Yanagihara, R., and Gajdusek, D. C. (1991*b*). Immuno-localization of scrapie amyloid (PrP 27-30) in chronic wasting disease of Rocky Mountain elk and hybrids of captive mule deer and white-tailed deer. *Neuroscience Letters*, **126**, 195–198.

Guiroy, D. C., Williams, E. S., Song, K-.J., Yanagihara, R., and Gajdusek, D. C. (1993). Fibrils in brain of Rocky Mountain elk with chronic wasting disease contain scrapie amyloid. *Acta Neuropathologica*, **86**, 77–80.

Hadlow, W. J., and Karstad, L. (1968). Transmissible encephalopathy of mink in Ontario. *Canadian Veterinary Journal*, **9**, 193–196.

Hadlow, W. J., Kennedy, R. C., and Race, R. E. (1982). Natural infection of Suffolk sheep and scrapie virus. *Journal of Infectious Diseases*, **146**, 657–664.

Hadlow, W. J., Kennedy, R. C., Race, R. E., and Eklund, C. M. (1980). Virologic and neuro-histologic findings in dairy goats affected with natural scrapie. *Veterinary Pathology*, **17**, 187–199.

Hadlow, W. J., Race, R. E., and Kennedy, R. C. (1987a). Temporal distribution of transmissible mink encephalopathy virus in mink inoculated subcutaneously. *Journal of Virology*, **61**, 3235–3240.

Hadlow, W. J., Race, R. E., and Kennedy, R. C. (1987b). Experimental infection of sheep and goats with transmissible mink encephalopathy virus. *Canadian Journal of Veterinary Research*, **51**, 135–144.

Hanson, R. P., Eckroade, R. J., Marsh, R. F., Zu Rhein, G. M., Kanitz, C. L., and Gustafson, D. P. (1971). Susceptibility of mink to sheep scrapie. *Science*, **172**, 859–861.

Hartsough, G. R. and Burger, D. (1965). Encephalopathy of mink. I. Epizootiologic and clinical observations. *Journal of Infectious Diseases*, **115**, 387–392.

Hoinville, L. J. (1994). Decline in the incidence of BSE in cattle born after the introduction of the 'feed ban'. *Veterinary Record*, **134**, 274–275.

Hope, J., Reekie, L. J. D., Hunter, N., Multhaup, G., Beyreuther, K., White, H., *et al.* (1988). Fibrils from brains of cows with new cattle disease contain scrapie-associated protein. *Nature*, **336**, 390–392.

Hourrigan, J. Klingsporn, A., Clark, W. W., and de Camp, M. (1979). Epidemiology of scrapie in the United States. In *Slow transmissible diseases of the nervous system* (ed. S. B. Prusiner and W. J. Hadlow), Vol. 1, pp. 331–356. Academic Press, London.

Hunter, N., Foster, J. D., Dickinson, A. G., and Hope, J. (1989). Linkage of the gene for the scrapie-associated fibril protein (PrP) to the *Sip* gene in Cheviot sheep. *Veterinary Record*, **124**, 364–366.

Hunter, N., Foster, J. D., Dickinson, A. G., and Hope, J. (1991). Restriction fragment length polymorphisms of the scrapie-associated fibril protein (*PrP*) gene and their association with susceptibility in natural scrapie in British sheep. *Journal of General Virology*, **72**, 1287–1292.

Hunter, N., Foster, W. Smith, G., and Hope, J. (1994). Frequencies of *PrP* gene variants in healthy cattle and cattle with BSE in Scotland. *Veterinary Record*, **135**, 400–403.

Ikegami, Y., Ito, M., Isomura, H., Momotani, E., Sasaki, K., Muramatsu, Y., *et al.* (1991). Pre-clinical and clinical diagnosis of scrapie by detection of PrP protein in tissues of sheep. *Veterinary Record*, **128**, 271–275.

Jeffrey, M. and Halliday, W. G. (1994). Numbers of neurons in vacuolated and non-vacuolated neuroanatomical nuclei in bovine spongiform encephalopathy-affected brains. *Journal of Comparative Pathology*, **110**, 287–293.

Jeffrey, M. and Wells, G. A. H. (1988). Spongiform encephalopathy in a nyala (*Tragelaphus angasi*). *Veterinary Pathology*, **25**, 398–399.

Jeffrey, M., Halliday, W. G. and Goodsir, C. M. (1992). A morphometric and immunohisto-chemical study of the vestibular nuclear complex in bovine spongiform encephalopathy. *Acta Neuropathologica*, **84**, 651–657.

Kimberlin, R. H. (1979). Early events in the pathogenesis of scrapie in mice: biological and biochemical studies. In *Slow transmissible diseases of the nervous system*, (ed. S. B. Prusiner and W. J. Hadlow), Vol. 2, pp. 33–54. Academic Press, London.

Kimberlin, R. H. (1981). Scrapie. *British Veterinary Journal*, **137**, 105–112.

Kimberlin, R. H. (1986). Scrapie: how much do we really understand? *Neuropathology and Applied Neurobiology*, **12**, 131–147.

Kimberlin, R. H. (1992). Bovine spongiform encephalopathy. *Revue Scientifique et Technique Office International des Epizooties*, **11**, 347–390.

Kimberlin, R. H. (1994). A scientific evaluation of research into bovine spongiform encephalopathy (BSE). In *Transmissible spongiform encephalopathies* (Proceedings of a consultation on BSE with the Scientific Veterinary Committee of the Commission of the European Communities held in Brussels, 14–15 September 1993) (ed. R. Bradley and B. Marchant), pp. 455–477. CEC, Brussels.

Kimberlin, R. H. and Walker, C. A. (1988). Pathogenesis of experimental scrapie. In *Novel infectious agents and the central nervous system* (Ciba Foundation Symposium No. 135) (ed. G. Bock and J. Marsh), pp. 37–62. Wiley, Chichester.

Kimberlin, R. H. and Walker, C. A. (1989a). Pathogenesis of scrapie in mice after intragastric infection. *Virus Research*, **12**, 213–220.

Kimberlin, R. H. and Walker, C. A. (1989b). The role of the spleen in the neuroinvasion of scrapie in mice. *Virus Research*, **12**, 201–212.

Kimberlin, R. H. and Wilesmith, J. W. (1994). Bovine spongiform encephalopathy: Epidemiology, low dose exposure and risks. *Annals of the New York Academy of Sciences*, **724**, 210–220.

Kimberlin, R. H., Cole, S., and Walker, C. A. (1987). Temporary and permanent modifications to a single strain of mouse scrapie on transmission to rats and hamsters. *Journal of General Virology*, **68**, 1875–1881.

Kirkwood, J. K. and Cunningham, A. A. (1994a). Epidemiological observations on spongiform encephalopathies in captive wild animals in the British Isles. *Veterinary Record*, **135**, 296–303.

Kirkwood, J. K. and Cunningham, A. A. (1994b). Spongiform encephalopathies in captive wild animal in Britain: epidemiological observations. In *Transmissible spongiform encephalopathies* (Proceedings of a consultation on BSE with the Scientific Veterinary Committee of the Commission of the European Communities held in Brussels, 14–15 September 1993) (ed. R. Bradley and B. Marchant), pp. 29–47. CEC, Brussels.

Kirkwood, J. K., Wells, G. A. H., Wilesmith, J. W., Cunningham, A. A., and Jackson, S. I. (1990). Spongiform encephalopathy in an Arabian oryx (*Oryx leucoryx*) and a greater kudu (*Tragelaphus strepsiceros*). *Veterinary Record*, **127**, 418–420.

Kirkwood, J. K. Wells, G. A. H., Cunningham, A. A., Jackson, S. I., Scott, A. C., Dawson, M., *et al.* (1992). Scrapie-like encephalopathy in a greater kudu (*Tragelaphus strepsiceros*) which had not been fed ruminant-derived protein. *Veterinary Record*, **130**, 365–367.

Kirkwood, J. K., Cunningham, A. A., Austin, A. R., Wells, G. A. H., and Sainsbury, A. W. (1994). Spongiform encephalopathy in a greater kudu (*Tragelaphus strepsiceros*) introduced into an affected group. *Veterinary Record*, **134**, 167–168.

Laplanche, J.-L, Chatelain, J., Beaudry, P., Dussaucy, M., Bounneau, C., and Launay J.-M. (1993). French autochthonous scrapied sheep without the 136Val *PrP* polymorphism. *Mammalian Genome*, **4**, 463–464.

Leggett, M. M., Dukes, J., and Pirie, H. M. (1990). A spongiform encephalopathy in a cat. *Veterinary Record*, **127**, 586–588.

Leopoldt, J. G. (1759). *Nützliche und auf die Erfahrung gegründete Einleitung zu der Landwirtschaft*, Part 5, Chapter 12, pp. 344–360. Glogau, Berlin.

Liberski, P. P., and Yanigihara, R., Wells, G. A. H., Gibbs C. J., Jr, and Gajdusek, D. C. (1992). Comparative ultrastructural neuropathology of naturally occurring bovine spongiform encephalopathy and experimentally induced scrapie and Creutzfeldt–Jakob disease. *Journal of Comparative Pathology*, **106**, 361–381.

MAFF (1994). *Bovine spongiform encephalopathy in Great Britain: a progress report.* MAFF, Tolworth.

Marsh, R. F. and Bessen, R. A. (1994). Physicochemical and biological characterizations of distinct strains of the transmissible mink encephalopathy agent. *Philosophical Transactions of The Royal Society of London*, **343**, 413–414.

Marsh, R. F. and Hadlow, W. J. (1992). Transmissible mink encephalopathy. *Revue Scientifique et Technique Office International des Epizooties*, **11**, 539–550.

Marsh, R. F. and Hanson, R. P. (1979). On the origin of transmissible mink encephalopathy. In *Slow transmissible diseases of the nervous system*, Vol. 1 (ed. S. B. Prusiner and W. J. Hadlow), pp. 451–60. Academic Press, New York.

Marsh, R. F., Burger, D., and Hanson, R. P. (1969a). Transmissible mink encephalopathy: behaviour of the disease agent in mink. *American Journal of Veterinary Research*, **30**, 1637–1642.

Marsh, R. F., Burger, D., Eckroade, R., Zu Rhein, G. M., and Hanson, R. P. (1969b). A preliminary report of the experimental host range of the transmissible mink encephalopathy agent. *Journal of Infectious Diseases*, **120**, 713–719.

Marsh, R. F., Bessen, R. A., Lehmann, S., and Hartsough, G. R. (1991). Epidemiological and experimental studies on a new incident of transmissible mink encephalopathy. *Journal of General Virology*, **72**, 589–594.

McGill, I. S. and Wells, G. A. H. (1993). Neuropathological findings in cattle with clinically suspect but histologically unconfirmed bovine spongiform encephalopathy (BSE). *Journal of Comparative Pathology*, **108**, 241–260.

Merz, P. A., Rohwer, R. G., Kascsak, R., Wisniewski, H. M., Somerville, R. A., Gibbs, Jr, C. J., and Gajdusek, D. C. (1984). Infection-specific particle from the unconventional slow virus diseases. *Science*, **225**, 437–440.

Merz, P. A., Somerville, R. A., Wisniewski, H. M., and Iqbal, K. (1981). Abnormal fibrils from scrapie-infected brain. *Acta Neuropathologica*, **54**, 63–74.

Mitrová, E. and Mayer, V. (1977). Neurohistology of early preclinical lesions in experimental subacute spongiform encephalopathy. *Biológia (Bratislava)*, **32**, 663–671.

Mohri, S., Farquhar, C. F., Somerville, R. A., Jeffrey M., Foster, J., and Hope, J. (1992). Immunodetection of a disease specific PrP fraction in scrapie-affected sheep and BSE-affected cattle. *Veterinary Record*, **131**, 537–539.

O'Rourke, K. I., Huff, T. P., Leathers, C. W., Robinson, M. M., and Gorham, J. R. (1994). SCID mouse spleen does not support scrapie agent replication. *Journal of General Virology*, **75**, 1511–1514.

Parry, H. B. (1983). *Scrapie disease in sheep*. Historical, clinical, epidemiological and practical aspects of the natural disease (ed. D. R. Oppenheimer), 192 pp. Academic Press, London.

Pattison, I. H., Hoare, M. N., Jebbett, J. N., and Watson, W. A. (1972). Spread of scrapie to sheep and goats by oral dosing with foetal membranes from scrapie-affected sheep. *Veterinary Record*, **90**, 465–468.

Pattison, I. H., Hoare, M. N., Jebbett, J. N., and Watson, W. A. (1974). Further observations on the production of scrapie in sheep by oral dosing with foetal membranes from scrapie-affected sheep. *British Veterinary Journal*, **130**, lxv–lxvii.

Pearson, G. R., Wyatt, J. M., Gruffydd-Jones, T. J., Hope, J., Chong, A., Higgins, R. J., et al. (1992). Feline spongiform encephalopathy: fibril and PrP studies. *Veterinary Record*, **131**, 307–310.

Pearson, G. R., Wyatt, J. M., Gruffydd-Jones, T. J. (1993). Feline spongiform encephalopathy: a review. *Veterinary Annual*, **33**, 1–10.

Peet, R. J. (1992). Spongiform encephalopathy in an imported cheetah (*Acinonyx jubatus*). *Australian Veterinary Journal*, **69**, 171.

Perrin, G. G., Perrin, G. J., and Benoit, C. (1991). Detection of scrapie-associated fibrils in scrapie in goats. *Veterinary Record*, **129**, 432.

Poidinger, M., Kirkwood, J., and Almond, W. (1993). Sequence analysis of the PrP protein from two species of antelope susceptible to transmissible spongiform encephalopathy. *Archives of Virology*, **131**, 193–199.

Race, R., Ernst, D., Jenny, A., Taylor W., Sutton, D., and Caughey, B. (1992). Diagnostic implications of detection of proteinase K-resistant protein in spleen, lymph nodes, and brain of sheep. *American Journal of Veterinary Research*, **53**, 883–889.

Robinson, M. M., Hadlow, W. J., Huff, T. P., Wells, G. A. H., Dawson, M., Marsh, R. F., *et al.* (1994). Experimental infection of mink with bovine spongiform encephalopathy. *Journal of General Virology*, **75**, 2151–2155.

Sarradet, M. (1883). Un cas de tremblante sur un boef. *Revue Veterinaire*, **7**, 310–312.

Scott, A. C., Wells, G. A. H., Chaplin, M. J., and Dawson, M. (1992). Bovine spongiform encephalopathy: detection of fibrils in the central nervous system is not affected by autolysis. *Research in Veterinary Science*, **52**, 332–336.

Stack, M. J., Scott, A. C., Done, S. H., and Dawson, M. (1991). Natural scrapie: detection of fibrils in extracts from the central nervous system of sheep. *Veterinary Record*, **128**, 539–540.

Stamp, J. T., Brotherston, J. G., Zlotnik, I., MacKay, J. M. K., and Smith, W. (1959). Further studies on scrapie. *Journal of Comparative Pathology*, **69**, 268–280.

Synge, B. A., and Waters, J. W. (1991). Spongiform encephalopathy in a Scottish cat. *Veterinary Record*, **129**, 320.

Taylor, D. M., Dickinson, A. G., Fraser, H., and Marsh, R. F. (1986). Evidence that transmissible mink encephalopathy agent is biologically inactive in mice. *Neuropathology and Applied Neurobiology*, **12**, 207–215.

Taylor, K. C. (1994). Bovine spongiform encephalopathy control in Great Britain. *Livestock Production Science*, **38**, 17–21.

Wells, G. A. H. and McGill, I. S. (1992). Recently described scrapie-like ephalopathies of animals: case definitions. *Research in Veterinary Science*, **53**, 1–10.

Wells, G. A. H., Scott, A. C., Johnson, C. T., Gunning, R. F., Hancock, R. D., Jeffrey, M., *et al.* (1987). A novel progressive spongiform encephalopathy in cattle. *Veterinary Record*, **121**, 419–420.

Wells, G. A. H., Hancock, R. D., Cooley, W. A., Richards, M. S., Higgins, R. J., and David, G. P. (1989). Bovine spongiform encephalopathy: diagnostic significance of vacuolar changes in selected nuclei of the medulla oblongata. *Veterinary Record*, **125**, 521–524.

Wells, G. A. H., Wilesmith, J. W., and McGill, I. A. (1991). Bovine spongiform encephalopathy: a neuropathological perspective. *Brain Pathology*, **1**, 69–78.

Wells, G. A. H., Dawson, M., Hawkins, S. A. C., Green, R. B., Dexter, I., Francis, M. E., *et al.* (1994*a*). Infectivity in the ileum of cattle challenged orally with bovine spongiform encephalopathy. *Veterinary Record*, **135**, 40–41.

Wells, G. A. H., Spencer, Y. I., and Haritani, M. (1994*b*). Configurations and topographic distribution of PrP in the central nervous system in bovine spongiform encephalopathy: an immunohistochemical study. *Annals of the New York Academy of Sciences*, **724**, 350–352.

Wells, G. A. H., Scott, A. C., Wilesmith, J. W., Simmons, M. M., and Matthews, D. (1994*c*). Correlation between the results of a histopathological examination and the detection of abnormal brain fibrils in the diagnosis of bovine spongiform encephalopathy. *Research in Veterinary Science*, **56**, 346–351.

Westaway, D., Goodman, P. A., Mirenda, C. A., McKinley, M. P., Carlson, G. A., and Prusiner, S. B. (1987). Distinct prion proteins in short and long scrapie incubation period mice. *Cell*, **51**, 651–662.

Westaway, D., Zuliani, V., Cooper, C. M., Da Costa, M., Neuman, S., Jenny, A. L., *et al.* (1994). Homozygosity for prion protein alleles encoding glutamine-171 renders sheep susceptible to natural scrapie. *Genes and Development*, **8**, 959–969.

Wilesmith, J. W. (1994). An epidemiologist's view of bovine spongiform encephalopathy. *Philosophical Transactions of the Royal Society of London B*, **343**, 357–361.

Wilesmith, J. W. and Ryan, J. B. M. (1992). Bovine spongiform encephalopathy: recent observations on the age-specific incidences. *Veterinary Record*, **130**, 491–492.

Wilesmith, J. W., Ryan, J. B. M., and Atkinson, M. J. (1991). Bovine spongiform encephalopathy: epidemiological studies on the origin. *Veterinary Record*, **128**, 199–203.

Wilesmith, J. W., Wells, G. A. H., Cranwell, M. P. and Ryan, J. B. M. (1988). Bovine spongiform encephalopathy: epidemiological studies. *Veterinary Record*, **123**, 638–644.

Wilesmith, J. W. and Wells, G. A. H. (1991). Bovine spongiform encephalopathy. *Current Topics in Microbiology and Immunology*, **172**, 21–38.

Wilesmith, J. W., Hoinville, L. J., Ryan, J. B. M., and Sayers, A. R. (1992). Bovine spongiform encephalopathy: aspects of the clinical picture and analyses of possible changes 1986–1990. *Veterinary Record*, **130**, 197–201.

Williams, E. S. and Young, S. (1980). Chronic wasting disease of captive mule deer: a spongiform encephalopathy. *Journal of Wildlife Diseases*, **16**, 89–98.

Williams, E. S. and Young, S. (1982). Spongiform encephalopathy of Rocky Mountain elk. *Journal of Wildlife Diseases*, **18**, 465–471.

Williams, E. S. and Young, S. (1992). Spongiform encephalopathies in Cervidae. *Revue Scientifique et Technique Office International des Epizooties*, **11**, 551–567.

Williams, E. S. and Young S. (1993). Neuropathology of chronic wasting disease of mule deer (*Odocoileus hemionus*) and elk (*Cervus elaphus nelsoni*). *Veterinary Pathology*, **30**, 36–45.

Willoughby, K., Kelly, D. F., Lyon, D. G., and Wells, G. A. H. (1992). Spongiform encephalopathy in captive puma (*Felis concolor*). *Veterinary Record*, **131**, 431–434.

Wood, J. L. N. and Done, S. H. (1992). Natural scrapie in goats: neuropathology. *Veterinary Record*, **131**, 93–96.

Wood, J. L. N., Lund, L. J. and Done, S. H. (1992*a*). The natural occurence of scrapie in moufflon. *Veterinary Record*, **130**, 25–27

Wood, J. L. N., Done, S. H., Pritchard, G. C., and Wooldridge, M. J. A. (1992*b*). Natural scrapie in goats: case histories and clinical signs. *Veterinary Record*, **131**, 66–68.

Wyatt, J. M., Pearson, G. R., Smerdon, T., Gruffydd-Jones, T. J., and Wells, G. A. H. (1990). Spongiform encephalopathy in a cat. *Veterinary Record*, **126**, 513.

Wyatt, J. M., Pearson, G. R., Smerdon, T. N., Gruffydd-Jones, T. J., Wells, G. A. H., and Wilesmith, J. W. (1991). Naturally occurring scrapie-like spongiform encephalopathy in five domestic cats. *Veterinary Record*, **129**, 233–236.

5 Cell biology and transgenic models of prion diseases

STANLEY B. PRUSINER

Introduction

Transgenic mice expressing foreign or mutant PrP genes have, in recent years, led to an impressive amount of new knowledge about prions and the diseases they cause. Transgenic mice now allow us to study most aspects of prions diseases and have created a framework for future investigations. From such studies, coupled with studies on the synthesis of PrP^{Sc} in cultured cells and on the molecular properties in PrP^{Sc}, we have gained information about the synthesis of prions, the determinants of neuropathology in prion diseases, the control of scrapie incubation times, the genetic mechanisms of prion diseases, and the mechanisms involved in the propagation of distinct isolates or strains of prions. Scrapie-infected murine neuroblastoma cells have provided much evidence that the conversion of PrP^{C} to PrP^{Sc} is a post-translational process that probably occurs in the endocytic pathway and is likely to involve a conformational change. The results of all the studies described in this chapter support the hypothesis that prion diseases are disorders of protein conformation. As the prion hypothesis of disease causation becomes more widely recognized, so too is there an increasing awareness that this phenomenon may not be restricted to the biology of prion diseases and that many other areas of biochemistry and cell biology may involve the same process of template-driven conformational change.

The following convention has been used to designate transgenic strains throughout this chapter. All transgenic animals commence with the prefix Tg, followed in parenthesis by the gene for which they are transgenic. For example, the Syrian hamster PrP gene is represented as SHaPrP, while the natural variants of mouse PrP are designated $Prnp^a$ or $Prnp^b$. Human mutations introduced onto the mouse gene, such as the proline to leucine variation at codon 101, are designated in the manner MoPrP-P101L, while chimeric mouse–hamster prion genes are represented by combinations of M and H depending on the order of gene fragments. Following the parenthesis is the transgenic line number. Different lines vary with respect to transgene copy and amount of protein expressed. In some cases high and low expression levels are further indicated by the suffix **H** or **L**. Within a particular section where the meaning is clear the names may be further abbreviated to just Tg followed by the line number.

Scrapie prion replication: requirement for homologous isoforms

Three lines of mice were made transgenic for Syrian hamster PrP by pronuclear injection of SHaPrP gene onto a (C57BL/6J × SLJ)F_1 background. The resulting lines therefore contained both the normal mouse PrP gene and the introduced hamster gene. Southern blot analysis of these lines suggested that the transgenes were integrated at one chromosomal site in a tandem array as has been reported for many transgenic mice harbouring other foreign genes (Scott *et al.* 1989). Northern blots showed that Tg(SHaPrP)69 mice with two to four copies of the transgene expressed the lowest levels of SHaPrP mRNA while Tg(SHaPrP)71 with a similar number of transgenes expressed slightly higher levels of SHaPrP mRNA. Tg(SHaPrP)81 mice with 30–50 copies of the transgene expressed substantially higher levels of SHaPrP mRNA. The hierarchy of SHaPrP mRNA levels which were found for the three transgenic lines reflected the transgene copy number (Prusiner *et al.* 1990).

Further lines were established by microinjections into (C57BL/6J × LT/Sv)F_1 fertilized eggs. Tg(SHaPrP)7 mice from this series carry about 60 copies of the transgene. The Tg(SHaPrP)20 line produced in the same series, however, expressed neither SHaPrP^C nor SHaPrP mRNA. Digestion with *XbaI* yielded an aberrant 3 kb hybridizing fragment rather than the 3.8 kb fragment seen in Tg(SHaPrP)7 and in Syrian hamsters. Whether a rearrangement or deletion within the SHaPrP insert in Tg(SHaPrP)20 mice is responsible for the lack of expression is unknown.

Western immunoblots showed a correlation between the translation product SHaPrP^C and SHaPrP mRNA levels in the four transgenic lines (Prusiner *et al.* 1990). While the levels of SHaPrP^C increased as the steady-state levels of SHaPrP mRNA rose in the four lines, the level of MoPrP^C was unaltered. Steady-state levels of SHaPrP^C in the brains of the four Tg(SHaPrP) Mo lines were also determined by ELISA (Fig. 5.1). The levels of SHaPrP^C as determined by ELISA are in reasonable agreement with those estimated by western immunoblotting. For example, the levels of SHaPrP^C in Tg(SHaPrP)69, Tg 71, and Syrian hamsters appear similar by western blotting, at 38, 56, and 52 μg SHaPrP per g protein by ELISA, respectively. The scrapie incubation times after inoculation with SHa prions were inversely related to the SHaPrP^C concentration in the brains of the four Tg(SHaPrP)lines (Fig. 5.1). When the data were fitted to an exponential function, a correlation coefficient of about 0.95 was found (Prusiner *et al.* 1990).

These mice expressing both hamster and murine PrP were used to test the hypothesis that the species barrier for transmission of disease is due to differences in the primary structure of PrP. Crossing the species barrier is a slow and inefficient process (Pattison 1965). Ordinarily scrapie prions propagated in mice cannot easily be transmitted to hamsters. Equally prions propagated in hamsters cannot be transmitted into normal mice. However, when the transgenic lines were inoculated with prions from infected Syrian hamster brains, the mice developed disease. For the four Tg(SHaPrP)Mo lines expressing SHaPrP mRNA there was a range of scrapie

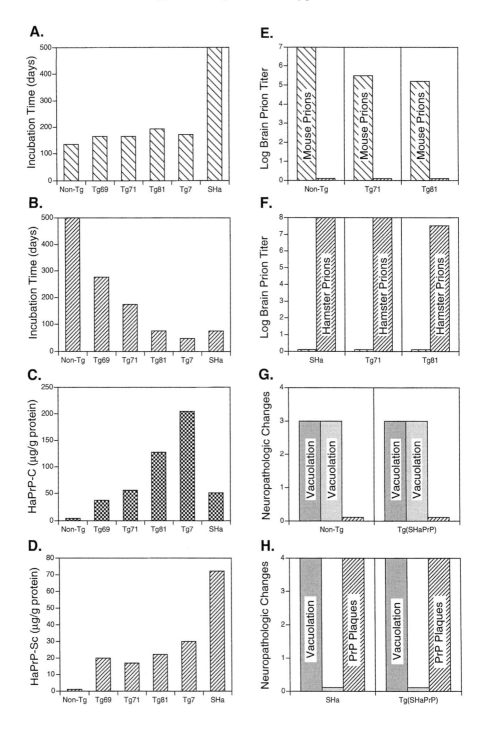

incubation times varying from 277 ± 6.7 days to 48 ± 1.0 days (Fig. 5.1). The mice with the lowest steady-state levels of SHaPrP mRNA, Tg(SHaPrP)69, had the longest incubation times while those with the highest levels of SHaPrP mRNA, Tg(SHaPrP)7, had the shortest incubation times. The Tg(SHaPrP)71 and Tg81 mice had intermediate levels of SHaPrP mRNA and displayed the incubation times of intermediate length. The Tg(SHaPrP)20 mice which failed to express SHaPrP mRNA have scrapie incubation times after inoculation with SHa prions exceeding 300 days. These observations demonstrate an inverse relationship between the level of transgene SHaPrP mRNA and the length of the incubation time after inoculation with SHa prions. The barrier to transmission is therefore abrogated by expression of PrP of the same sequence as that of the inoculating prions, and the efficacy of disease progression is facilitated by increasing the level of expression of that sequence.

While normal, non-transgenic mice developed scrapie between 128 and 148 days after inoculation with mouse (Mo) prions, Tg(SHaPrP)69 and Tg71 mice exhibited incubation times of 166 ± 4.7 days and 165 ± 3.4 days, respectively. Even greater prolongation of the incubation times after Mo prion inoculation was seen with Tg(SHaPrP)81 and Tg7 mice where periods of 194 ± 3.5 and 173 ± 4.8 days were observed, respectively. Tg(SHaPrP)20 mice developed scrapie 134 ± 3.1 days after inoculation with Mo prions consistent with their failure to express the SHaPrP transgene. These observations argue that expression of the SHaPrP transgene impedes Mo prion synthesis.

Fig. 5.1 Transgenic mice expressing Syrian hamster (SHa) prion protein exhibit species-specific scrapie incubation times, infectious prion synthesis, and neuropathology. (**A**) Scrapie incubation times in non-transgenic mice (Non-Tg) and four lines of transgenic mice expressing SHaPrP and Syrian hamsters inoculated intracerebrally with about 10^6 ID_{50} units of Chandler Mo prions serially passaged in Swiss mice. The four lines of transgenic Tg mice have different numbers of transgene copies: Tg69 and Tg71 mice have two to four copies of the SHaPrP transgene, whereas Tg81 have 30 to 50, and Tg7 mice have more than 60. Incubation times are number of days from inoculation to onset of neurological dysfunction. (**B**) Scrapie incubation times in mice and hamsters inoculated with about 10^7 ID_{50} units of Sc237 prions serially passaged in Syrian hamsters and as described in (**A**). (**C**) Brain SHaPrP^C in Tg mice and hamsters. SHaPrP^C levels were quantitated by an enzyme-linked immunoassay. (**D**) Brain SHaPrP^{Sc} in Tg mice and hamsters. Animal were killed after exhibiting clinical signs of scrapie, and SHaPrP^{Sc} levels determined by immunoassay. (**E**) Prion titres in brains of clinically ill animals after inoculation with Mo prions. Brain extracts from Non-Tg, Tg71, and Tg81 mice were bioassayed for prions in mice (left bar of each pair) and hamsters (right bars). (**F**) Prion titres in brains of clinically ill animals after inoculation with SHa prions. Brain extracts from Syrian hamsters as well as Tg71 and Tg81 mice were bioassayed for prions in mice (left bars) and hamsters (right bars). (**G**) Neuropathology in non-Tg mice and Tg(SHaPrP) mice with clinical signs of scrapie after inoculation with Mo prions. Vacuolation in grey (left bars) and white matter (centre bars); PrP amyloid plaques (right bars). Vacuolation score: 0, none; 1, rare; 2, modest; 3, moderate; 4, intense. (**H**) Neuropathology in Syrian hamsters and transgenic mice inoculated with SHa prions. Degree of vacuolation and frequency of PrP amyloid plaques as described in (**G**). (Adapted from Prusiner 1991.)

Having demonstrated that disease transmission was dependent upon the presence of homologous PrP sequences it was then possible to ask whether the prions generated in the inoculated transgenic animals were of hamster or mice type or whether they were a mixture of the two. In the absence of antibodies which unambiguously distinguish between the two isoforms a bioassay was used in which brain material from the inoculated animal was further passaged into normal mice or hamsters to determine the species range of the prions produced in the transgenic mice. As shown in Fig. 5.1, inoculation of either Tg(SHaPrP)71 or Tg81 mice with SHa prions produced high levels of SHa prions, but virtually no Mo prions were detected by bioassay. Conversely, inoculation with Mo prions generated substantial levels of Mo prions, but virtually no SHa prions were found. These findings argue that the origin of the prion inoculum determines whether SHa or Mo prions are produced by Tg(SHaPrP) mice which are capable of supporting the replication of either prion. Development of scrapie in non-transgenic mice after inoculation with SHa prions is a stochastic process presumably due to the relative incompatibility between SHaPrP^{Sc} and MoPrP^{C}. Only a few non-transgenic mice inoculated with SHa prions eventually develop scrapie after greatly extended incubation periods (Scott *et al.* 1989).

Our results also show that the scrapie prion titres in the brains of transgenic mice were independent of the length of the incubation time. For example, Tg(SHaPrP)71 and Tg81 mice had SHa prion titres of about 10^8 ID$_{50}$ per g of brain, yet the incubation time after inoculation with SHa prions for the Tg(SHaPrP)71 mice was 161 ± 1.3 days compared with incubation times of 75 ± 0.9 days for Tg(SHaPrP)81 mice. Since the titres of SHa prions in the brains of Tg(SHaPrP)71 and Tg81 mice at the time of illness were similar, we surmised that it was likely that the levels of the Tg(SHaPrP)would also be similar. Indeed, the brain levels of SHaPrP^{Sc} in all four lines of Tg(SHaPrP) mice were similar at the time of illness (Fig. 5.1). These findings are in accord with earlier observations showing that the scrapie prion titre at the time of clinical illness is independent of the incubation time (Kimberlin and Walker 1977, 1978; Prusiner 1987), whereas the concentration of PrP^{Sc} is directly proportional to the prion titre (McKinley *et al.* 1983). As shown in Fig. 5.1, SHaPrP^{Sc} levels in the brains of transgenic mice with clinical signs of scrapie ranged between 25 and 50% of those found in Syrian hamster brains. Differences in SHaPrP^{Sc} levels of two- to four-fold would not be expected to be reflected as measurable changes in prion titres.

Not only did species-specific inocula dictate whether SHa or Mo prions are produced in Tg(SHaPrP) mice (Fig. 5.1), but they also determined the distribution of spongiform change as well as the formation of PrP amyloid plaques. Tg(SHaPrP) mice inoculated with SHa prions developed an intense spongiform change confined to grey matter of the hippocampus, thalamus, cerebral cortex, and brainstem, sparing the white matter. Numerous PrP amyloid plaques reactive with the SHaPrP-specific monoclonal antibody (mAb) 135A5 (Barry and Prusiner 1986) were found in the subcallosal and periventricular regions. Interestingly, the mean size of the PrP amyloid plaques was proportional to the level of PrP transgene expression. The distribution of spongiform changes and the PrP amyloid plaques resembled those found in Syrian hamsters inoculated with SHa prions (DeArmond *et al.* 1987). Astrocytic gliosis was a prominent feature of the brains of all Tg(SHaPrP) mice developing clinical signs of scrapie. Neither the distribution nor the extent of gliosis was altered by the scrapie inoculum.

Tg(SHaPrP)69, Tg71, and Tg81 mice inoculated with Mo prions had widespread spongiform change in both the grey and white matter but the degree of vacuolation was less than that found when the same mice were inoculated with SHa prions. Only a few PrP amyloid plaques were found in these mice inoculated with Mo prions. These plaques reacted with SHa-specific monoclonal antibodies (Barry and Prusiner 1986). In non-transgenic mice (*Prnp*ᵃ) inoculated with Mo prions, spongiform change in the grey and white matter is commonly seen. SHaPrP reactive plaques were not seen in non-transgenic mice developing scrapie after inoculation with Mo prions.

Transgenic mice and incubation time

Incubation times for mice inoculated with scrapie is dependent in part on the PrP genotype. Long and short incubation time mice have been found which differ in their PrP sequence (Westaway *et al.* 1987; Race *et al.* 1990). Short incubation time mice such as NZW have a leucine at position 108 and a threonine at 189 (*Prnp*ᵃ), while long incubation time mice such as I/Ln have a phenylalanine at 108 and a valine at 189 (*Prnp*ᵇ). When long and short incubation time mice are crossed (*Prnp*ᵃ × *Prnp*ᵇ) the resultant F_1 mice have a long incubation time indicating that the *Prnp*ᵇ allele is dominant (Carlson *et al.* 1986).

To further clarify the effects of the PrP sequence on incubation times, and to address the claims of some researchers that incubation time was determined by a gene distinct from PrP (*Prn-i*), transgenic mice were generated by microinjection of the long incubation time allele from an I/Ln genomic clone onto a short incubation time background (Westaway *et al.* 1991). The cosmid used, cos6.I/LnJ-4, encompassed about 6 kb of 5′ and 12.5 kb 3′ flanking sequences. Three founders from this microinjection, Tg(*Prnp*ᵇ)93, Tg94, and Tg117, were followed up. The gene array in lines Tg(*Prnp*ᵇ)94 and Tg(*Prnp*ᵇ)117 remained stable but the line Tg(*Prnp*ᵇ)93 gave rise to both high and low copy number arrays, Tg(*Prnp*ᵇ)93H and Tg(*Prnp*ᵇ)93L. The transgene copy numbers per haploid genome are two, about 52, about 31, and about 36 for the Tg(*Prnp*ᵇ)93L, 93H, Tg94, and Tg117 lines, respectively.

Reverse transcription polymerase chain reaction (PCR) analysis of mRNA from the brains of these mice, followed by digestion with the restriction endonuclease *Bst*EII, was used to establish the levels of expression of the two alleles. Tg93L mice produced the same *a:b* ratio as *Prnp*ᵃ × *Prnp*ᵇ F_1 mice, while the diagnostic *b* fragment predominated in Tg117 and Tg94 mice, indicating overexpression of *Prnp*ᵇ. All four lines of mice produced higher levels of PrP^C as determined by

ELISA assay of serial dilutions of membrane-bound brain protein. Overexpression ranged from two- to four-fold for Tg93L, to approximately eight-fold for Tg94 and Tg117 (Westaway *et al.* 1991).

When non-transgenic littermates were inoculated with an isolate of Chandler strain of murine scrapie passaged in NZW mice, the incubation times were between 125 and 137 days. However, all four transgenic lines exhibited significantly shorter incubation times (Table 5.1). Incubation times from inoculation to onset of illness were 79, 75, and 78 days for each of the lines Tg93H, Tg94, and Tg117 respectively. Tg93L had a longer incubation time of 97 days, though this is still 30 days shorter than non-transgenic controls. The time interval between onset of disease and death was 6.9 days in Tg93H and 17.2 days in Tg93L. All the Tg($Prnp^b$)Mo lines showed clinical signs and characteristic pathological features of scrapie disease in $Prnp^a$ mice (Carlson *et al.* 1989), including spongiform degeneration and reactive astrocytic gliosis (Westaway *et al.* 1991). The spongy degeneration tended to be bilaterally symmetrical and focal, concentrated in the hippocampus and thalamus. There was a delicate spongy degeneration in the white matter. No amyloid plaques were detected with either the trichrome staining or by immunohistochemistry with PrP-directed antisera.

Table 5.1   Incubation times of $Prnp^b$ transgenic lines

Mice	Illness[1]		Death[2]	
	Incubation times in days ± SE			
Tg93L[3]	96.7 ± 3.0	(12)	107.1 ± 5.0	(3)
non-Tg[4]	125.3 ± 2.8	(16)	135.8 ± 3.3	(10)
Tg93H	79.4 ± 2.9	(14)	86.3 ± 3.0	(6)
non-Tg	129.9 ± 3.7	(9)	145.4 ± 5.7	(7)
Tg94	75.5 ± 1.8	(15)	83.4 ± 1.7	(10)
non-Tg	137.0 ± 2.1	(21)	145.9 ± 2.4	(15)
Tg117	78.5 ± 1.9	(13)	85.8 ± 2.7	(8)
non-Tg[5]	129.5 ± 4.6	(15)	140.5 ± 4.2	(11)

[1]Mice were inoculated intracerebrally with ~10^7 ID_{50} units of RML extract prepared from the brains of NZW mice. In parentheses are the number of animals developing clinical signs of scrapie.

[2]In parentheses are the number of mice dying of scrapie. Mice sacrificed for pathologic examination were excluded in these calculations.

[3]One mouse with sickness and death times of 124 and 138 days, respectively, was presumably a mistyped non-Tg animal, but no tissues were available for retyping.

[4]One mouse with sickness and death times 93 and 96 days, respectively, was presumably a mistyped Tg animal, but no tissues were available for retyping.

[5]One mouse with sickness and death times of 77 and 85 days, respectively, was presumably a mistyped Tg animal, but no tissues were available for retyping.

(Reprinted from Westaway *et al.* 1991.)

Passage from the brains of clinically ill Tg(*Prnp*ᵇ) animals into normal CD-1 mice showed no change in the incubation times seen in CD-1 passaged scrapie inoculations. This indicates that the Tg(*Prnp*ᵇ) mice had not selected a more rapidly replicating prion variant and that the alterations in incubation time are probably due to changes in the level of expression of prion protein in the transgenic mice.

Transgenic mice expressing a mutant MoPrP gene

The first demonstration of linkage of familial prion disease to the prion protein was made in a family with Gerstmann–Sträussler–Scheinker syndrome (GSS) in which there was a mutation at codon 102 of the PrP gene resulting in the substitution of leucine for proline (Hsiao *et al.* 1989) and is present in families with GSS from different ethnic backgrounds (Doh-ura *et al.* 1989). Studies showing that SHaPrP transgenes modify virtually all aspects of experimental scrapie in mice suggested that the dominantly inherited GSS phenotype might be manifest in transgenic mice expressing mutant PrP. To test this hypothesis, MoPrP genes containing a codon 101 substitution of leucine for proline denoted 'P101L' were microinjected into fertilized oocytes to produce Tg mice. Codon 101 in MoPrP is homologous to codon 102 in the human PrP gene (*PRNP*).

Three transgenic founder lines were initially created—Tg(MoPrP-P101L)174**H**, Tg(MoPrP-P101L)180, Tg(MoPrP-P101L)196**L**. All animals were housed in rooms which had not been exposed to animal scrapie to avoid the possibility of contamination. The haploid transgene copy numbers in each line were determined by comparison of the intensities of a radiolabelled 0.6 kb *Bst*EII-*Eco*RI fragment near the 3′ end of exon III (containing the open reading frame) (ORF) hybridized to mouse DNA of varying dilutions. Tg(MoPrP-P101L)174, Tg180, and Tg196 mice harboured approximately 60, five, and five haploid transgene copies, respectively. The male Tg(MoPrP-P101L)174**H** founder mouse readily produced offspring, but the Tg(MoPrP-P101L)180 founder was sterile and the female Tg(MoPrP-P101L)196**L** founder was slow to produce progeny. PrPᶜ expression in Tg(MoPrP-P101L)174**H** brains was about eight-fold higher than controls as determined by intensities of immunoblots on nitrocellulose of varying dilutions of brain extracts. The approximately 60 nucleotide hamster-biased probe hybridized to 0.1 μg transgenic brain RNA but not to 20 μg non-transgenic brain RNA confirming expression of the transgene. The mutant transgenes were inherited in a manner consistent with a single autosomal site of insertion, since it was present in approximately half (87 of 176) of Tg(MoPrP-P101L)174**H** progeny and could be transmitted by males.

The Tg(MoPrP-P101L)174**H** mice express high levels of MoPrP(P101L)ᶜ while Tg(MoPrP-P101L)196**L** mice express low levels. Ninety-eight Tg(MoPrP-P101L)174**H** mice appeared healthy until symptoms of ataxia, lethargy, and rigidity developed between seven and 39 weeks of age. The mean age of the 98 animals that developed neurological dysfunction was 180 ± 6 days (± SEM). The oldest Tg(MoPrP-P101L)**H** mouse to develop disease was 287 days old, and the youngest was 49 days old. The youngest mouse was the offspring of two transgenic mice and may have been homozygous for the MoPrP-P101L transgene. Once affected, the animals deteriorated over three to 36 days until death. Although initially it was a formal possibility that the site of MoPrP-P101L transgene insertion alone was the cause of spontaneous neurodegeneration in Tg(MoPrP-P101L)174**H** mice, additional lines of Tg(MoPrP-P101L) mice that spontaneously develop CNS degeneration argue against the site of insertion being important.

Neurodegeneration

Clinically sick Tg(MoPrP-P101L)174**H** mice, both immersion-fixed and perfusion-fixed, had the same pathological features. Numerous 5–15 μm vacuoles (spongiform degeneration) were present in both the grey and white matter (Fig. 5.2B). Vacuoles in perfusion-fixed animals appeared to contain a pale-staining, amorphous substance which was absent from most, but not all, of the vacuoles in immersion-fixed animals. The vacuoles were found in most grey an white matter structures of the cerebral hemispheres and brainstem. There was a mild to moderate degree of reactive astrocytic gliosis in a patchy distribution in both grey and white matter. A prominent Bergmann radial gliosis was present in much of the molecular layer of the cerebellar cortex. The vacuolation and gliosis induced by inoculation of Swiss CD-1 mice with scrapie prions (Fig. 5.2A) was virtually indistinguishable from that found in the uninoculated Tg(MoPrP-P101L)**H** mice (Fig. 5.2B).

Like GSS in humans, amyloid plaques were found in the brains of affected Tg(MoPrP-P101L)**H** mice as shown by periodic acid–Schiff staining (Fig. 5.2C); immunostaining demonstrated that these plaques are PrP positive (Fig. 5.2D). In our initial report (Hsiao *et al.* 1990), we stated that no plaques were found by the Gomori trichrome method or with PrP antiserum R073 (Serban *et al.* 1990). We probably failed to observe the plaques because they are relatively infrequent. PrP amyloid plaques are a constant feature of GSS in humans, but they are infrequent in familial Creutzfeldt–Jakob disease (CJD) (Ghetti *et al.* 1989; Hsiao *et al.* 1989, 1991; Owen *et al.* 1989). It is noteworthy that PrP amyloid plaques are relatively rare in mice inoculated with most isolates of Mo prions. Only the 87V 'strain' of prions induces large numbers of PrP amyloid plaques and these are confined to *Prnp*[b] mice (Fraser and Bruce 1973).

Even though the PrP amyloid plaques were found which presumably contain PrP^{Sc} in the brains of Tg(MoPrP-P101L)174**H** mice, only very low levels of proteinase K-resistant prion proteins could be demonstrated by Western blots of brain extracts. Because Tg(MoPrP-P101L)174**H** mice express high levels of MoPrP(P101L)^{C}, we assumed that some or all of the low levels of protease-resistant PrP detected on western blots were residual PrP^{C} rather than PrP^{Sc} (Hsiao *et al.* 1990). With Tg(SHaPrP) mice, uncertainties about low levels of protease-resistant SHaPrP on immunoblots were resolved by ELISA using SHaPrP monoclonal antibodies (Prusiner *et al.* 1990) but no monoclonal antibodies to MoPrP are currently available. Although the accumulation of PrP^{Sc} seems to be responsible for both clinical dys-

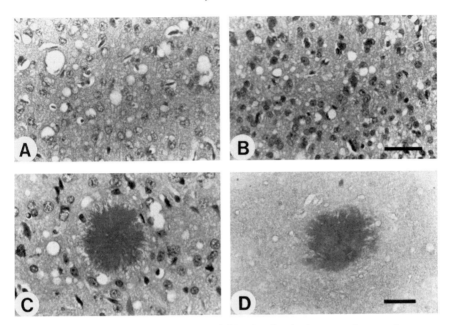

Fig. 5.2 Neuropathology of Tg(MoPrP-P101L) mice developing neurodegeneration spontaneously. **(A)** Vacuolation in cerebral cortex of a Swiss CD-1 mouse that exhibited signs of neurological dysfunction at 138 days after intracerebral inoculation with about 10^6 ID_{50} units of RML scrapie prions. **(B)** Vacuolation in cerebral cortex of Tg(MoPrP-P101L) mouse that exhibited signs of neurological dysfunction at 252 days old. **(C)** Kuru-type PrP amyloid plaque stained with periodic acid–Schiff in the caudate nucleus of a Tg(MoPrP-P101L) mouse that exhibited signs of neurological dysfunction. **(D)** PrP amyloid plaques stained with anti-PrP antiserum (RO73) in the caudate nucleus of a Tg(MoPrP-P101L) mouse that exhibited signs of neurological dysfunction. Bar in **B** (also applies to **A**) is 50 μm. Bar in **D** (also applies to **C**) is 25 μm. (From Prusiner 1993*b*.)

function and neuropathological lesions in scrapie, mutant MoPrP(P101L)^C may through an inborn error of PrP metabolism produce neurological disease without the generation of infectivity (Hsiao and Prusiner 1990).

   To assess whether brains of affected Tg(MoPrP-P101L)174**H** mice synthesize infectious prions *de novo*, 10% (w/v) brain homogenates from clinically ill Tg(MoPrP-P101L)174**H** mice and from non-transgenic controls were injected intracerebally into Swiss CD-1, Tg(SHaPrP)7, Tg(*Prnp*^{b})117, and Tg(MoPrP-P101L)196**L** mice as well as Syrian golden hamsters. Subsequently, we learned that uninoculated Tg(SHaPrP)7 and Tg(*Prnp*^{b})117 mice develop spontaneous neurodegeneration after 300–500 days of age. This finding forced us to abandon studies with these two transgenic lines, but studies with the other three inoculated hosts seem valid. We found that three of 17 extracts prepared from ill Tg(MoPrP-P101L)174**H** mice produced neurological disease in nine of 112 Syrian hamsters between 221 and 441 days, while 24 extracts from non-transgenic controls failed to produce disease. Eleven of 16 extracts transmitted CNS disease to 61 of 160 Tg(MoPrP-P101L)196L mice between 226 and 549 days. The Tg(MoPrP-P101L)196L mice expressing MoPrP(P101L)^C at low levels did not develop disease either spontaneously or after inoculation with nine extracts prepared from non-transgenic control brains. Neither 17 extracts prepared from clinically ill Tg(MoPrP-P101L)174H mice nor 14 extracts from non-transgenic controls produced disease in 260 Swiss CD-1 mice that were observed for more than 500 days.

Murine model of inherited prion disease

Our clinical and neuropathological observations on spontaneous disease in Tg(MoPrP-P101L)174H mice support the hypothesis that the PrP codon 101 leucine change is the cause of their neurological disease and, by inference, the *PRNP* codon 102 leucine mutation is responsible for GSS in humans. Although the neurological disorder in Tg(MoPrP-P101L)174H mice is clinically and pathologically similar to scrapie, the low levels of protease-resistant PrP distinguish these animals from those developing scrapie after inoculation with prions.

The broad range in the age of onset and the duration of disease in Tg(MoPrP-P101L)174H mice is in contrast to the narrow range in the incubation period and disease duration observed in mice inoculated with prions (Carlson *et al.* 1986, 1988; Hunter *et al.* 1987; Race *et al.* 1990). However, it resembles that observed in human GSS and argues that PrP primary structure is not the sole determinant of age of onset and disease duration. Genes both linked and unlinked to PrP can also have a major influence on incubation times. Since Tg(MoPrP-P101L)174 mice were not inbred, being derived from (C57BL/6 × SJL)F$_2$ fertilized oocytes, some of the variation may be due to modifier genes.

The development of spontaneous spongiform neurodegeneration in Tg(MoPrP-P101L)174H mice established, for the first time, that a neurodegenerative process similar to a human disease could be genetically modelled in an animal. The argument that the P102L point mutation in humans and Tg(MoPrP-P101L)174H mice are potent susceptibility genes for a ubiquitous, but as yet unidentified pathogen, remains a formal interpretation of our results (Weissmann 1989). However, multiple lines of investigation on the physical and biological properties of the infectious agent consistently converge upon PrP^{Sc}, and fail to reveal additional essential components (Prusiner 1989, 1993*a*).

Artificial prions in Tg mice expressing chimeric Mo–SHa PrP genes

It follows from the observation that mice transgenic for hamster prion protein become susceptible to hamster scrapie that this change in host responsiveness must be a consequence of the differences in sequence between mouse and hamster prion proteins. There are 16 amino acid differences between mouse and hamster of which five lie in the signal sequences cleaved during synthesis. PrP can be subdivided arbitrarily into five regions corresponding to fragments generated by four internal restriction endonuclease sites at positions 151, 283, 392, and 563 of the hamster PrP gene. By exchanging the four DNA fragments to the 3′ side of the restriction site at position 151 with the corresponding sequences from the mouse gene, chimeric mouse–hamster proteins can be produced. Since the following constructs are combinations of four sections, the resulting protein is defined by the order of mouse and hamster fragments. For example MHM2 implies that the first fragment is mouse, as are the final two, while the second fragment is hamster (Fig. 5.3).

Several chimeric PrP gene cassettes were constructed in this way (Scott *et al.* 1992). One chimeric construct, MHM2 PrP (Taraboulos *et al.* 1990*a*; Rogers *et al.* 1991; Scott *et al.* 1992), contains two amino acid substitutions from Syrian hamsters—a leucine to methionine at position 108, and a valine to methionine at position 111 (Fig. 5.3). MHM2 PrP appears to behave similarly to murine PrP; it forms recombinant MHM2 PrP^{Sc} when expressed in murine neuroblastoma (N$_2$a) cells infected with RML isolate of mouse prions. Another chimeric ORF, MH2M PrP, contains a total of five amino acid substitutions from Syrian hamsters. In addition to the two represented in MHM2 PrP, MH2M PrP contains an isoleucine to methionine substitution at position 138, a tyrosine to asparagine at position 154, and a serine to asparagine at position 169. The presence of 108 methionine and 111 methionine in both of these constructs provides an epitope for a SHa-specific monoclonal antibody, mAb 3F4 (Kascsak*et al.* 1987), which allows the recombinant proteins to be easily discriminated from endogenous murine PrP. When expressed in scrapie-infected (Sc) N$_2$a cells, MH2M PrP also appears to be eligible for formation of PrP^{Sc}, but at much lower efficiency than MHM2 PrP (M. Scott, unpublished). In contrast, SHaPrP does not form PrP^{Sc} when expressed in these same cells. Because of this, we considered that MH2M PrP might represent a new, artificial 'species' of PrP which would be intermediate between that of hamsters and mice.

To test this hypothesis, transgenic mice expressing MHM2 PrP and MH2M PrP were constructed. The recombinant SHa–Mo PrP ORFs were transferred into the transgene expression vector cosSHa.Tet (Scott *et al.* 1992). This vector was derived by manipulation of a 45 kb segment of SHa DNA which encompasses the entire SHaPrP gene and was designed to allow exact replacement of the ORF, without disruption of any neighbouring regions. Following transfer of the recombinant ORFs into cosSHa.Tet, the recombinant transgenes were used to construct transgenic mice as described previously (Scott *et al.* 1989). Of three founders originally constructed harbouring the MH2M PrP transgene, only one—Tg(MH2M PrP)92—proved suitable for further analysis. One line expressed the recombinant protein at low levels, and the other could not be bred. The level of expression of the transgene product in the brains of Tg(MH2M PrP)92 mice is similar to that of Tg(SHaPrP)81, a transgenic mouse line harbouring the SHaPrP gene (Scott *et al.* 1989; Prusiner *et al.* 1990). We also obtained three lines expressing MHM2 PrP, designated Tg(MHM2 PrP)285, Tg(MHM2 PrP)294, and Tg(MHM2 PrP)321. Tg(MHM2 PrP)285 mice contain similar levels of transgene product as Tg(SHaPrP)81 and

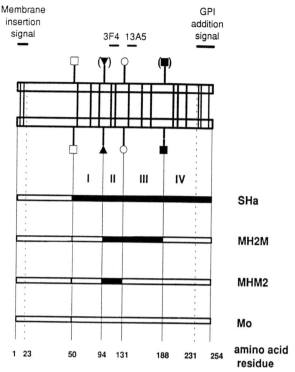

Fig. 5.3 Construction and expression of chimeric Mo/SHaPrP transgenes: the relationship of chimeric PrP constructs to SHa and MoPrP open reading frames (ORFs). At the top is a schematic of the SHa and MoPrP ORFs. The approximate locations of amino acid sequence differences are depicted as vertical bars which correspond to Syrian hamster codons 5, 14, 53, 71, 79, 108, 111, 138, 154, 169, 202, 204, 215, 232, 233, and 252. Those occurring in the 22-amino acid N-terminal signal peptide and in the glycoinositol phospholipid anchor signal are depicted within these lines. Also shown are the approximate locations of restriction enzyme cleavage sites used to construct chimeric molecules. These are, together with the distance in nucleotides between their cleavage sites and the start of the SHaPrP ORF: □, *Oxa*NI (151); ▲, *Kpn*I (283); ○, *Bgl*I (392, this site is not unique within the SHaPrP and MoPrP ORFs); ■ *Bst*EII (563). Parentheses indicate that enzyme sites do not exist in the native DNA sequence but were introduced by site-directed mutagenesis without disrupting the amino acid sequence. The bottom half of the diagram depicts the relationship of various chimeric ORFs. Black regions were derived from SHaPrP, white regions from MoPrP. The region shown in grey is homologous between SHa and MoPrP. The names of the ORFs are shown at right. The amino acid positions of boundaries defined in this diagram are shown at bottom. (From Scott *et al.* 1993.)

Tg(MH2M PrP)92 mice. These transgenic mice express two- to four-fold more PrP per mg of total brain protein than normal hamsters (Scott *et al.* 1993).

In order to define clearly the transmission history of prion inocula, we created a scheme for naming the prions (Scott *et al.* 1993). For example, the Sc237 prion isolate previously passaged in Syrian hamsters and inoculated into the same animals again are designated SHa(Sc237)SHa or abbreviated SHa(Sc237). Passage of Sc237 prions from Syrian hamsters through Tg(MH2M PrP) mice twice and back into Syrian hamsters is denoted SHa(Sc237)MH2MMH2MSHa or abbreviated MH2M(Sc237)MH2MSHa where the host for the last passage is written first and the isolate designation is last. We prefer this expression since it places the most recent passage last which seems to be the least ambiguous.

Scrapie incubation times in mice expressing chimeric PrP^C

By comparing transgenic lines with similar levels of foreign PrP expression, we sought to minimize the influence of gene dosage on incubation time, which has been described for Tg(SHaPrP) mice (Prusiner *et al.* 1990). When Tg(MH2M PrP)92 mice were inoculated with SHa(Sc237) or Mo(RML) prions, the animals developed scrapie at about 140 days (Scott *et al.* 1993). In contrast, all three lines of Tg(MHM2 PrP) mice behaved like non-transgenic mice and were resistant to infection with SHa(Sc237) prions, showing no evidence of disease after more than 350 days. Brains of Tg(MH2M PrP)92 animals inoculated with SHa(Sc237) prions contained large quantities of protease-resistant MH2M PrP^{Sc}, at levels similar to TG(SHa PrP)81 mice, which develop scrapie about 70 days after inoculation with SHa(Sc237) prions, and Tg(SHa PrP)7 mice which develop scrapie about 50 days after inoculation with SHa(Sc237) prions. The presence of MH2M PrP^{Sc} suggests that MH2M(Sc237) prions are produced in these animals as well. That Tg(MH2M PrP) and Tg(MHM2 PrP) mice display markedly different susceptibility to infection with SHa(Sc237) prions argues that the larger region of identity with SHaPrP contained in MH2M PrP as compared to MHM2 PrP is apparently able to confer sensitivity to SHa prions. These studies and those reported previously (Prusiner *et al.* 1990) suggest that initiation of prion infection may require a homotypic interaction between PrP^{Sc} in the infecting prion and PrP^C synthesized by the host. Since MHM2 and MH2M PrP differ at only three amino acid locations, it seems reasonable to conclude that some or all three of these amino acid residues influence this putative interaction.

All the transgenic mouse lines were susceptible to infection with Mo(RML) prions and succumbed to the disease at 110–150 days. The presence of the endogenous MoPrP gene should ensure that these mice are permissive for Mo(RML) infection. In previous studies using Tg(SHaPrP) mice, however, expression of SHaPrP caused a prolongation of the incubation period after inoculation with Mo(RML) scrapie prions. The most pronounced effects were with lines expressing the highest levels of SHaPrP; those same lines exhibited the shortest incubation periods following inoculation with SHa(Sc237) prions (Prusiner *et al.* 1990). In contrast to the Tg(SHaPrP) mice, Tg(MH2M PrP), and Tg(MHM2 PrP) mice exhibited shorter incubation times after inoculation with Mo(RML) prions than their non-transgenic littermate controls. This was especially evident in Tg(MHM2 PrP)294 mice, which express the highest levels of the chimeric PrP. Furthermore, the brains of Tg(MHM2 PrP)285 and Tg(MHM2 PrP)294 mice infected with Mo(RML) prions contained high levels of MHM2 PrP^{Sc} when analysed using a monospecific antiserum. The resistance to infection with SHa prions, the acceleration rather than inhibition of Mo(RML) prion replication, and the efficient formation of MHM2 PrP^{Sc} in Mo(RML)-infected Tg(MHM2 PrP) mice all suggest that MHM2 PrP is similar to MoPrP, differing only by virtue of a fortuitous epitope 'tag'. In contrast, SHaPrP does not efficiently form SHaPrP^{Sc} following infection with Mo(RML) prions. Taken together these observations provide further evidence that the inhibition of Mo(RML) prion replication in Tg(SHaPrP) mice arises because SHaPrP^{C} in some unknown manner inhibits the conversion of MoPrP^{C} to MoPrP^{Sc}, perhaps via competitive inhibition.

If MH2M PrP contains all of the SHa residues needed for these PrP molecules to behave as SHaPrP, then these mice should resemble Tg(SHaPrP) mice in all respects. After inoculation of Tg(MH2M PrP)92 mice with Mo(RML) prions, the incubation times were similar to those found in non-transgenic littermate controls, with no evidence of the prolongation observed for Tg(SHaPrP) mice. Additionally, MH2M PrP^{Sc} was readily detected in the brains of Mo(RML)-infected Tg(MH2M PrP)92 mice, in quantities similar to those observed in the brains of Tg(MHM2 PrP)285 inoculated with Mo(RML) prions. Protease-resistant SHaPrP^{Sc} was not observed in Tg(SHaPrP) mice infected with Mo prions as judged by measuring protease-resistant SHaPrP on immunoblots. Thus Tg(MH2M PrP) mice clearly differ from Tg(SHaPrP) mice, and resemble Tg(MHM2 PrP) mice when inoculated with Mo prions. The incubation period for Tg(MH2M PrP)92 following inoculation with Mo(RML) prions was similar to that observed for Tg(MHM2 PrP)285 mice, which express similar levels of chimeric PrP. The chimeric MH2M PrP^{Sc} was indistinguishable in these animals where they were inoculated with Mo(RML) or SHa(Sc237) prions.

Chimeric prions with artificial properties

Previous studies with three species of hamsters showed that individual prion isolates have distinct properties which are highly dependent on the host (Lowenstein *et al.* 1990; Hecker *et al.* 1992). Brain extracts of Tg(MH2M PrP)92 mice containing MH2M(Sc237) prions were serially passaged in Tg(MH2M PrP)92 and Syrian hamsters (Table 5.2). The incubation period for the homologous transmission shortened from about 140 days for the initial passage from hamsters to Tg(MH2M)92 to about 70 days. After a second passage of MH2M(Sc237)MH2M prions, the incubation was reduced to about 65 days (Table 5.2) but this is not a significant change. As expected, MH2M PrP^{Sc} was detected in the brains of these animals after both passages. In contrast, when MH2M(Sc237) prions were transmitted to hamsters, the incubation period was about 120 days, which is significantly longer than a homologous passage of SHa(Sc237) prions in hamsters with an incubation period of about 70 days. After a second passage in Tg(MH2M PrP)92 mice, the MH2M(Sc237)MH2M inoculum gave an even longer incubation period of about

Table 5.2 Incubation times of chimeric prions passaged in Tg(MH2M PrP)92
mice or Syrian hamsters

Inoculum	Host	(n/n_0)	Scrapie incubation times Illness (days ± SE)	$(n/n_0)^1$	Death (days ± SE)
SHa(Sc237)	Tg(MH2M PrP)92	34/34	133.8 ± 3.6	26/26	141.7 ± 4.4
MH2M(SHa (Sc237))	Tg(MH2M PrP)92	22/22	72.8 ± 0.7	2/12	85.3 ± 1.2
MH2M(MH2M (SHa(Sc237)))	Tg(MH2M PrP)92	10/10	63.9 ± 1.9	8/8	75.5 ± 2.9
SHa(Sc237)	Syrian hamsters	48/48	77 ± 1.1^2	48/48	89 ± 1.7
MH2M(SHa (Sc237))	Syrian hamsters	23/23	116.0 ± 1.9	10/10	136.2 ± 3.5
MH2M(MH2M (SHa(Sc237)))	Syrian hamsters	6/6	161.0 ± 3.8	4/4	187.0 ± 2.4
SHa(MH2M (SHa(Sc237)))	Syrian hamsters	8/8	76.9 ± 0.6	4/4	84.8 ± 1.2

[1]The reduced number of animals in the death column reflects sacrifice of some animals for immunoblotting and neuropathology.
(Reprinted from Scott *et al.* 1989.)

155 days when introduced into hamsters. The presence of SHaPrP^{Sc} in the recipient hamsters was confirmed by western blotting.

The abbreviated incubation times of MH2M(Sc237) prions compared to SHa(Sc237) prions passaged in Tg(MH2M PrP)92 mice did not permanently alter the characteristic incubation time of the Sc237 isolate. Re-introduction into hamsters followed by serial transmission in hamsters, that is MH2M(Sc237)SHaSHa, produced incubation times of about 70 days which are characteristic of SHa(Sc237) prions. To characterize further the properties of Sc237 prions passaged through Tg(MH2M PrP)92 mice and back into Syrian hamsters, the patterns of PrP^{Sc} accumulation were determined by histoblotting (Taraboulos *et al.* 1992a).

The distribution of PrP^{Sc} in Syrian hamsters inoculated with MH2M(Sc237) prions passaged in Tg(MH2M PrP)92 mice was similar to that in Syrian hamsters inoculated with SHa(Sc237) prions. The only differences in the patterns of PrP^{Sc} accumulation were in the intensity of immunostaining. For example, the hippocampus and medial hypothalamus were less intensely immunostained with SHa(Sc237) prions than with MH2M(Sc237) prions. The intensity and extent of PrP^{Sc} deposition in the subependymal and subpial regions were reversed—there were more with

SHa(Sc237) prions than with MH2M(Sc237) prions. Thus the histoblot patterns were qualitatively similar but different quantitatively.

Distinct prion isolates passaged in Tg(MH2M PrP)92 mice

Similar results were obtained when Tg(MH2M PrP)92 mice were inoculated with a second distinct isolate or 'strain' of Syrian hamster-adapted scrapie prions, 139H (Kimberlin *et al.* 1989; Hecker *et al.* 1992), with the mice developing disease at about 110 days, slightly shorter than with Sc237. Western blotting experiments confirmed the presence of MH2M PrP^{Sc}. Interestingly, the SHa(139H) isolate showed somewhat different behaviour during serial transmission in Tg(MH2M PrP)92 mice. Passage of SHa(139H) prions in Tg(MH2M PrP)92 mice gave a slightly shorter incubation time of about 105 days on second passage. These incubation times contrast with those produced by the SHa(Sc237) isolate. On first passage in Tg(MH2M PrP)92 mice, SHa(Sc237) prions gave incubation times of about 140 days, while second passage was about 70 days (Table 5.2). It will be important to learn whether the properties of the SHa(139H) isolate are permanently altered by repeated passage through Tg(MH2M PrP)92 mice by subsequent passaging back into Syrian hamsters.

We also serially passaged extracts from Tg(MH2M PrP)92 mice infected with Mo(RML) prions into Tg(MH2M PrP)92 mice. Although the significance of these data is clouded by the presence of endogenous MoPrP, some shortening of incubation period was detected during the homologous passage. Passage of MH2M(RML) prions into Syrian hamsters also produced a unique pattern of PrP^{Sc} deposition, as determined by histoblotting. The three most obvious differences between the distribution of PrP^{Sc} and that found with SHa(Sc237) or MH2M(Sc237) prions were:

(1) the intensity and thickness of PrP^{Sc} deposition in the region of the hippocampal fissure and the molecular layer of the dentate gyrus of the hippocampus;
(2) the prominent subpial deposition of PrP^{Sc}, particularly in the molecular layer of the cerebral cortex;
(3) the absence of PrP^{Sc} deposition in the subependyma.

Constrasting neuropathology of prion isolates in Syrian hamsters

We observed other striking differences in the neuropathology of Syrian hamsters infected with MH2M(RML) or MH2M(Sc237) prions. With MH2M(Sc237) prions, a delicate vacuolation occurred in the hippocampus throughout the apical dendrite portion (stratum radiatum) of the pyramidal cells of the CA1 region. These vacuoles varied in diameter from 5 to 15 μm and corresponded spatially with the small amount of PrP^{Sc} in that region. With MH2M(RML) prions, a similar very delicate vacuolation occurred in most of the stratum radiatum; however, intense spongiform degeneration with more vacuoles of greater size, up to 50 μm in diameter, occurred in the deeper layers of the CA1 region coincident with the intense PrP^{Sc} signal in the region of the hippocampal fissure. We have not seen this pattern before, which supports the view that the properties of the MH2M(RML) isolate may be unique in hamsters.

In the cerebellum, additional difference in the distribution of vacuolation were seen. Scrapie caused by SHa(Sc237)MH2M prions was characterized by very large vacuoles with diameters as great as 60 μm in the deep cerebellar nuclei but none in the granule cell layer of the cerebellar cortex. In contrast, Mo(RML)MH2M prions caused 25 μm vacuoles in the granule cell layer of the cerebellar cortex but no vacuoles in the deep cerebellar nuclei.

In Syrian hamsters inoculated with SHa(Sc237) prions, numerous amyloid plaques are found, particularly in the subcallosal region. These plaques stained strongly with anti-PrP antiserum designated RO73, less strongly with the anti-PrP mAb designated 13A5, and not at all with anti-PrP mAb designated 3F4. Whether this lack of staining with 3F4 is due to limited proteolysis where the N-terminal PrP residues containing the 3F4 epitope (Rogers *et al.* 1991) are hydrolysed, or because the epitope remains buried *in situ* even after denaturation, remains to be established. Similarly, when SHa(Sc237) prions were inoculated into Tg(MH2M PrP)92 mice, kuru-type amyloid plaques developed which were strongly RO73 immunopositive.

Surprisingly, although passage of SHa(Sc237) prions in Tg(MH2M PrP)92 mice produced cerebral amyloid plaques, brain extracts from Tg(MH2M PrP)92 mice inoculated with SHa(Sc237) failed to produce amyloid plaques upon a second passage in Tg(MH2M PrP)92 mice or upon passage back into Syrian hamsters. However, upon a second passage through Syrian hamsters the Prp amyloid plaques were found, indicating that the properties of the Sc237 prions were changed by passage through Tg(MH2MPrP)92 mice.

No PrP amyloid plaques were found in the brains of Tg(MH2M PrP)92 mice inoculated with Mo(RML) prions. A few weakly antigenic amyloid plaques were found in one of three Tg(MH2M PrP)92 mice inoculated with MH2M(RML) prions derived by a single passage in Tg(MH2M PrP)92 mice. However, the MH2M(RML) prions, when passaged in Syrian hamsters, produced multiple amyloid plaques which were RO73 immunopositive.

Homophilic interactions feature in prion propagation

The unique host range of MH2M prions, especially those derived by infection with SHa(Sc237) prions, has several important implications for understanding scrapie prion replication. Homologous transmissions, back into Tg(MH2M PrP)92 animals, are clearly favoured, although the chimeric prions may also be passaged into Syrian hamsters and mice (Scott *et al.* 1993). We conclude this by observing the lengthening and shortening of incubation period during homologous or heterologous transmissions (Table 5.2). This preference for infection of animals expressing a homologous PrP demonstrates that prion infection requires an interaction of PrP^{Sc} molecules in the inoculum with the PrP^C in cells of the host.

Further evidence for the unique tropism of MH2M(Sc237) prions was obtained following serial transmission to normal CD-1 mice. When Tg(SHaPrP) mice infected with SHa(Sc237) prions were serially passaged into mice, no evidence for transmission of the SHa prions was observed. In contrast, MH2M(Sc237) prions were able to infect mice efficiently, with an incubation period of about 200 days for the first passage (Table 5.2). As expected, mice inoculated with MH2M(Sc237) prions contained PrP^{Sc} when analysed by western blot.

Extracts of brains from Tg(MH2M PrP) mice inoculated with Mo(RML) prions transmitted to Syrian hamsters in about 240 days. Since Tg(MH2M PrP)92 mice contain an endogenous MoPrP gene, we would expect that the inocula would also contain MoPrP^{Sc} in addition to the MH2M PrP^{Sc} observed by Western blotting. Unfortunately, no MoPrP-specific antibody exists which could be used to confirm this proposal. However, since previous studies have clearly shown that Mo(RML) prions cannot infect hamsters (Scott *et al.* 1989; Prusiner *et al.* 1990), it seems reasonable to conclude that MH2M(RML) prions are responsible for the transmission to hamsters observed in this experiment. It will be important to perform a detailed analysis of SHa(RML) prions in comparison with other known Syrian hamster prion isolates, such as Sc237 and 139H (Hecker *et al.* 1992). In addition, construction of Tg(MH2M PrP) mice in a background lacking an endogenous MoPrP gene (Büeler *et al.* 1992) will clarify the results of transmission experiments using Mo(RML) prions, as well as those of other Mo prion isolates. A similar approach to study the other chimeric PrP gene (MHM2 PrP) described in this chapter, will presumably be required to establish the host range of MHM2 prions.

Prion replication and diversity

Although conversion of PrP^{C} to PrP^{Sc} might involve a conformational change and the transgenetic data reported here implicate homotypic interactions between PrP^{C} and PrP^{Sc} during prion replication, the diversity of scrapie prions (Bruce and Dickinson 1987; Dickinson and Outram 1988) poses a conundrum. Some investigators invoke the participation of a hitherto unidentified nucleic acid genome to explain distinct isolates or 'strains' of prions. Since no scrapie-specific polynucleotide has been found and a wealth of data refutes the existence of such a molecule, alternative hypotheses merit consideration. The finding that the pattern of PrP^{Sc} accumulation in the CNS is characteristic for a particular prion isolate led us to propose a mechanism for the propagation of distinct prion isolates (Hecker *et al.* 1992). In this model, different scrapie strains would be either confined to or targeted to different cells depending on the disposition of covalent structures attached to the PrP backbone, the best candidate being the asparagine-linked oligosaccharides. As we have shown here, small variations in the primary structure of PrP can create dramatic variations in the susceptibility of the host animal to scrapie prions presumably through alterations in the tertiary structure of PrP^{Sc}. Variations in the asparagine-linked oligosaccharides might influence either the specificity of the homophilic interactions between PrP^{C} and PrP^{Sc}, or the targeting of PrP^{Sc} to specific sets of neurones.

If different sub-populations of cells with distinct variations in covalent modifications of PrP exist, it follows that prions derived from these cells could be more efficiently able to infect cells of the same cell type as those from which they were originally derived, because of the requirement for a specific interaction between PrP^C and PrP^{Sc}. This model yields an interesting prediction. The proposed interaction of PrP^C and PrP^{Sc} would be dependent on both the PrP sequence and the putative structures responsible for 'strain'–specific behaviour. If this were true, it might be expected that the susceptibility of the host to infection with prions derived from another species would vary depending on the particular 'strain' being studied. This phenomenon is mirrored in experiments described here which indicate a marked difference in the relative efficiency of transmission of the Sc237 and 139H isolates between hamsters and Tg(MH2M PrP)92 mice (Scott *et al.* 1993). Indeed, it appears that Tg(MH2M PrP)92 mice are more susceptible to SHa(139H) prions than to SHa(Sc237). Adaptation of the Sc237 to the MH2M background required at least two serial transmissions, shortening the incubation period from about 135 days to about 70 days, whereas the 139H isolate did not appreciably change its incubation period (about 115 days) following the first passage. Although the data seem consistent, it is noteworthy that PrP^{Sc} synthesis can occur in absence of asparagine-linked glycosylation in scrapie-infected cultured cells (Taraboulos *et al.* 1990*a*). Since prion replication in the absence of asparagine-linked glycosylation has not been demonstrated, further studies are needed to determine the molecular basis of the cellular tropism exhibited by prions. Since no other covalent modifications of PrP have been described which could effect this diversity, it is also conceivable that an as yet unrecognized tightly bound ligand might modify scrapie prion interaction with the host in a cell-specific manner (Weissmann 1991).

From these experiments, it appears likely that the Mo(RML) and SHa(Sc237) inocula probably represent different isolates or 'strains'. This is suggested by the contrasting incubation periods and neuropathology observed when these isolates were transmitted to homologous hosts. Although Syrian hamsters are generally preferred as hosts for biochemical studies on scrapie prions, most studies on scrapie 'strains' have been performed in mice. Transgenic mice expressing MH2M PrP may contribute to the analysis of scrapie prion 'strains' by virtue of their ability to act as a bridge across the species barrier between hamsters and mice, allowing murine scrapie 'strains' to be adapted to Syrian hamsters. Similar experiments, using chimeric PrP genes derived from other species, might facilitate the development of murine models for human prion diseases, scrapie of sheep and transmissible bovine spongiform encephalopathy.

These data demonstrate that it is possible to manipulate the properties of scrapie prions, the clinical manifestation of the disease, and the susceptibility of the host by changing the side-chains of a few amino acids encoded by the PrP gene. In concert with biochemical studies on purified proteins, it may become feasible to reconcile the effects of PrP gene manipulation directly with the biochemical characteristics of the genetically engineered prion proteins, suggesting a new approach where artificial prions with contrived properties may be used to unravel the complexities of scrapie replication.

Gene-targeted mice with ablated PrP genes

In an attempt to determine the function of the normal prion protein Büeler *et al.* (1992) constructed mice in which the prion protein was not expressed. To do this a molecular clone, containing the third exon of the *Prnp* gene, was modified by removing 183 codons of PrP and substituting the neomycin phosphotransferase gene. This modified PrP gene was introduced into ES cells derived from agouti 129/SV mice by electroporation and recombinants were selected in the presence of neomycin. Resistant ES cells were injected into the blastocysts of 16–32 cell embryos and chimeric offspring identified by agouti coat colour characteristic for the ES cell genotype. Chimeric mice were mated to C57BL6 mice and mice heterozygous for the *Prnp* ablation were identified by hybridization of *Neo* and *Prnp* probes to the PCR product of the hybrid *Neo/Prnp* gene.

The heterozygous (Prnp$^{0/+}$) ablated mice were mated to each other to produce offspring homozygous (Prnp$^{0/0}$) for ablation of the *Prnp* gene (Büeler *et al.* 1992). The absence of PrP expression was established by measurements of PrP mRNA and PrP^C. Development of the Prnp$^{0/0}$ mice was normal and behavioural evaluation failed to show any differences among the wild-type (wt), Prnp$^{0/+}$, and Prnp$^{0/0}$ mice. Morphological studies of brain, muscle, and spleen also failed to show any differences among the three groups of mice. Similarly, the results of lymphocyte activation studies were also similar for all three groups; it had previously been suggested that PrP^C functions as a lymphocyte-activation molecule because of its cell surface localization and changes in mitogenesis induced by anti-PrP antibodies (Cashman *et al.* 1990). That Prnp$^{0/0}$ mice develop normally and remain healthy for more than 600 days argues that CNS dysfunction in scrapie results from the accumulation of PrP^{Sc} rather than an inhibition of PrP^C function.

Wild-type (Prnp$^{+/+}$), Prnp$^{0/+}$, and Prnp$^{0/0}$ mice were inoculated with Mo(RML) prions passaged in Swiss CD-1 mice (Büeler *et al.* 1993). By 184 days after inoculation, all of the Prnp$^{+/+}$ littermates developed clinical signs of scrapie while the Prnp$^{0/0}$ mice remained alive and well at more than 450 days after inoculation (Prusiner *et al.* 1993). Prnp$^{0/+}$ mice, heterozygous for the PrP gene ablation, remained well until about 400 days after inoculation when they began to exhibit signs of CNS dysfunction. Prnp$^{0/0}$ mice sacrificed at intervals after inoculation failed to show evidence of significant prion titres by bioassay of brain and spleen extracts inoculated into CD-1 mice, while Prnp$^{+/+}$ littermates showed propagation of prions to high levels in brain (Büeler *et al.* 1993). The results of these studies are in accord with a wealth of data which argue that PrP^{Sc} is necessary for both transmission of prion infectivity and pathogenesis of disease.

Overexpression of wild-type prion proteins

We had generated mice for different experiments containing high copy numbers of prion protein transgenes, and observed that older mice in these groups developed a spontaneous neurological disease. Mice expressing hamster, sheep, and mouse PrP—Tg(SHaPrP)7, Tg(SHaPrP)1855, Tg(SHaPrP)B3669, Tg($Prnp^b$)94, and Tg($Prnp^b$)117—developed truncal ataxia, hindlimb paralysis, and tremors (Table 5.3). They exhibited a profound necrotizing myopathy involving skeletal muscle, a demyelinating polyneuropathy, and focal vacuolation of the CNS (Westaway *et al.* 1994).

Two colonies of uninoculated Tg(SHaPrP)7 mice in separate animal colonies both developed progressive disorders characterized by tremors, ataxia, head bobbing, and an abnormal hunched posture. Between 5 and 10% of the animals also developed rear limb ataxia. The earliest age of onset was 220 days with a mean of 468 ± 8 days. The duration of disease was generally more than two months but was quite variable. Of 94 mice containing two transgene arrays (homozygous, 120 gene copies), only 12 died without symptoms of neurological dysfunction. Nine mice out of 20 that were hemizygous for the array (60 gene copies) developed disease after periods in excess of 650 days. No disease was seen in mice containing fewer transgene copies (8 to 30). Nor was disease seen in non-transgenic mice or mice overexpressing a human Alzheimer amyloid precursor protein (APP) transgene.

Uninoculated mice containing about 30 copies of the mouse PrP-B gene Tg($Prnp^b$)94 developed paresis of the rear limbs with a mean onset of 567 ± 43 days. This progressed to total paralysis. A minority of animals developed kyphosis, a phenotype predominant in Tg(SHaPrP)7 mice. Spontaneous neurological dysfunction was not seen in Tg($Prnp^b$)15 mice carrying just three copies of the transgene during an observation period of over 720 days.

CNS lesions in the Tg7, Tg94, and Tg117 mice (including the spinal cord) seemed insufficient to account for the profound clinical signs. However, striking pathological changes were found in both peripheral nerves and skeletal muscle. Myopathic features in Tg($Prnp^b$)94 and Tg(SHaPrP)7 animals was most intense in the quadriceps. Myopathy was found in all skeletal muscle groups including the diaphragm and intercostal muscles, while smooth and cardiac muscle were unaffected. In clinically ill mice the quadriceps femoris muscle contained scatterd degenerating fibres, increased numbers of fibres with central nuclei, and fibres undergoing phagocytosis, and showed mild to moderate endomysial fibrosis. Extensive neurogenic rearrangement (fibre-type grouping) was found indicating that a contiguous set of muscle fibres were denervated then reinnervated by axon sprouts from single neurones or neurones of the same type. The myopathic features appear to have predated the neurogenic changes as 90-day-old Tg(SHaPrP)7 mice had occasional degenerating fibres but no fibre-type grouping.

Consistent with the neurogenic rearrangement, sciatic nerves of Tg(SHaPrP)7 mice showed significant changes. There were large numbers of thinly myelinated axons and mild loss of large myelinated axons. Although thinly myelinated axons usually indicate demyelination followed by remyelination, the absence of onion bulb formations suggests that there were no repeated cycles of demyelination and remyelination in these mice.

Table 5.3 PrP transgenic lines: disease presentation and pathology

Construct	Transgenic lines	Transgenic status	Copy number	Reference	Clinical signs	Age at onset (days)	CNS vacuolation	Necrotizing myopathy	Peripheral myopathy
SHaPrP cosmid	Tg(SHaPrP$^{+/+}$)7	Homozygous	120	Prusiner et al. 1990	Tremor, kyphosis, gait abnormalities	220–600	Yes	Yes	Yes
SHaPrP cosmid	Tg(SHaPrP$^{+/0}$)7	Hemizygous	60	Prusiner et al. 1990	Similar to above	>650	Yes	ND	ND
MoPrP^b cosmid	Tg(MoPrP-B$^{+/0}$)94	Hemizygous	31	Westaway et al. 1991	Hind-limb paresis, paralysis, kyphosis	524–733	Yes	Yes	Yes
MoPrP^b cosmid	Tg(MoPrP-B$^{+/0}$)117	Hemizygous	36	Westaway et al. 1991	Hind-limb paresis, paralysis, kyphosis	540–643	Yes	ND	ND
MoPrP^b cosmid	Tg(MoPrP-B$^{+/0}$)15	Hemizygous	3	Carlson et al. 1993	None observed	NA	None observed	None observed	None observed
SHaPrP cosmid	Tg(SHaPrP$^{+/0}$) A1855, B3669	Hemizygous	High	Westaway et al. 1994	Truncal ataxia, tremor	100–146	Yes	ND	ND
SHaPrP cosmid	Tg(SHaPrP$^{+/0}$) 217, A1855M	Hemizygous	Intermediate	Westaway et al. 1994	None observed	NA	ND	ND	ND
SHaPrP cosmid	Tg(SHaPrP$^{+/0}$) 1847, 1849	Hemizygous	Single copy	Westaway et al. 1994	None observed	NA	None observed	ND	ND
APP$_{695}$ cDNA	Tg(HuAPP$_{695}$)5	Hemizygous	2–3	Beer et al. 1991	None observed	NA	None observed	None observed	None observed

ND, not determined; NA, not applicable.
Copy numbers for the Tg(SHaPrP) lines were estimated from slot blot analysis of mouse tail DNA and Tg217 DNA as single copy and intermediate copy number standards, respectively.

Focal spongiform degeneration of the grey matter in Tg(SHaPrP)7 and Tg($Prnp^b$) mice was found localized to the stratum lacunosum moleculare of the hippocampus, the superior colliculus, and midbrain tegmentum. The spongiform change was less intense than that of experimental scrapie but was also associated with moderate astrogliosis. In addition dystrophic mineral deposits staining for iron but not calcium were found in six out of 17 clinically ill animals examined histopathologically.

To determine whether this disease was associated with the abnormal isoform of the prion protein, PrP^{Sc} immunoblots were performed of protease-K treated tissue samples. PrP in the quadriceps of three clinically ill Tg(SHaPrP)7 mice was protease sensitive indicating that there was no pathogenic PrP^{Sc} present in these mice. Spontaneous neuromyopathy is therefore not caused by prion infection.

Cell biology of prion protein

PrP^{Sc} synthesis in cultured cells

Metabolic labelling studies of scrapie-infected cultured cells have shown that PrP^C is synthesized and degraded rapidly while PrP^{Sc} is synthesized slowly by a post-translational process (Fig. 5.4) (Caughey *et al.* 1989; Borchelt *et al.* 1990, 1992; Caughey and Raymond 1991). Both PrP isoforms appear to transit through the Golgi apparatus where their asparagine-linked oligosaccharides are modified and sialylated (Bolton *et al.* 1985; Manuelidis *et al.* 1985; Endo *et al.* 1989, Haraguchi *et al.* 1989; Rogers *et al.* 1990). PrP^C is presumably transported within secretory vesicles to the external cell surface where it is anchored by the glycosyl phosphatidylinositol (GPI) moiety (Stahl *et al.* 1987; 1992; Safar *et al.* 1990). In contrast, PrP^{Sc} accumulates primarily within cells where it is deposited in cytoplasmic vesicles, many of which appear to be secondary lysosomes (Caughey *et al.* 1991; McKinley *et al.* 1991*b*; Borchelt *et al.* 1992; Taraboulos *et al.* 1990*b*, 1992*b*).

Whether PrP^C is the substrate for PrP^{Sc} formation or a restricted subset of PrP molecules are precursors for PrP^{Sc} remains to be established. Several experimental results argue that PrP molecules destined to become PrP^{Sc} exit to the cell surface, as does PrP^C (Stahl *et al.* 1987), before their conversion into PrP^{Sc}. Interestingly, the GPI anchors of both PrP^C and PrP^{Sc}, which presumably feature in directing the subcellular trafficking of these molecules, are sialylated (Fig. 5.4) (Stahl *et al.* 1992). It is unknown whether sialylation of the GPI anchor participates in some aspect of PrP^{Sc} formation.

Studies with brefeldin A indicate that PrP^{Sc} synthesis does not occur in the endoplasmic reticulum–Golgi and that transport down the secretory pathway is required for this synthesis (Taraboulos *et al.* 1992*b*). Experiments with monensin demonstrate that PrP^{Sc} precursor transverses the mid-Golgi in the same time frame as PrP^C. These PrP molecules continue along the secretory pathway to the cell surface where they are bound by a glycosylinositol phospholipid anchor (Caughey and

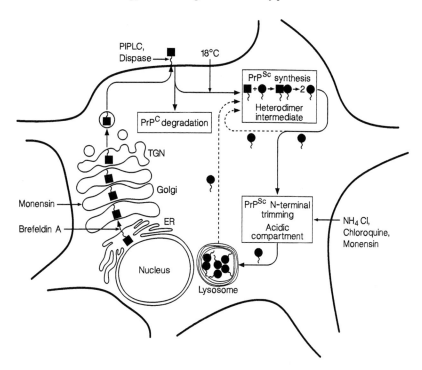

Fig. 5.4 Pathways of prion protein synthesis and degradation in cultured cells. PrP^{Sc} is denoted by circles; squares designate PrP^{C} and the PrP^{Sc} precursor, which may be indistinguishable. Rectangular boxes denote as yet unidentified subcellular compartments. Before becoming protease resistant, the PrP^{Sc} precursor transits through the plasma membrane and is sensitive to dispase or phosphatidyl inositol-specific phospholipase C (PIPLC) added to the medium. PrP^{Sc} synthesis probably occurs in a compartment accessible from the plasma membrane, such as caveolae or endosomes; PrP^{Sc} formation is blocked at 18°C. PrP^{Sc} synthesis probably occurs through the interaction of PrP^{Sc} precursor with existing PrP^{Sc}; the dotted lines denote possible feedback pathways for the reflection of PrP^{Sc} in the active site. Acidic pH within vesicles is not obligatory for PrP^{Sc} synthesis. About 1–2 h after PrP^{Sc} formation, it is N-terminally trimmed by an acidic protease; PrP^{Sc} then accumulates primarily in secondary lysosomes. The inhibition of PrP^{Sc} synthesis by brefeldin A demonstrates that the endoplasmic reticulum–Golgi is not competent for its synthesis and that transport of PrP down the secretory pathway is required for the formation of PrP^{Sc}. (From Taraboulos *et al.* 1992.)

Raymond 1991; Borchelt *et al.* 1992). A minority of these PrP molecules are then converted to PrP^{Sc}, presumably either in the endocytic pathway or on the plasma membrane. Brefeldin A is the first compound found to inhibit the synthesis of PrP^{Sc}.

Those PrP molecules that are destined to become PrP^{Sc} appear transiently on the cell surface and can be released with phosphatidyl inositol-specific phospholipase C (PIPLC) (Borchelt *et al.* 1992) or hydrolysed by dispase. The synthesis of PrP^{Sc} was dramatically reduced when nascent PrP^C was digested with PIPLC at 18°C, but digestion of nascent PrP^{Sc} with PIPLC at 37°C did not reproducibly diminish the synthesis of PrP^{Sc} by more than a factor of two. Digestion of nascent PrP^C with dispase significantly reduced the synthesis of PrP^{Sc}, and this phenomenon could be partially prevented by delaying the exposure of cells to dispase. While trypsin digestion (2 mg/ml for 20 min at 37°C) of nascent PrP^C did on occasion cause a large decrease in PrP^{Sc} synthesis, as reported by others (Caughey and Raymond 1991), these conditions were so harsh that we could not determine if the reduction in PrP^{Sc} synthesis was due to digestion of cell surface protein or to nonspecific effects of the treatment, such as the dislodging and reattachment of the cells. Dispase proved to be a more gentle protease that did not dislodge cells from culture vessels.

Is PrP^{Sc} derived from a specific precursor pool?

Whether PrP^{Sc} is synthesized from a subset of PrP molecules or all PrP^C molecules are eligible for conversion remains to be established. Less than 10% of the radiolabelled nascent PrP molecules that have been synthesized by the end of a 1 hour metabolic radiolabelling pulse are converted into PrP^{Sc}. At present, we and others have not been able to identify any differences between those PrP molecules which are destined to become PrP^{Sc} and the pool of PrP^C molecules. Both the PrP^{Sc} precursor molecules and PrP^C can be released from the surface of cells by PIPLC digestion or hydrolysed by dispase. Furthermore, both PrP^C and those PrP molecules destined to become PrP^{Sc} appear to be susceptible to cellular degradation.

Although most of the difference in the mass of PrP 27–30 predicted from the amino acid sequence and that observed after post-translational modification is due to complex-type oligosaccharides, these sugar chains are not required for PrP^{Sc} synthesis in scrapie-infected cultured cells based on experiments with the asparagine-linked glycosylation inhibitor tunicamycin and site-directed mutagenesis studies (Taraboulos *et al.* 1990a). ScN$_2$a cells produce three species of PrP^{Sc} that differ in their degree of N-linked glycosylation. Since the formation of any particular PrP^{Sc} glycoform could not be uncoupled from another, all three species of PrP^{Sc} seem to traverse the same biosynthetic pathway.

Studies with cultured cells showed that unglycosylated PrP produced in the presence of tunicamycin was converted to unglycosylated PrP^{Sc}, but unglycosylated PrP^C was not readily detected at the cell surface. Recombinant PrP molecules lacking consensus sites for N-linked glycosylation were not detected on the cell surface, but could be converted to unglycosylated PrP^{Sc} in ScN$_2$a cells. Although these results suggest that unglycosylated PrP need not transit to the cell surface before conversion into PrP^{Sc}, we could not eliminate the possibility that a small fraction of PrP was transported to the cell surface in these experiments and was converted to PrP^{Sc} on re-entry into the cell. Alternatively, in the presence of tunicamycin, PrP may be transported directly from the endoplasmic reticulum or Golgi to the endocytic pathway where it may be converted to PrP^{Sc} before entering the lysosomes.

Where does PrP acquire protease resistance?

Since infectious prions are composed largely, if not entirely, of PrP^{Sc} molecules (Prusiner *et al.* 1990; Prusiner 1991), it is important to identify the site of PrP^{Sc} synthesis and define the molecular events involved in this process. Our observations argue that PrP^{Sc} synthesis occurs within the endocytic pathway. Exogenous prions could initiate infection by entry through the endocytic pathway to stimulate the conversion of PrP^{C} molecules from cell surface to PrP^{Sc}.

Multiple lines of evidence suggest that PrP may acquire protease resistance in the endocytic pathway. First, when ScN$_2$a cells were exposed to dispase immediately after the labelling pulse, no PrP^{Sc} was formed during the chase at 37°C (Fig. 5.4). In contrast, when ScN$_2$a cells were chased for 2 hours at 37°C before exposure to dispase, some PrP became inaccessible to the dispase and subsequently acquired resistance to proteinase K. Second, when ScN$_2$a cells were chased at 18°C but not at 37°C, PrP was released by PIPLC digestion and PrP^{Sc} synthesis was abolished (Borchelt *et al.* 1992). In our studies, PIPLC catalysed the release of PrP^{C} from the cell surface relatively slowly; we found that long digestions with PIPLC at 18°C were required to remove those molecules destined to become PrP^{Sc}. At 37°C, radiolabelled PrP molecules probably transit to the surface and are endocytosed too rapidly for PIPLC digestion to be completely effective. As noted above, our results with both PIPLC and trypsin differ from those reported by others and the basis for these discrepancies is unknown. Third, the formation of PrP^{Sc} in ScN$_2$a cells was inhibited when the chase was performed at 18°C, and PrP remained largely accessible to PIPLC throughout a long 18°C chase. As predicted from the work of other investigators, endocytosis and vesicular compartmentalization of membrane glycoproteins was retarded at 18°C in ScN$_2$a cells. Fourth, if ScN$_2$a cells were held at 37°C for 1–2 hours of chase prior to shifting to 18°C, then some PrP^{Sc} was formed at 18°C. Presumably, some PrP was endocytosed at 37°C and acquired protease resistance via a process that is less temperature dependent.

Inhibition of PrP^{Sc} synthesis at 18°C

The endosomal transport of membrane glycoproteins to lysosomes is inhibited at 18°C. ScN$_2$a cells were shown to behave in similar manner by demonstration that endocytosis of FITC-WGA (flouroscein isothiocyanote-wheat germ agglutin) occurred at 18°C but the formation of well-defined cytoplasmic vesicles was greatly inhibited as compared to 37°C. Thus, it seems likely that exposure to 18°C inhibited endosome function in ScN$_2$a cells, as reported for other types of cells, and that PrP^{Sc} acquires protease resistance in the endocytic pathway.

Most membrane glycoproteins are transported to lysosomes via endosomes, which act as receptacles for plasma membrane proteins that are destined for degradation or recycling (Dunn *et al.* 1980; Stoorvogel *et al.* 1991). After endosomes have received membrane glycoproteins from endocytic vesicles they appear to mature as they change from early to late endosomes before delivery of their contents to lysosomes (Stoorvogel *et al.* 1991).

Many membrane proteins are degraded after endocytosis and transit through endosomes to lysosomes (Dunn *et al.* 1980; Steinman *et al.* 1983; Wolkoff *et al.* 1984). Although PrP^{Sc} accumulates in cytoplasmic vesicles, many of which are secondary lysosomes (McKinley *et al.* 1991a), recent studies argue that PrP^{Sc} is formed before entry into lysosomes. First, while lysosomotropic amines block the digestion of the N-terminal 90 amino acids of PrP^{Sc}, they do not interfere with the formation of PrP^{Sc} (Caughey *et al.* 1991; Taraboulos *et al.* 1992b). Second, lysosomotropic amines do not alter substantially the degradation of PrP^{C}, suggesting that it might be degraded before reaching lysosomes. Third, kinetic studies indicate that PrP^{Sc} acquires protease resistance approximately 1 hour before exposure to lysosomal proteases and digestion of the N-terminus.

Several caveats force our conclusions to be tentative with respect to the site at which PrP^{C} is converted to PrP^{Sc}. First, although it is likely that PIPLC and dispase prevent PrP^{Sc} synthesis by digestion of PrP^{C} at the cell surface, we cannot exclude the entry of these enzymes into cells before digestion of PrP^{C}. Second, we cannot exclude the possibility that PrP^{C} is converted at the cell surface into PrP^{Sc}. Perhaps PrP enters the endocytic pathway as a result of an event that initiates PrP^{Sc} synthesis at the cell surface to produce a molecule that resists PIPLC and dispase digestion, but has not yet acquired all the properties of PrP^{Sc}. Third, multiple routes of PrP^{C} trafficking during conversion into PrP^{Sc} might occur (Taraboulos *et al.* 1990a). Fourth, we do not know how either PrP^{C} or the PrP^{Sc} precursor enters the endocytic pathway. Some GPI-anchored proteins are internalized via cholesterol-rich membrane patches called caveolae (Rothberg *et al.* 1990; Anderson *et al.* 1991). Alternatively, PrP^{C} could enter the endocytic pathway via free-flow endocytosis. While each of these issues requires further resolution, the current studies argue that the conversion of PrP^{C} into PrP^{Sc} is likely to occur in the endocytic pathway.

Conclusions

Studies with transgenic mice have contributed a wealth of new knowledge about the synthesis of prion particles and the pathogenesis of both the genetic and infectious forms of the prion diseases. Transgenetic studies argue persuasively that the 'species barrier' is due to differences in PrP gene sequences among mammals. Furthermore, during the propagation of prions, PrP^{C} and PrP^{Sc} form a complex as PrP^{C} molecules are converted into PrP^{Sc}. This complex or replication intermediate involves a homophilic interaction between the substrate PrP^{C} and the pathogenic

PrP^{Sc} molecule. Physical and chemical analyses of PrP^{Sc} contend that the conversion of PrP^{C} into PrP^{Sc} involves a conformational change. Spectroscopic and electron microscopic studies suggest that the post-translational synthesis of PrP^{Sc} involves an unfolding of α-helical domains followed by refolding into β-sheets.

Transgenetic studies have established that the PrP gene can drastically modify the length of the scrapie incubation time. Investigations with transgenic mice have also demonstrated that the pattern of PrP^{Sc} accumulation and the distribution of neuropathological lesions depend on the PrP^{Sc} molecules which are synthesized. Both neuronal vacuolation and astrocytic gliosis appear to be a consequence of PrP^{Sc} deposition. Furthermore, PrP amyloid plaques are dependent on the PrP sequence as well as the 'strain' of prion which initiates the infection.

These studies on the synthesis and distribution of PrP^{Sc} have given new insights into the replication of scrapie prion 'strains' or isolates. Each isolate appears to induce a unique pattern of PrP^{Sc} deposition which suggests that each isolate may replicate in a distinct set of cells. The molecular basis of this cellular trophism remains to be established but has been suggested that it may reside either in the N-linked oligosaccharides of PrP^{Sc} or the tertiary structure of PrP^{Sc}.

The modelling of GSS in Tg(MoPrP-P101L) mice argues that PrP gene mutations in humans cause prion diseases. These results are in accord with studies showing that nucleotide changes which result in non-conservative amino acid substitutions are genetically linked to the development of an inherited prion disease. These findings also offer an explanation for the sporadic prion diseases such as CJD: a somatic mutation of the *PRNP* gene rather than exogenous infection may initiate the formation of PrP^{Sc}.

The study of prion diseases seems to be emerging as a unique area of investigation at the interface of such disciplines as genetics, cell biology, and virology (Prusiner 1991). Advances in the purification and characterization of both PrP^{C} and PrP^{Sc} appear to have identified the central event in PrP^{Sc} synthesis and prion propagation—the unfolding of α-helical domains followed by refolding into β-sheets. These findings underscore the fundamental features of prion structure and propagation that differentiate prions from other transmissible pathogens. All these studies taken together offer a compelling view that prions are composed largely, if not entirely, of PrP^{Sc} molecules. In addition, prion diseases seem to be diseases of protein conformation and arise through either infectious or genetic mechanisms.

Acknowledgement

I thank M. Baldwin, D. Borchelt, G. Carlson, F. Cohen, C. Cooper, S. DeArmond, R. Fletterick, D. Foster, J.-M. Gabriel, M. Gasset, R. Gabizon, D. Groth, L. Hood, K. Hsiao, V. Lingappa, M. McKinley, W. Mobley, B. Oesch, D. Riesner, M. Scott, A. Serban, N. Stahl, A. Taraboulos, M. Torchia, C. Weissmann, and D. Westaway for their help in these studies. Special thanks to L. Gallagher who assembled this manuscript. Supported by grants from the National Institute of Health (NS14069,

AG08967, AG02132, and NS22786) and the American Health Assistance Foundation, as well as by gifts from Sherman Fairchild Foundation, Bernard Osher Foundation, and National Medical Enterprises.

References

Anderson, R., Kamen, B., Rothberg, K., and Lacey, S. (1991). Potocytosis: sequestration and transport of small molecules by caveolae. *Science*, **255**, 410–411.

Barry, R. A. and Prusiner, S. B. (1986). Monoclonal antibodies to the cellular and scrapie prion proteins. *Journal of Infectious Diseases*, **154**, 518–521.

Beer, J., Salbaum, J. M., Schlichtmann, E., Hoppe, P., Early, S., Carlson, G. A., *et al.* (1991). Transgenic mice and Alzheimer's disease. In *Alzheimer's disease; basic mechanisms, diagnosis, and therapeutic strategies*, (ed. K. Iqbal, D. R. C. McLachlan, B. Winblad, and H. M. Wisniewski), pp. 473–478. Wiley, New York.

Bolton, D. C., Meyer, R. K., and Prusiner, S. B. (1985). Scrapie PrP 27–30 is a sialoglyco-protein. *Journal of Virology*, **53**, 596–606.

Borchelt, D. R., Scott, M., Taraboulos, A., Stahl, N., and Prusiner, S. B. (1990). Scrapie and cellular prion proteins differ in their kinetics of synthesis and topology in cultured cells. *Journal of Cell Biology*, **110**, 743–752.

Borchelt, D. R., Taraboulos, A., and Prusiner, S. B. (1992). Evidence for synthesis of scrapie prion proteins in the endocytic pathway. *Journal of Biological Chemistry*, **267**, 16188–16199.

Bruce, M. E. and Dickinson, A. G. (1987). Biological evidence that scrapie agent has an independent genome. *Journal of General Virology*, **68**, 79–89.

Büeler, H., Fischer, M., Lang, Y., Bluethmann, H., Lipp, H.-P., DeArmond, S. J., *et al.* (1992). Normal development and behaviour of mice lacking the neuronal cell-surface PrP protein. *Nature*, **356**, 577–582.

Büeler, H., Aguzzi, A., Sailer, A., Greiner, R.-A., Autenreid, P., Aguet, M., *et al.* (1993). Mice devoid of PrP are resistant to scrapie. *Cell*, **73**, 1339–1347.

Carlson, G. A., Kingsbury, D. T., Goodman, P. A., Coleman, S., Marshall, S. T., DeArmond, S., *et al.* (1986). Linkage of prion protein and scrapie incubation time genes. *Cell*, **46**, 503–511.

Carlson, G. A., Goodman, P. A., Lovett, M., Taylor, B. A., Marshall, S. T., Peterson, T. M., *et al.* (1988). Genetics and polymorphism of the mouse prion gene complex: control of scrapie incubation time. *Molecular and Cellular Biology*, **8**, 5528–5540.

Carlson, G. A., Westaway, D., DeArmond, S. J., Peterson, T. M., and Prusiner, S. B. (1989). Primary structure of prion protein may modify scrapie isolate properties. *Proceedings of the National Academy of Science of the USA*, **86**, 7475–7479.

Carlson, G. A., Ebeling, C., Torchia, M., Westaway, D., and Prusiner, S. B. (1993). Delimiting the location of the scrapie prion incubation time gene on chromosome 2 of the mouse. *Genetics*, **133**, 979–988.

Cashman, N. R., Loertscher, R., Nalbantoglu, J., Shaw, I., Kascsak, R. J., Bolton, D. C., *et al.* (1990). Cellular isoform of the scrapie agent protein participates in lymphocyte activation. *Cell*, **61**, 185–192.

Caughey, B. and Raymond, G. J. (1991). The scrapie-associated form of PrP is made from a cell surface precursor that is both protease- and phospholipase-sensitive. *Journal of Biological Chemistry*, **266**, 18217–18223.

Caughey, B., Race, R. E., Ernst, D., Buchmeier, M. J., and Chesebro, B. (1989). Prion protein biosynthesis in scrapie-infected and uninfected neuroblastoma cells. *Journal of Virology*, **63**, 175–181.

Caughey, B., Raymond, G. J., Ernst, D., and Race, R. E. (1991). N-terminal truncation of the scrapie-associated form of PrP by lysosomal protease(s): implications regarding the site of conversion of PrP to the protease-resistant state. *Journal of Virology*, **65**, 6597–6603.

DeArmond, S. J., Mobley, W. C., Demott, D. L., Barry, R. A., Beckstead, J. H., and Prusiner, S. B. (1987). Changes in the localization of brain prion proteins during scrapie infection. *Neurology*, **37**, 1271–1280. [erratum in *Neurology* (1987), **37**, 1770.]

Dickinson, A. G. and Outram, G. W. (1988). Genetic aspects of unconventional virus infections: the basis of the virino hypothesis. *Ciba Foundation Symposium*, **135**, 63–83.

Doh-ura, K., Tateishi, J., Sasaki, H., Kitamoto, T., and Sakaki, Y. (1989). Pro–Leu change at position 102 of prion protein is the most common but not the sole mutation related to Gerstmann–Sträussler syndrome. *Biochemical and Biophysical Research Communications*, **163**, 974–979.

Dunn, W., Hubbard, A., and Aronson, N. (1980). Low temperature selectively inhibits fusion between pinocytic vesicles and lysosomes during heterophagy of 125-I-asialofetuin by the perfused rat liver. *Journal of Biological Chemistry*, **255**, 5971–5978.

Endo, T., Groth, D., Prusiner, S. B., and Kobata, A. (1989). Diversity of oligosaccharide structures linked to asparagines of the scrapie prion protein. *Biochemistry*, **28**, 8380–8388.

Fraser, H. and Bruce, M. (1973). Argyrophilic plaques in mice inoculated with scrapie from particular sources. *Lancet*, **i**, 617–618.

Ghetti, B., Tagliavini, F., Masters, C. L., Beyreuther, K., Giaccone, G., Verga, L., *et al.* (1989). Gerstmann–Sträussler–Scheinker disease. II. Neurofibrillary tangles and plaques with PrP-amyloid coexist in an affected family. *Neurology*, **39**, 1453–1461.

Haraguchi, T., Fisher, S., Olofsson, S., Endo, T., Groth, D., Tarentino, A., *et al.* (1989). Asparagine-linked glycosylation of the scrapie and cellular prion proteins. *Archives of Biochemistry and Biophysics*, **274**, 1–13.

Hecker, R., Taraboulos, A., Scott, M., Pan, K. M., Yang, S. L., Torchia, M., *et al.* (1992). Replication of distinct scrapie prion isolates is region specific in brains of transgenic mice and hamsters. *Genes and Development*, **6**, 1213–1228.

Hsiao, K. and Prusiner, S. B. (1990). Inherited human prion diseases. *Neurology*, **40**, 1820–1827.

Hsiao, K., Baker, H. F., Crow, T. J., Poulter, M., Owen, F., Terwilliger, J. D., *et al.* (1989). Linkage of a prion protein missense variant to Gerstmann–Sträussler syndrome. *Nature*, **338**, 342–345.

Hsiao, K. K., Scott, M., Foster, D., Groth, D. F., DeArmond, S. J., and Prusiner, S. B. (1990). Spontaneous neurodegeneration in transgenic mice with mutant prion protein. *Science*, **250**, 1587–1590.

Hsiao, K. K., Cass, C., Schellenberg, G. D., Bird, T., Devine, G. E., Wisniewski, H., *et al.* (1991). A prion protein variant in a family with the telencephalic form of Gerstmann–Sträussler–Scheinker syndrome. *Neurology*, **41**, 681–684.

Hunter, N., Hope, J., McConnell, I., and Dickinson, A. G. (1987). Linkage of the scrapie-associated fibril protein (PrP) gene and *Sinc* using congenic mice and restriction fragment length polymorphism analysis. *Journal of General Virology*, **68**, 2711–2716.

Kascsak, R. J., Rubenstein, R., Merz, P. A., Tonna, D. M., Fersko, R., Carp, R. I., *et al.* (1987). Mouse polyclonal and monoclonal antibody to scrapie-associated fibril proteins. *Journal of Virology*, **61**, 3688–3693.

Kimberlin, R. H. and Walker, C. (1977). Characteristics of a short incubation model of scrapie in the golden hamster. *Journal of General Virology*, **34**, 295–304.

Kimberlin, R. H. and Walker, C. A. (1978). Pathogenesis of mouse scrapie: effect of route of inoculation on infectivity titres and dose–response curves. *Journal of Comparative Pathology*, **88**, 39–47.

Kimberlin, R. H., Walker, C. A., and Fraser, H. (1989). The genomic identity of different strains of mouse scrapie is expressed in hamsters and preserved on reisolation in mice. *Journal of General Virology*, **70**, 2017–2025.

Lowenstein, D. H., Butler, D. A., Westaway, D., McKinley, M. P., DeArmond, S. J., and Prusiner, S. B. (1990). Three hamster species with different scrapie incubation times and neuropathological features encode distinct prion proteins. *Molecular and Cellular Biology*, **10**, 1153–1163.

Manuelidis, L., Valley, S., and Manuelidis, E. E. (1985). Specific proteins associated with Creutzfeldt–Jakob disease and scrapie share antigenic and carbohydrate determinants. *Proceedings of the National Academy of Sciences of the USA*, **82**, 4263–4267.

McKinley, M. P., Bolton, D. C., and Prusiner, S. B. (1983). A protease-resistant protein is a structural component of the scrapie prion. *Cell*, **35**, 57–62.

McKinley, M. P., Meyer, R. K., Kenaga, L., Rahbar, F., Cotter, R., Serban, A., *et al.* (1991*a*). Scrapie prion rod formation in vitro requires both detergent extraction and limited proteolysis. *Journal of Virology*, **65**, 1340–1351.

McKinley, M. P., Taraboulos, A., Kenaga, L., Serban, D., Stieber, A., DeArmond, S. J., *et al.* (1991*b*). Ultrastructural localization of scrapie prion proteins in cytoplasmic vesicles of infected cultured cells. *Laboratory Investigation*, **65**, 622–630.

Owen, F., Poulter, M., Lofthouse, R., Collinge, J., Crow, T. J., Risby, D., *et al.* (1989). Insertion in prion protein gene in familial Creutzfeldt–Jakob disease. *Lancet*, **i**, 51–52.

Pattison, I. H. (1965). Experiments with scrapie and with special reference to the nature of the agent and the pathology of the disease. In *Slow latent and temperate virus infections*, *NINDB Monograph 2*. (ed. D. C. Gajdusek, C. J. Gibbs, and M. P. Alpers), pp. 249–257. US Government Printing, Washington DC.

Prusiner, S. B. (1987). Prions and neurodegenerative diseases. *New England Journal of Medicine*, **317**, 1571–1581.

Prusiner, S. B. (1989). Scrapie prions. *Annual Reviews of Microbiology*, **43**, 345–374.

Prusiner, S. B. (1991). Molecular biology of prion diseases. *Science*, **252**, 1515–1522.

Prusiner, S. B. (1993*a*). Chemistry and biology of prions. *Biochemistry*, **31**, 12278–12288.

Prusiner, S. B. (1993*b*). Transgenetics and cell biology of prion diseases: investigations of PrP^{Sc} synthesis and diversity. *British Medical Bulletin*, **49**, 873–912.

Prusiner, S. B., Scott, M., Foster, D., Pan, K. M., Groth, D., Mirenda, C., *et al.* (1990). Transgenetic studies implicate interactions between homologous PrP isoforms in scrapie prion replication. *Cell*, **63**, 673–686.

Prusiner, S. B., Groth, D., Serban, A., Koehler, R., Foster, D., Torchia, M., *et al.* (1993). Ablation of the prion protein (PrP) gene in mice prevents scrapie and facilitates production of anti-PrP antibodies. *Proceedings of the National Academy of Sciences of the USA*, **90**, 10608–10612.

Race, R. E., Graham, K., Ernst, D., Caughey, B., and Chesebro, B. (1990). Analysis of linkage between scrapie incubation period and the prion protein gene in mice. *Journal of General Virology*, **71**, 493–497.

Rogers, M., Taraboulos, A., Scott, M., Groth, D., and Prusiner, S. (1990). Intracellular accumulation of the cellular prion protein after mutagenesis of its Asn-linked glycosylation sites. *Glycobiology*, **1**, 101–109.

Rogers, M., Serban, D., Gyuris, T., Scott, M., Torchia, T., and Prusiner, S. B. (1991). Epitope mapping of the Syrian hamster prion protein utilizing chimeric and mutant genes in a vaccinia virus expression system. *Journal of Immunology*, **147**, 3568–3574.

Rothberg, K., Ying, Y., Kolhouse, J., Kamen, B., and Anderson, R. (1990). The glycophospholipid linked folate receptor internalizes folate without entering the clathrin coated pit endocytic pathway. *Journal of Cell Biology*, **110**, 627–649.

Safar, J., Ceroni, M., Piccardo, P., Liberski, P. P., Miyazaki, M., Gajdusek, D. C., *et al.* (1990). Subcellular distribution and physicochemical properties of scrapie-associated precursor protein and relationship with scrapie agent. *Neurology*, **40**, 503–508.

Scott, M., Foster, D., Mirenda, C., Serban, D., Coufal, F., Walchli, M., *et al.* (1989). Transgenic mice expressing hamster prion protein produce species-specific scrapie infectivity and amyloid plaques. *Cell*, **59**, 847–857.

Scott, M. R., Kohler, R., Foster, D., and Prusiner, S. B. (1992). Chimeric prion protein expression in cultured-cells and transgenic mice. *Protein Science*, **1**, 986–997.

Scott, M., Groth, D., Foster, D., Torchia, M., Yang, S. L., Dearmond, S. J., *et al.* (1993). Propagation of prions with artificial properties in transgenic mice expressing chimeric PrP genes. *Cell*, **73**, 979–988.

Serban, D., Taraboulos, A., DeArmond, S. J., and Prusiner, S. B. (1990). Rapid detection of Creutzfeldt–Jakob disease and scrapie prion proteins. *Neurology*, **40**, 110–117.

Stahl, N., Borchelt, D. R., Hsiao, K., and Prusiner, S. B. (1987). Scrapie prion protein contains a phosphatidylinositol glycolipid. *Cell*, **51**, 229–240.

Stahl, N., Baldwin, M. A., Hecker, R., Pan, K. M., Burlingame, A. L., and Prusiner, S. B. (1992). Glycosylinositol phospholipid anchors of the scrapie and cellular prion proteins contain sialic-acid. *Biochemistry*, **31**, 5043–5053.

Steinman, R., Mellman, I., Muller, W., and Cohn, Z. (1983). Endocytosis and the recycling of plasma membrane. *Journal of Cell Biology*, **96**, 1–27.

Stoorvogel, W., Strous, G., Geuze, H., Oorschot, V., and Schwartz, A. (1991). Late endosomes derive from early endosomes by maturation. *Cell*, **65**, 417–427.

Taraboulos, A., Rogers, M., Borchelt, D. R., McKinley, M. P., Scott, M., Serban, D., *et al.* (1990*a*). Acquisition of protease resistance by prion proteins in scrapie-infected cells does not require asparagine-linked glycosylation. *Proceedings of the National Academy of Sciences of the USA*, **87**, 8262–8266.

Taraboulos, A., Serban, D., and Prusiner, S. B. (1990*b*). Scrapie prion proteins accumulate in the cytoplasm of persistently infected cultured cells. *Journal of Cell Biology*, **110**, 2117–2132.

Taraboulos, A., Jendroska, K., Serban, D., Yang, S. L., Dearmond, S. J., and Prusiner, S. B. (1992*a*). Regional mapping of prion proteins in brain. *Proceedings of the National Academy of Sciences of the USA*, **89**, 7620–7624.

Taraboulos, A., Raeber, A. J., Borchelt, D. R., Serban, D., and Prusiner, S. B. (1992*b*). Synthesis and trafficking of prion proteins in cultured-cells. *Molecular Biology of the Cell*, **3**, 851–863.

Weissmann, C. (1989). Prions. Sheep disease in human clothing. *Nature*, **338**, 298–299.

Weissmann, C. (1991). A 'unified theory' of prion propagation. *Nature*, **352**, 679–683.

Westaway, D., Goodman, P. A., Mirenda, C. A., McKinley, M. P., Carlson, G. A., and Prusiner, S. B. (1987). Distinct prion proteins in short and long scrapie incubation period mice. *Cell*, **51**, 651–662.

Westaway, D., Mirenda, C. A., Foster, D., Zebarjadian, Y., Scott, M., Torchia, M. *et al.* (1991). Paradoxical shortening of scrapie incubation times by expression of prion protein transgenes derived from long incubation period mice. *Neuron*, **7**, 59–68.

Westaway, D., DeArmond, S. J., Cayetano, C. J., Groth, D., Foster, D., Yang, S. L., *et al.* (1994). Degeneration of skeletal muscle, peripheral nerves, and the central nervous system in transgenic mice overexpressing wild-type prion proteins. *Cell*, **76**, 117–129.

Wolkoff, A., Klausner, R., Ashwell, G., and Harford, J. (1984). Intracellular segregation of asialoglycoproteins and their receptor: A prelysosomal event subsequent to dissociation of the ligand–receptor complex. *Journal of Cellular Biology*, **98**, 375–381.

6 Neurophysiology of prion disease

JOHN G. R. JEFFERYS

PrP^C is found in high concentrations in neuronal membranes, is highly conserved in mammals, and may be present in all vertebrates (Harris *et al.* 1993). This conservation suggests that it has an important role in neural function. Until recently this role remained a mystery. Proposals linking PrP^C with cholinergic function now appear unlikely (Brenner *et al.* 1992; Harris *et al.* 1993). The neurological symptoms of prion diseases give clues on possible functions of normal PrP. This chapter will first review the pathophysiology of these diseases, and then discuss recent evidence on the physiological consequences of the presence and absence of PrP^C based on work on gene-targeted mice lacking prion protein.

Pathophysiology

The clinical consequences of prion diseases are devastating, and ultimately lethal. The most obvious symptoms of Creutzfeldt–Jakob disease (CJD) are the rapidly progressing dementia and myoclonus. In addition about 80% of patients develop abnormal periodic electroencephalogram (EEG) complexes or sharp waves at some stage in the disease. These complexes recur at 0.5–2 s and are widely synchronized in both hemispheres (Brechet *et al.* 1980; Brown *et al.* 1986; Brown 1993), and also involve subcortical structures such as the thalamus, caudate nucleus, globus pallidus, and hypothalamus (Traub and Pedley 1981). The high (up to 10%) incidence of generalized seizures in CJD patients (Cathala and Baron 1987) further reinforces the idea that the activity of the brains of these patients is prone to excessive synchronization. The neurological signs of classical Gerstmann–Sträussler Syndrome (GSS) differ from those of CJD, with a prominent cerebellar ataxia, but as these two diseases otherwise are closely related in their molecular and pathological features (Collinge *et al.* 1989) it is likely that their clinical differences reflect the relative involvement of different regions in the brain.

Hypersynchronous EEGs have been reported in several prion diseases of domestic and laboratory animals. There is some variability in the results for different species, but this may not be so surprising given the range of symptoms seen in humans. Even within the mouse the anatomical distribution of PrP^{Sc} differs markedly for different 'strains' of scrapie (DeArmond *et al.* 1993). Sheep with natural scrapie have EEG complexes similar to those seen in CJD, although they are not regular enough to be called periodic (Strain *et al.* 1986); they also are prone to seizures (Craig *et al.* 1993). It is unclear if similar abnormalities are seen in cattle with bovine spongiform encephalopathy (BSE). Many species have been inoculated with pathogenic prions, and some of them have been investigated electrophysiologically. A minority of squirrel monkeys inoculated with transmissible mink encephalopathy agent prions developed periodic complexes on their EEGs (Grabow *et al.* 1973). A similar study on mink with encephalopathy revealed some EEG abnormalities, but no periodic complexes (Grabow *et al.* 1971*a,b*). Squirrel monkeys receiving intracerebral CJD agent developed EEG abnormalities, including epileptiform activity, before they developed clinical signs (Cathala *et al.* 1981). Rats infected with scrapie show EEG disturbances that precede gross neurological signs (Bassant *et al.* 1984). One of the most detailed electrophysiological studies *in vivo* was performed on rats receiving intracerebral inoculates of a rat-adapted scrapie strain. They started to develop EEG abnormalities after three months; by eight months they had pronounced periodic polyspikes or spindle-shaped bursts of EEG spikes during quiet wakefulness, and sometimes paroxysmal bursts occurred in the cortex (Bassant *et al.* 1987). At this stage parallels have been drawn (Bassant *et al.* 1987) with the feline generalized penicillin epilepsy model, which is a model of absence seizures that depends on abnormal interactions between the thalamus and cortex (Gloor and Fariello 1988). As scrapie progresses in the rat, the amplitudes of EEG events and of evoked potentials decrease, and evidence of thalamic involvement increases. During these later stages, the neurological dysfunction becomes pronounced, especially the ataxia and dyskinesia, and large numbers of neurones are lost. The rats generally die 16–17 months after inoculation (Bassant *et al.* 1987).

Several hypotheses exist on the cellular pathology responsible for the EEG abnormalities found in CJD and in other prion diseases:

1. *Electrical coupling of neurones.* The common hispathological expression of the prion diseases is the spongy appearance of the brain in histological section. The holes in the sponge are intracellular (mainly intradendritic) and are formed from the cisternae of the smooth endoplasmic reticulum (Baker *et al.* 1990). The swollen neuronal processes may fuse (Kidson *et al.* 1978), and this could lead to excessive electrotonic coupling, which would allow the spread of excitation across the population of coupled cells and hence could contribute to the EEG abnormalities found in CJD (Traub and Pedley 1981).

2. *Altered synaptic connectivity.* Measurements of synaptic proteins suggests that synapses are lost early in the course of these diseases, before the gross loss of neurones and before the onset of spongiform pathology (Clinton *et al.* 1993). The altered neuronal circuitry could promote excessive neuronal synchrony. Experimental deafferentation and other lesions lead to epileptiform activity in neocortex and hippocampus (Ashwood and Wheal 1986; Buzsáki *et al.* 1989; Prince and Tseng 1993).

3. *Loss of synaptic inhibition.* Binding studies in scrapie-infected mice reveal a loss of $GABA_A$ receptors (or, more strictly, muscimol binding sites) (Quinn and Somerville

1984). Reductions in seizure threshold in scrapie-infected hamsters also suggest impaired inhibition, although these animals had normal numbers of muscimol binding sites (Pocchiari *et al.* 1985). This hypothesis was promoted as a likely mechanism for the abnormal EEGs seen in scrapie-infected rats (Bassant *et al.* 1987).

4. *Other transmitter systems* are also disrupted. This has been suggested by Goudsmit *et al.* (1981) and Rohwer *et al.* (1981), but how these would contribute to the EEG abnormalities remains unclear.

5. *Other cellular changes.* Other cellular changes occur, such as the accumulation of abnormal cytoskeletal protein, but again the significance they have for the EEG remains unclear.

Experimental neurophysiology

To distinguish between these and other potential cellular and local network mechanisms of the electrophysiological abnormalities of prion diseases, we have used the brain slice preparation, which has already had a major impact on studies of epilepsy and the normal functioning of the brain. This kind of work will tell us little about mechanisms of infection. Rather it addresses the functional changes in the brain throughout the course of prion disease, and is directly relevant to the cellular mechanisms of symptoms such as cognitive impairments, EEG abnormalities (general periodic complexes), and myoclonus. This kind of analysis also provides the basis for the development of rational therapies for controlling some of the symptoms and perhaps also the progression of prion diseases. The ideal experimental model should be reproducible, reasonably quick, and not too expensive. Several mouse models of spongiform encephalopathies could fit the bill. For instance there are transgenic mice that are susceptible to sheep or hamster-adapted scrapie (Scott *et al.* 1989; Hunter 1991; Prusiner 1991; Hecker *et al.* 1992) and at least one that spontaneously expresses a disease similar to GSS (Hsiao *et al.* 1990).

Mice transgenic for Syrian hamster PrP

The Tg(SHaPrP)81 transgenic mouse expresses multiple copies of the normal prion protein gene of hamster, and is one of the lines most highly susceptible to hamster-adapted strains of scrapie, such as Sc237. The clinical and pathological progress of this disease has been charted in some detail (Scott *et al.* 1989; Hecker *et al.* 1992). In short, the heterozygous mice show the classical histopathology by 70 days after inoculation, develop neurological signs characteristic of scrapie by 81 ± 2 days and die by 83 ± 3 days (Hecker *et al.* 1992), while the homozygous Tg(SHaPrP)81[+/+] mice develop neurological signs by about 50 days (Prusiner *et al.* 1993). We prepared coronal brain slices from the latter for electrophysiological studies *in vitro* (Jefferys *et al.* 1994*a,b*). These appeared normal up to 30 days after inoculation. From 30 days on, the whole of the cortex in these slices generated both spontaneous and evoked activity, which resembled the epileptic activity that can be induced by a variety of acute and chronic convulsants (Brener *et al.* 1991). The epileptic activity in the scrapie-infected mice was all or none, that is threshold stimuli would either evoke a small, brief, normal response, or it would trigger the full-scale synchronous discharge lasting several seconds (which is extremely long for the circuitry preserved in the brain slice preparation; Fig. 6.1A) (Jefferys *et al.* 1994*a*). Abnormal responses also occurred in the hippocampus, but were restricted to the CA1 region. Normally it is the CA3 region that is most susceptible to epileptic activity (Jefferys 1993, 1994), but it is likely that the selectivity for CA1 seen here is due to the localization of this strain of PrP^{Sc} (DeArmond *et al.* 1993). Between 30 and about 45–50 days, these epileptiform discharges were the most dramatic manifestation of the disease. At least during the first half of this period spongiform histopathology was minimal or absent, and neurological signs were equivocal, limited to the animals clasping rather than splaying their hind limbs when picked up by their tails. From about 55 days until death at about 60 days, the mice developed progressively more intense neurological signs, notably ataxia and dyskinesia. Spongiform histopathology became progressively more widespread and dramatic. The brain slices continued to show the synchronous epileptiform activity, but they also revealed changes in the intrinsic properties of about one third of neurones impaled. Action potentials became grossly prolonged from their normal duration of less than 4 ms to 20–120 ms (Fig. 6.1C).

We are currently working on the cellular bases of the electrophysiological abnormalities of scrapie. Our preliminary studies (Jefferys *et al.* 1994*a*) suggest that inhibition may be weakened as proposed previously (Quinn and Somerville 1984; Pocchiari *et al.* 1985; Bassant *et al.* 1987). This does not exclude other mechanisms, such as synaptic recognization (Clinton *et al.* 1993) or cell fusion and electrotonic coupling (Traub and Pedley 1981) also have a role to play. Indeed the duration of the epileptic discharges suggests the cooperation of several mechanisms (Traub *et al.* 1993, 1994). Intrinsic neuronal properties also change during scrapie infection. This may be a contributory factor in the early epileptiform activity, but it is especially prominent in the terminal stages when action potentials become grossly prolonged. Preliminary pharmacological studies suggest that the prolonged action potentials are due to voltage-sensitive calcium channels, because they are sensitive to nitrendipine (Jefferys *et al.* 1994*a*). The same study also implicates abnormalities in potassium channels, which would normally curtail the action potential.

These physiological abnormalities have important functional implications. Firstly, the abnormal cortical synchrony will disrupt brain function from an early stage, some weeks before the appearance of spongiform pathology. This may explain human cases of dementia with molecular confirmation of prion disease, but lacking the classical histopathology (Collinge *et al.* 1990; Lantos 1992). Secondly, the excessive cortical activity will contribute to the loss of neurones and the progression of the disease as a result of the considerable release of glutamate that will occur during the synchronous discharges. In this context it is significant that antagonists of the NMDA class of glutamate receptor protect against PrP^{Sc} toxicity

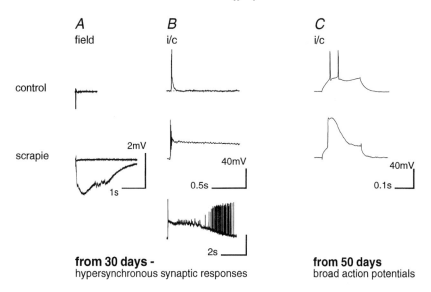

Fig. 6.1 Abnormal activity in cortical slices from Tg(SHaPrP)81 mice infected with scrapie. (*A*) 30–50 days after inoculation, the normal brief, graded extracellular field potential response to electrical stimulation of the incoming axons is replaced by a large, prolonged 'all-or-none' response indicating an abnormally synchronous discharge of the neuronal population in the slice. (*B*) Intracellular recordings under the same conditions reveal the strong depolarization and rapid discharge of cortical neurones during these abnormal responses. Recordings from layer II neocortical neurones and hippocampal CA1 neurones showed no obvious inhibitory postsynaptic potential, in marked contrast to normal cells (data not shown). (*C*) During the terminal stage (50–60 days after inoculation) action potentials, evoked by intracellular current injection, become abnormally prolonged in one third of cells. (Modified from Jefferys *et al.* 1994a).

in cortical neuronal lines (Müller *et al.* 1993). Thirdly, neuronal loss will be exacerbated by calcium entry both during the epileptiform activity and during the prolonged action potentials during the terminal stages. This fits with the observation that scrapie infection of cultured hamster brain cells makes them susceptible to damage when they were incubated in high concentrations (< 20 mM) of Ca^{2+} (Kristensson *et al.* 1993). Chronic scrapie infection of both cultured neuroblastoma cells and cultured hamster brain cells also disrupts the increases in intracellular Ca^{2+} normally evoked by bradykinin (Kristensson *et al.* 1993).

Mice lacking PrP

The consequences of infection with PrP^{Sc} have now been documented in some detail, and we are starting to understand its underlying cellular pathophysiology. Much progress has also been made on the molecular relationship between PrP^C and PrP^{Sc}. What has been much less clear until recently is what might be the role of the normal isoform, PrP^C. A major breakthrough in this area has been the development of genetically modified mice that fail to produce PrP. Accounts of at least two types of PrP knockout mice have now been published (Büeler *et al.* 1992; Manson *et al.* 1994). Given the high degree of conservation of PrP genes over evolution, and the high levels of the PrP^C found in neurones as well as in the spleen and lymph nodes, it is surprising that these mice survive at all. It is even more surprising that they appear to develop normally. Behavioural studies show that these mice can perform a range of learning tasks as well as controls, with only minor differences in some of the details of their behavioural responses (most notably greater perseverance when the goal was moved in a Morris swim task) (Büeler *et al.* 1992). These mice also have functional immune systems (Büeler *et al.* 1992). Furthermore no differences have been found in the development of their neuromuscular system (Brenner *et al.* 1992).

We used the transgenic mice developed by Büeler *et al.* (1992) in which the PrP gene had been ablated, to study the electrophysiology of brain slices. These PrP-null, or $PrP^{0/0}$, mice have two major abnormalities that we have identified so far, although we suspect there may be others.

1. Synaptic inhibition
The neurophysiology of these diseases, together with speculation that PrP could be involved in some form of membrane adhesion process based on the topology and biophysical properties of PrP, suggested that we should measure the strength of synaptic inhibition in these $PrP^{0/0}$ mice. Fast inhibitory postsynaptic potentials (IPSPs), which are mediated by $GABA_A$ receptors, are easily quantified. This is done by blocking all other classes of synapse likely to be activated by stimulation of the slice, and then applying a stimulus that can excite inhibitory neurones directly (Davies and Collingridge 1989; Davies *et al.* 1990). Then we can record a pure IPSP from pyramidal cells in the region, in this case the CA1 zone of the hippocampus (Fig. 6.2). IPSPs from the $PrP^{0/0}$ mice differed from controls in their reversal potentials and in their conductances (Collinge *et al.* 1994). The fast IPSP is in the normal hyperpolarizing direction in the control CA1 pyramidal cell, but that it is depolarizing in the $PrP^{0/0}$ case (Fig. 6.2A). Measurements are made using single-electrode voltage clamp, that is on responses where we hold the membrane potential of the postsynaptic cell at a preset value and measure the current that we need to inject into the cell to achieve that holding potential. This provides an estimate of the current flowing through the channels opened by, in this case, the synaptically released GABA.

A plot of the peak inhibitory postsynaptic current (IPSC) against the holding potential shows two important points. First, the intercept with the x-axis—the reversal potential at which the IPSP is zero—has shifted in the depolarizing direction in the $PrP^{0/0}$ mice, from –69 mV to –62 mV. Second, the gradient of the I–V curve, which estimates the conductance, or the strength of inhibition, is smaller in the $PrP^{0/0}$ mice (Fig. 6.2B). The changes are at least partly selective for fast IPSPs. Slow monosynaptic IPSPs, mediated by $GABA_B$ receptors, remain at control levels. The corresponding measurements of EPSPs are more difficult, but the pharmacologically

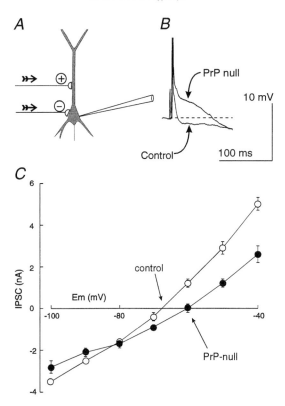

Fig. 6.2 (*A*) IPSPs recorded from hippocampal slices prepared from PrP$^{0/0}$ mice tend to depolarize rather than hyperpolarize hippocampal CA1 pyramidal cells (*B*). Measurements were made of pharmacologically isolated inhibitory postsynaptic currents under voltage clamp (by blocking excitatory synapses, (+) in A, and also slow IPSPs). The membrane potential set by the experimenter was plotted against the peak inhibitory postsynaptic current (*C*) and shows that the reversal potential (arrowed) for the IPSC is abnormally depolarized in slices from PrP$^{0/0}$ mice, and that the slope of the curve (the conductance) is markedly reduced. (*C* modified from Collinge *et al.* 1994.)

isolated NMDA component has the same amplitude as the controls, and the non-NMDA component is at least qualitatively unchanged (Collinge *et al.* 1994).

The subcellular basis of the abnormal IPSP remains unclear. The smaller mono-synaptic IPSP conductance in the PrP$^{0/0}$ mice probably reflects a change in the number or efficacy of inhibitory synapses, or in the properties or number of receptors on the postsynaptic membrane. The initial response of CA1 pyramidal cells to exogenous GABA differs between PrP$^{0/0}$ and control mice qualitatively in the same direction as the IPSPs, which implicates postsynaptic abnormalities. We know that normal hippocampal slices can also produce depolarizing GABA responses, for instance IPSPs recorded under 4-aminopyridine, barbiturates, or when exogenous

GABA is applied to the dendrites (Andersen *et al.* 1980; Lambert *et al.* 1991). The depolarizing response to dendritic applications of GABA is why we measure the initial component of the response to our somatic applications; the later components are dominated by the response to GABA diffusing from the site of application. These considerations lead to one hypothesis of the origin of the depolarized IPSP in slices from PrP$^{0/0}$ mice. If inhibitory synapses were structurally disrupted so that a significant fraction of GABA spilled over to activate extrasynaptic receptors, then the IPSP would become dominated by extrasynaptic receptors, as may occur with 4-aminopyridine. A second hypothesis is that the selectivity of the GABA$_A$ receptor is abnormal, being either of an extrasynaptic or an entirely aberrant type. An increased permeability to bicarbonate ions is quite feasible, and would shift the reversal potential in the depolarizing direction (Grover *et al.* 1993). The final hypothesis is that the chloride equilibrium potential is depolarized because intracellular chloride concentration is greater than normal, perhaps as a result of impaired ion transport.

2. *Synaptic plasticity*

We also measured a more subtle synaptic phenomenon on the basis that it could be more sensitive to molecular disruption than simple transmission across synapse. This study was performed in parallel with the measurements of synaptic inhibition, which is fortunate because we probably would not have made these measurements once we knew of the abnormal IPSPs in these mice. The remarkable result was that synaptic plasticity was greatly impaired.

The test we used for plasticity is the phenomenon of long-term potentiation (LTP). In this we stimulate presynaptic axons every 30 seconds, and measure the population response from the CA1 pyramidal cells. After a stable baseline response is established, we deliver a burst of 200 stimuli in 1 second (the conditioning train). This normally has a marked and persistent effect on the response to low-frequency stimulation. The control responses double their original amplitude, and remain at that level for at least 30 minutes (Fig. 6.3). The contrast with the PrP$^{0/0}$ mice is obvious. They peak at a lower level of potentiation, and are back at their control levels within 30 minutes. LTP could appear to be impaired in slices from PrP$^{0/0}$ mice because of some consequence of the systematic difference in IPSPs between them and the controls. However, the difference in LTP persists when inhibition is blocked as was the case for Fig. 6.3.

At first sight the impairment of LTP has little in common with the IPSP abnormalities found in the same mice. However, the two are linked through the properties of the NMDA class of glutamate receptor. NMDA receptors play a minimal role in excitatory synaptic transmission as normally measured in the hippocampus (Herron *et al.* 1986). The small contribution of the NMDA receptor is at least partly due to the block of its ion channel by an Mg^{2+} ion, but it is also severely attenuated by synaptic inhibition simultaneously activated by the electric stimuli normally used. The first functional role for the NMDA receptor was identified in the initiation of LTP; the conditioning train of stimuli unblocks NMDA receptors and triggers the chain of events that leads to LTP (Collingridge *et al.* 1983). We now know that activating NMDA receptors during low frequency stimulation before the

John G. R. Jefferys 171

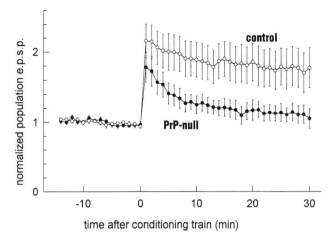

Fig. 6.3 Disrupted synaptic plasticity in PrP$^{0/0}$ mice. Evoked field potentials recorded from the synaptic layers of the CA1 region of hippocampal slices reveal a marked 'long-term potentiation' (LTP) following a 1 second train of 200 stimuli at time zero. In contrast the PrP$^{0/0}$ slices failed to produce LTP lasting over 30 minutes, but they did sustain short-term potentiation lasting about 15 minutes. e.p.s.p., excitatory postsynaptic potential. (Modified from Collinge *et al.* 1994.)

conditioning train attenuates subsequent LTP (Coan *et al.* 1989; Huang *et al.* 1992). We also know that unblocking inhibition increases the contribution of NMDA receptors to the excitatory postsynaptic potential (EPSP) (Herron *et al.* 1985). Therefore the weakened LTP in the PrP$^{0/0}$ mice could be a consequence of a primary defect of synaptic inhibition.

The impairment of LTP that is so obvious in Fig. 6.3 stands in marked contrast with the near-normal performance of the same line of knockout mice on a range of behavioural tasks that are thought to depend on hippocampal function (Büeler *et al.* 1992). This is troubling if one is to follow the conventional view that LTP has something to do with learning and memory. While one can argue that normal LTP in the face of impaired learning could be due to some other link in the physiological chain that produces the behavioural expression of learning (Brace *et al.* 1985), the preservation of learning ability in the absence of LTP is more of a problem. We have at least two potential ways of reconciling the behavioural and physiological data on these mice. The first is methodological. We could not give more than one train of stimuli during conditioning process without inducing repetitive firing of the pyramidal cells, because of the weakened inhibition. It may be that repeated trains are needed for the behaviourally relevant form of LTP. Longer-lived LTP, with a time course of days, appears to be more relevant to at least some behavioural tasks (Barnes 1979). The second is the proposal that it is short-term potentiation rather than LTP that is behaviourally relevant (Hannay *et al.* 1993). This kind of short-term potentiation resembles LTP in that it requires the activation of NMDA receptors and postsynaptic depolarization. It differs from LTP in that it only lasts a few minutes, much as does the potentiation we recorded in the PrP$^{0/0}$ mice. Similarities in the pharmacology of short-term and long-term potentiation mean that it is very difficult to distinguish their roles in learning and memory, so that the near-normal performance of PrP$^{0/0}$ mice on 'hippocampal' tasks could be due to short-term potentiation.

Rescue of PrP$^{0/0}$ phenotype

Whatever the cellular mechanism of the abnormality in the IPSPs of the PrP$^{0/0}$ mice, we are confident that it is the result of the absence of prion protein. PrP$^{0/0}$ mice (MoPrP$^{0/0}$) and transgenic mice with human PrP genes in addition to the wild-type mouse PrP gene (MoPrP$^{+/+}$, HuPrP+ve) were crossed. HuPrP+ve F$_1$ offspring were then crossed to produce F$_2$ litters which provided for our experiments:

- PrP$^{0/0}$ mice, which lacked any kind of PrP gene (MoPrP$^{0/0}$ HuPrP-ve)
- wild-type control mice (MoPrP$^{+/+}$ HuPrP-ve)
- mice lacking the mouse PrP gene, but with the human transgene (MoPrP$^{0/0}$ HuPrP+ve).

This experiment confirmed the impaired synaptic inhibition in the PrP$^{0/0}$ mice. It also showed that one line of HuPrP+ve mice rescued the phenotype and one did not. The successful transgenic mouse, HuPrP(Tg152), has a high copy number of the HuPrP transgene and produces high levels of PrP^C, while the unsuccessful transgenic mouse, HuPrP(Tg110), has a low copy number and produces low levels of human PrP^C (Whittington *et al.* 1995).

Conclusion

The weakened synaptic inhibition we found in PrP$^{0/0}$ mice resembles those suggested by our qualitative observations on scrapie infection in Tg(HaPrP)81 mice. Clearly the PrP$^{0/0}$ mice lack the marked neurological problems of scrapie. Nevertheless, we believe that these results re-open the question of whether scrapie is due to PrP^{Sc} accumulation or whether it is due to PrP^C deficiency. The less marked behavioural problems for the PrP$^{0/0}$ mice could be due to adaptive changes in response to the absence of PrP over the lifetime of the animals; symptoms might be much more disruptive if PrP were sequestered over a short period (Collinge *et al.* 1994). These speculations warrant further study. They also underline an important point about work on transgenic animals in general; they are abnormal from conception. At the most straightforward, the lack of the relevant protein could cause a phenotype detected in adults, or indeed in any postnatal stage. This is usually the result the experimenter is hoping for. However, the severity of the phenotype may be ameliorated by other processes that can substitute for the absent protein. Alternatively the phenotype could be a secondary response to the primary effects of the lack of the protein, which could, for instance, occur during embryonic development.

Prion proteins have a marked impact on the electrophysiological function of the nervous system. In both scrapie-infected and PrP$^{0/0}$ mice we have evidence of malfunction of synaptic inhibition, and also indications of other physiological dysfunctions. These studies provide some initial insights into the functional role of prion proteins, whether in their normal cellular or abnormal scrapie isoforms.

Note added in proof

The hippocampal phenotype of PrP$^{0/0}$ mice is proving controversial. Lledo *et al.* (1996) fail to replicate our two (larger) studies (Collinge *et al.* 1994; Whittington *et al.* 1995). Manson *et al.* (1995) confirm the impairment of LTP, while Colling *et al.* (1996) find changes in intrinsic properties of pyramidal cells.

References

Andersen, P., Dingledine, R., Gjerstad, L., Langmoen, I. A., and Laursen, A. M. (1980). Two different responses of hippocampal pyramidal cells to application of gamma-amino butyric acid. *Journal of Physiology*, **305**, 279–296.

Ashwood, T. J. and Wheal, H.V. (1986). Loss of inhibition in the CA1 region of the kainic acid lesioned hippocampus is not associated with changes in postsynaptic responses to GABA. *Brain Research*, **367**, 390–394.

Baker, H. F., Duchen, L. W., Jacobs, J. M., and Ridley, R. M. (1990). Spongiform encephalopathy transmitted experimentally from Creutzfeldt–Jakob and familial Gerstmann–Sträussler–Scheinker diseases. *Brain*, **113**, 1891–1909.

Barnes, C. A. (1979). Memory deficits associated with senescence: a neurophysiological and behavioural study in the rat. *Journal of Comparative Physiology and Psychology*, **93**, 74–104.

Bassant, M. H., Cathala, F., Court, L., Gourmelon, P., and Hauw, J. J. (1984). Experimental scrapie in rats: first electrophysiological observations. *Electroencephalography and Clinical Neurophysiology*, **57**, 541–547.

Bassant, M. H., Court, L., and Cathala, F. (1987). Impairment of the cortical and thalamic electrical activity in scrapie-infected rats. *Electroencephalography and Clinical Neurophysiology*, **66**, 307–316.

Brace, H. M., Jefferys, J. G. R., and Mellanby, J. (1985). Long-term changes in hippocampal physiology and in learning ability of rats after intrahippocampal tetanus toxin. *Journal of Physiology*, **368**, 343–357.

Brechet, R., Sicard, C., Moret-Chalmin, C., Olivesi, L., Cathala, F., Brown, P. *et al.* (1980). Etude électroencéphalographique de vingt-cinq cas de maladie de Creutzfeldt–Jakob. *Revue d'Electroencéphalographie et de Neurophysiologie Clinique*, **10**, 55–63.

Brener, K., Chagnac-Amitai, Y., Jefferys, J. G. R., and Gutnick, M. J. (1991). Chronic epileptic foci in neocortex: *in vivo* and *in vitro* effects of tetanus toxin. *European Journal of Neuroscience*, **3**, 47–54.

Brenner, H. R., Herczeg, A., and Oesch, B. (1992). Normal development of nerve–muscle synapses in mice lacking the prion protein gene. *Proceedings of the Royal Society of London (Biology)*, **250**, 151–155.

Brown, P. (1993). EEG findings in Creutzfeldt–Jakob disease. *Journal of the American Medical Association*, **269**, 3168.

Brown, P., Cathala, F., Castaigne, P., and Gajdusek, D. C. (1986) Creutzfeldt–Jakob disease: clinical analysis of a consecutive series of 230 neuropathologically verified cases. *Annals of Neurology*, **20**, 597–602.

Buzsáki, G., Ponomareff, G. L., Bayardo, F., Ruiz, R., and Gage, F. H. (1989). Neuronal activity in the subcortically denervated hippocampus: A chronic model for epilepsy. *Neuroscience*, **28**, 527–538.

Büeler, H., Fischer, M., Lang, Y., Bluethmann, H., Lipp, H.-P., DeArmond, S. J., *et al.* (1992). Normal development and behaviour of mice lacking the neuronal cell-surface PrP protein. *Nature*, **356**, 577–582.

Cathala, F., Court, L., Breton, P., Mestries, J. C., Gourmelon, P., Dormont, D., *et al.* (1981). Creutzfeldt–Jakob disease in the squirrel monkeys. *Revue Neurologique*, **137**, 785–805.

Cathala, F. and Baron, H. (1987). Clinical aspects of Creutzfeldt–Jakob disease. In *Prions: novel infectious pathogens causing scrapie and Creutzfeldt–Jakob disease*, (ed. S. B. Prusiner and M. P. McKinley), pp. 467–509. Academic Press, San Diego.

Clinton, J., Forsyth, C., Royston, M. C., and Roberts, G. W. (1993). Synaptic degeneration is the primary neuropathological feature in prion disease: a preliminary study. *Neuroreport*, **4**, 65–68.

Coan, E. J., Irving, A. J., and Collingridge, G. L. (1989). Low-frequency activation of the NMDA receptor system can prevent the induction of LTP. *Neuroscience Letters*, **105**, 205–210.

Colling, S. B., Collinge, J., and Jefferys, J. G. R. (1996). Hippocampal slices from prion protein null mice: disrupted Ca^{2+}-activated K^+ currents. *Neuroscience Letters*, **209**, 49–52.

Collinge, J., Harding, A. E., Owen, F., Poulter, M., Lofthouse, R., Boughey, A. M., *et al.* (1989). Diagnosis of Gerstmann–Sträussler syndrome in familial dementia with prion protein gene analysis. *Lancet*, **ii**, 15–17.

Collinge, J., Owen, F., Poulter, M., Leach, M., Crow, T. J., Rossor, M. N., *et al.* (1990). Prion dementia without characteristic pathology. *Lancet*, **336**, 7–9.

Collinge, J., Whittington, M. A., Sidle, K. C. L., Smith, C. J., Palmer, M. S., Clarke, A. R., *et al.* (1994). Prion protein is necessary for normal synaptic function. *Nature*, **370**, 295–297.

Collingridge, G. L., Kehl, S. J., and McLennan, H. (1983). Excitatory amino acids in synaptic transmission in the Schaffer collateral-commissural pathway of the rat hippocampus. *Journal of Physiology*, **334**, 33–46.

Craig, A. M., Blackstone, C. D., Huganir, R. L., and Banker, G. (1993). The distribution of glutamate receptors in cultured rat hippocampal neurons: postsynaptic clustering of AMPA-selective subunits. *Neuron*, **10**, 1055–1068.

Davies, C. H., Davies, S. N., and Collingridge, G. L. (1990). Paired-pulse depression of monosynaptic GABA-mediated inhibitory postsynaptic responses in rat hippocampus. *Journal of Physiology*, **424**, 513–531.

Davies, S. N. and Collingridge, G. L. (1989) Role of excitatory amino acid receptors in synaptic transmission in area CA1 of rat hippocampus. *Proceedings of the Royal Society of London (Biology)*, **236**, 373–384.

DeArmond, S. J., Yang, S.-L., Lee, A., Bowler, R., Taraboulos, A., Groth, D., *et al.* (1993). Three scrapie prion isolates exhibit different accumulation patterns of the prion protein scrapie isoform. *Proceedings of the National Academy of Sciences of the USA*, **90**, 6449–6453.

Gloor, P. and Fariello, R. G. (1988). Generalized epilepsy: some of its cellular mechanisms differ from those of focal epilepsy. *Trends in Neuroscience*, **11**, 63–68.

Goudsmit, J., Rohwer, R. G., Silbergeld, E. K., and Gajdusek, D. C. (1981). Hypersensitivity to central serotonin receptor activation in scrapie-infected hamsters and the effect of serotonergic drugs on scrapie symptoms. *Brain Research*, **220**, 372–377.

Grabow, J. D., Eckroade, R. J., and Hanson, R. P. (1971a). Serial electroencephalographic studies in experimental mink encephalopathy. *Electroencephalography and Clinical Neurophysiology*, **30**, 160.

Grabow, J. D., Eckroade, R. J., and Hanson, R. P. (1971*b*). Serial electroencephalographic studies of experimentally induced transmissible mink encephalopathy. *American Journal of Veterinary Research*, **32**, 457–464.

Grabow, J. D., ZuRhein, G. M., Eckroade, R. J., Zollman, P. E., and Hanson, R. P. (1973). Transmissible mink encephalopathy agent in squirrel monkeys: serial electroencephalographic, clinical and pathologic studies. *Neurology*, **23**, 820–832.

Grover, L. M., Lambert, N. A., Schwartzkroin, P. A., and Teyler, T. J. (1993). Role of HCO_3^- ions in depolarizing $GABA_A$ receptor-mediated responses in pyramidal cells of rat hippocampus. *Journal of Neurophysiology*, **69**, 1541–1555.

Hannay, T., Larkman, A., Stratford, K., and Jack, J. (1993). A common rule governs the synaptic locus of both short-term and long-term potentiation. *Current Biology*, **3**, 832–841.

Harris, D. A., Lele, P., and Snider, W. D. (1993). Localization of the mRNA for a chicken prion protein by *in situ* hybridization. *Proceedings of the National Academy of Sciences of the USA*, **90**, 4309–4313.

Hecker, R., Taraboulos, A., Scott, M., Pan, K.-M., Yang, S.-L., Torchia, M., *et al.* (1992). Replication of distinct scrapie prion isolates is region specific in brains of transgenic mice and hamsters. *Genes and Development*, **6**, 1213–1228.

Herron, C. E., Williamson, R., and Collingridge, G. L. (1985). A selective *N*-methyl-D-aspartate antagonist depresses epileptiform activity in rat hippocampal slices. *Neuroscience Letters*, **61**, 255–260.

Herron, C. E., Lester, R. A., Coan, E. J., and Collingridge, G. L. (1986). Frequency-dependent involvement of NMDA receptors in the hippocampus: a novel synaptic mechanism. *Nature*, **322**, 265–268.

Hsiao, K. K., Scott, M., Foster, D., Groth, D. F., DeArmond, S. J., and Prusiner, S. B. (1990). Spontaneous neurodegeneration in transgenic mice with mutant prion protein. *Science*, **250**, 1587–1590.

Huang, Y. Y., Colino, A., Selig, D. K., and Malenka, R. C. (1992). The influence of prior synaptic activity on the induction of long-term potentiation. *Science*, **255**, 730–733.

Hunter, N. (1991). Scrapie and GSS—the importance of protein. *Trends in Neuroscience*, **14**, 389–390.

Jefferys, J. G. R. (1993). The pathophysiology of epilepsies. In *The epilepsies* (ed. J. Laidlaw, A. Richens, and D. W. Chadwick) 4th edn, pp. 241–276. Churchill Livingstone, Edinburgh.

Jefferys, J. G. R. (1994). Experimental neurobiology of epilepsies. *Current Opinions in Neurology*, **7**, 113–122.

Jefferys, J. G. R., Empson, R. M., Whittington, M. A., and Prusiner, S. B. (1994*a*). Scrapie infection of transgenic mice leads to network and intrinsic dysfunction of cortical and hippocampal neurons. *Neurobiology of Disease*, **1**, 25–30.

Jefferys, J. G. R., Whittington, M. A., and Empson, R. M. (1994*b*). Thin film isolator for the preparation of, and making electrophysiological recording from, *in vitro* brain slices from scrapie-infected mice and other biological hazards. *Journal of Physiology*, **476**, 9P.

Kidson, C., Moreau, M. C., Asher, D. M., Brown, P. W., Coon, H. G., Gajdusek, D. C., *et al.* (1978). Cell fusion induced by scrapie and Creutzfeldt–Jakob virus-infected brain preparations. *Proceedings of the National Academy of Sciences of the USA*, **75**, 2969–2971.

Kristensson, K., Feuerstein, B., Taraboulos, A., Hyun, W. C., Prusiner, S. B., and DeArmond, S. J. (1993). Scrapie prions alter receptor-mediated calcium responses in cultured cells. *Neurology*, **43**, 2335–2341.

Lambert, N. A., Borroni, A. M., Grover, L. M., and Teyler, T. J. (1991). Hyperpolarizing and depolarizing $GABA_A$ receptor-mediated dendritic inhibition in area CA1 of the rat hippocampus. *Journal of Neurophysiology*, **66**, 1538–1548.

Lantos, P. L. (1992). From slow virus to prion: a review of transmissible spongiform encephalopathies. *Histopathology*, **20**, 1–11.

Lledo, P.- M., Tremblay, P., DeArmond, S. J., Prusiner, S. B., and Nicoll, R. A. (1996). Mice deficient for prion protein exhibit normal neuronal excitability and synaptic transmission in the hippocampus. *Proceedings of the National Academy of Sciences of the USA*, **93**, 2403–2407.

Manson, J. C., Clarke, A. R., Hooper, M. L., Aitchison, L., McConnell, I., and Hope, J. (1994). 129/Ola mice carrying a null mutation in PrP that abolishes mRNA production are developmentally normal. *Molecular Neurobiology*, **8**, 121–127.

Manson, J. C., Hope, J., Clarke, A. R., Johnstone, A., Black, C., and MacLeod, N. (1995). PrP gene dosage and long term potentiation (letter). *Neurodegeneration*, **4**, 113–114.

Müller, W. E. G., Ushijima, H., Schröder, H. C., Forrest, J. M. S., Schatton, W. F. H., Rytik, P. G., *et al.* (1993). Cytoprotective effect of NMDA receptor antagonists on prion protein (Prion^{Sc})-induced toxicity in rat cortical cell cultures. *European Journal of Pharmacology and Molecular Pharmacology*, **246**, 261–267,

Pocchiari, M., Masullo, C., Lust, W. D., Gibbs, C. J., Jr, and Gajdusek, D. C. (1985). Isonicotinic hydrazide causes seizures in scrapie-infected hamsters with shorter latency than in control animals: a possible GABAergic defect. *Brain Research*, **326**, 117–123.

Prince, D. A. and Tseng, G.-F. (1993) Epileptogenesis in chronically injured cortex: *in vitro* studies. *Journal of Neurophysiology*, **69**, 1276–1291.

Prusiner, S. B. (1991). Molecular biology of prion diseases. *Science*, **252**, 1515–1522.

Prusiner, S. B., Groth, D., Serban, A., Koehler, R., Foster, D., Torchia, M., *et al.* (1993). Ablation of the prion protein (PrP) gene in mice prevents scrapie and facilitates production of anti-PrP antibodies. *Proceedings of the National Academy of Sciences of the USA*, **90**, 10608–10612.

Quinn, M. R. and Somerville, R. A. (1984). Decreased high-affinity binding of [^{3}H]muscimol to cerebral synaptic membranes of scrapie-infected mice. *Journal of Neurochemistry*, **42**, 290–293.

Rohwer, R. G., Goudsmit, J., Neckers, L. M., and Gajdusek, D. C. (1981). Hamster scrapie: evidence for alterations in serotonin metabolism. *Advances in Experimental Medical Biology*, **134**, 375–384.

Scott, M., Foster, D., Mirenda, C., Serban, D., Coufal, F., Wälchli, M., *et al.* (1989). Transgenic mice expressing hamster prion protein produce species-specific infectivity and amyloid plaques. *Cell*, **59**, 847–857.

Strain, G. M., Olcott, B. M., and Braun, W. F., Jr (1986) Electroencephalogram and evoked potentials in naturally occurring scrapie in sheep. *American Journal of Veterinary Research*, **47**, 828–836.

Traub, R. D. and Pedley, T. A. (1981). Virus-induced electrotonic coupling: hypothesis on the mechanism of periodic EEG discharges in Creutzfeldt–Jakob disease. *Annals of Neurology*, **10**, 405–410.

Traub, R. D., Miles, R., and Jefferys, J. G. R. (1993). Synaptic and intrinsic conductances shape picrotoxin-induced synchronized after-discharges in the guinea-pig hippocampal slice. *Journal of Physiology*, **461**, 525–547.

Traub, R. D., Jefferys, J. G. R., and Whittington, M. A. (1994). Enhanced NMDA conductance can account for epileptiform activity induced by low Mg^{2+} in the rat hippocampal slice. *Journal of Physiology*, **478**, 379–393.

Whittington, M. A., Sidle, K. C. L., Gowland, I., Meads, J., Hill, A., Palmer, M. S., *et al.* (1995). Rescue of neurophysiological phenotype seen in PrP$^{0/0}$ mice by transgene encoding human prion protein. *Nature Genetics*, **9**, 197–201.

7 Structural properties of the prion protein

CORINNE SMITH AND ANTHONY R. CLARKE

Properties of the infectious agent

Resolution of the many puzzles associated with prion diseases rests, at least in part, on gaining an understanding of the structural nature of the prion protein (PrP) in both its normal and disease-associated forms, and on understanding the nature of molecular interactions of PrP which occur *in vivo*. Although molecular characterization of the infectious agent of prion diseases has been attempted over the last 30 years, we are only now beginning to see structural details of the prion protein emerge. In this chapter we review what is known of the prion protein structure, its association with other molecules, and its pathogenic properties.

The idea of a protein-only infectious agent was first proposed by Griffiths (1967). However, it was not until the co-purification of prion protein with hamster scrapie infectivity that Prusiner (1982) was able to describe the infectious agent as a proteinaceous infectious particle or 'prion' in order to distinguish it from a virion or virus. The 'protein-only' hypothesis suggests that replication occurs without the requirement of informational input from DNA, and has been a point of dispute ever since. Extensive searches have been made for an informational DNA molecule which could modify the process of prion infectivity but these have so far been unsuccessful. Detailed investigations by Kellings *et al.* (1994) on DNA fragments isolated from prion preparations have not shown any homogeneous population of fragments specific for these diseases associated with infectivity. Heterogeneous populations obtained by return refocusing gel electrophoresis of hamster scrapie preparations include molecules up to 1100 nucleotides. However, if the hypothetical scrapie-specific nucleic acid were to be homogeneous in size then, on the basis of the mass of DNA observed, it would have to be less than 80 nucleotides in length.

Estimates on the number of PrP^{Sc} molecules associated with each infectious unit suggest that it is in the order of 10^5 molecules. What remains to be determined is whether this reflects the minimum amount of PrP^{Sc} necessary for infectivity or whether this is merely associated with the real infectious unit, whose molecular number to infectivity ratio is closer to one and which may be either DNA or an alternative isoform of the prion protein for which there is as yet no assay. Until alternative molecules or isoforms are isolated, the main emphasis of structural studies remains to elucidate the structure of PrP^C and PrP^{Sc}.

Mass spectrometry on PrP

According to the protein-only hypothesis, the abnormal, infectious form of the prion protein, PrP^{Sc}, is derived from the normal cellular form, PrP^{C}, by a post-translational event. This might be a covalent modification of amino acid side-chains, a novel cleavage or processing of the molecule, or might represent differences in aggregation state or conformation. The structural difference would have to account for both the biological properties, such as infectivity, and the physical properties, such as resistance to proteolytic degradation, that characterize the alternative forms of the prion protein. Mass spectrometry has been used to determine whether there are covalent modifications which distinguish PrP^{C} from PrP^{Sc}. PrP^{Sc} is a relatively insoluble molecule in normal aqueous buffers and requires denaturation in guanidine hydrochloride (GdHCl) before it can be analysed. In the most comprehensive study of PrP^{Sc} by mass spectrometry (Stahl *et al.* 1993), PrP^{Sc} was purified from infected hamster brains. Protein was solubilized in 6 M GdHCl, the disulphide bonds reduced, and cysteine residues alkylated before being precipitated from ethanol and resuspended in 0.1% sodium dodecyl sulphate (SDS). The solubilized PrP^{Sc} could then be digested with **endoproteinase-Lys-C** to generate peptide fragments that could be isolated by reverse-phase high-performance liquid chromatography and subjected to Edman sequencing. Peptides were also analysed by liquid secondary-ion mass spectrometry and electrospray mass spectrometry.

The results of these procedures were consistent with the interpretation that PrP^{Sc} contains the same amino acid sequence as that expected of PrP^{C}, following removal of the amino- and carboxy-terminal signal sequences, and that there was no covalent modification of amino acids within the sequence. However, because PrP^{C} is present at very low levels and is less easy to purify, the same experiments have not been performed on PrP^{C} itself. It is therefore possible that PrP^{C} is the covalently modified form and that loss or failure of this modification leads to PrP^{Sc} formation. The techniques applied in this study would not have been sufficiently sensitive to detect a minor subpopulation of modified PrP^{Sc}, if it existed, which could be the actual infectious form. This study also showed that, if PrP^{Sc} preparations are labelled with the hydrophobic derivative 3-(triflouromethyl)-3-(*m*-iodophenyl)diazarine (TID), the label remains associated with a macromolecule in the sample well and stacking gel of SDS-polyacrylamide gels. Although this molecule was not fully characterized it appears to be a glycosaminoglycan derivative covalently attached to lipid. This could explain why when PrP^{Sc} is re-extracted from SDS-polyacrylamide gels it appears to have only one mole of fatty acid per mole of protein compared with the four moles found before gel electrophoresis.

The results of this study have been taken to imply that there is no covalent post-translational modification which accounts for the properties of PrP^{Sc} and that there must therefore be a difference in the conformation of the two proteins.

Primary structure of PrP

To date there is no information on the three-dimensional structure of the prion protein, though the amino acid sequence determined from the gene sequence predicts certain secondary structures and possible domains (Oesch *et al.* 1985). The principle modifications of PrP nascent protein are shown in Fig. 7.1. These include amino- and carboxy-terminal signal sequences which are cleaved in the endoplasmic reticulum following synthesis. At the amino signal site there are two lysines which mark the site of signal cleavage, leaving Lys23 and Lys24 as the first two residues of the mature protein. At the carboxy terminus the cleavage occurs between serine 236 and serine 237. The remaining Ser236 is then attached to a glycosylated phosphatidylinositol (GPI) anchor (Stahl *et al.* 1987). The GPI anchor exists in six different glycoforms (Baldwin *et al.* 1990; Stahl *et al.* 1992). Two of these contain N-acetylneuraminic acid (sialic acid) which has not been seen on other GPI anchors. There are two phosphoethanolamine residues, one of which attaches the protein to the carbohydrate residues. The protein is anchored to the extracellular membrane by this anchor and can be released from the cell surface by digestion with phosphatidyl inositol-specific phospholipase C (PIPLC) (Stahl *et al.* 1990).

As the protein passes through the Golgi complex, it is progressively glycosylated on two sites, asparagine 181 and asparagine 197 (Endo *et al.* 1989; Somerville and Ritchie 1990). Sequential exoglycosidase digestion and methylation analysis shows that there is a combination of bi-, tri-, and tetra-antennary complex-type sugar chains. Nine core structures were identified of which six are further modified by sialylation to give 20 possible structures per asparagine residue, or 400 different protein structures. Studies in cell culture experiments have shown that the formation of protease-resistant PrP is not dependent on the presence of either the N-linked oligosaccharides or the GPI anchor (Taraboulos *et al.* 1990). Following cleavage of the signal sequences there remain two cysteine residues which form an internal disulphide bond. These are at positions 179 and 214, the glycosylation sites both lying within this domain.

Within the sequence there are a number of other regions of interest, although since there is no homology with amino acid sequences in the protein databases it is not clear what role any of these regions might have. At the amino-terminal end there are two series or repeats. There are two copies of a six amino acid sequence—GGS/NRYP—immediately preceding a region known as the octapeptide-repeat region. In humans this is actually a nonapeptide followed by four identical octapeptides. In the mouse there are five octapeptides here, and in sheep and goats there is a nonapeptide, three octapeptides, and a further nonapeptide. Cattle show allelic variation with either three or four octapeptides flanked by two nonapeptides. The conserved octapeptide sequence is PHGGGWGQ. The 29 amino acids preceding these repeat motifs contain six basic amino acids (three lysines and three arginines), four of which are within the first five amino acids of the molecule, and which might therefore form a domain of concentrated positive charge.

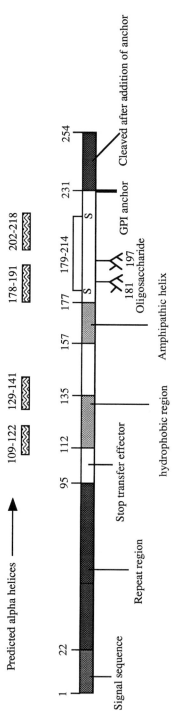

Fig. 7.1 Elements of Syrian hamster prion protein primary structure. 1–22 amino-terminal signal peptide which is removed during biosynthesis; 23–95, proline/glycine-rich region which contains four identical tandem octapeptide repeats with one similar nonapeptide; 96–112, region controlling topology of PrP called the stop transfer effector; 112–135, hydrophobic region with features of a typical transmembrane domain; 157–177, region predicted to encode an amphipathic helix; 232–254 hydrophobic signal sequence removed on addition of the glycosylated phosphatidyl inositol (GPI) anchor at serine 231. Also shown (above) are the α-helices used in the prediction of the four-helix bundle model for PrP. (Based on Prusiner *et al.* 1992.)

A 24 amino acid sequence between residues 112 and 135 is highly conserved between all species including chicken, the most divergent of all the species in which PrP has been sequenced so far (Harris *et al.* 1991). This region is comprised entirely of hydrophobic amino acids and looks like a conventional transmembrane helix. The fact that PrP can be released from cells with PIPLC suggests that this domain does not function as a transmembrane helix. However, expression of PrP in a wheat-germ cell-free translation system produced a membrane-inserted form of PrP which spanned the membrane twice. In a comparable rabbit reticulocyte expression system, the protein produced was fully translocated into lipid vesicles (Lopez *et al.* 1990). The chain translocation process has been shown to be affected by the positively charged residues adjacent to the hydrophobic domain, known as the stop transfer effector (Yost *et al.* 1990). Studies in *Xenopus* oocytes have shown that the form of PrP which spans the membrane twice exists transiently before becoming fully translocated into the lumen of the endoplasmic reticulum (De Fea *et al.* 1994) (Fig. 7.2). Expression systems in which the PrP stop transfer effector has been introduced next to other well characterized membrane domains have been

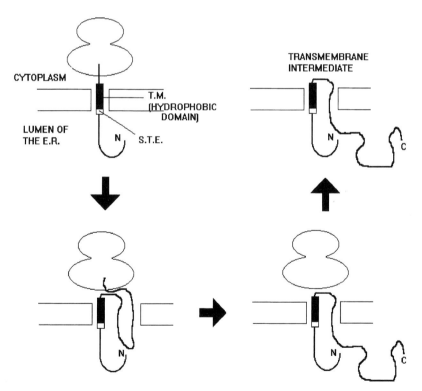

Fig. 7.2 Diagram to show the mechanism by which the stop transfer effector (STE) and the hydrophobic domains cause newly synthesized PrP to span the membrane twice. (After De Fea *et al.* 1994.) ER, endoplasmic reticulum; TM, transmembrane domain.

used to demonstrate that this region is also responsible for providing the signals necessary to complete the translocation of PrP following its transient association with the membrane. This mechanism may explain why no transmembrane isoform of PrP has been detected in normal cells but may also provide a route by which a second isoform of PrP could be generated. If the transmembrane form is normally a transient intermediate in the PrP transport process, but in some circumstances the protein becomes trapped in the membrane, then it is possible that this form will accumulate to an extent which is cytotoxic.

Octapeptide-repeat region

The N-terminal octapeptide-repeat domain of the prion protein has been an obvious target for structural studies because of its unique sequence motif and its relation to known properties of the molecule. Some patients with inherited prion disease have insertions of multiple copies of the octapeptide repeat with up to nine extra copies (Collinge and Palmer 1994), equivalent to a 72 amino acid insertion, associated with disease. However, the 27–30 kDa protease-resistant core of PrP^{Sc}, which retains infectivity, lacks the sequence containing the repeat region. This suggests that, while mutations in different parts of the molecule (including the repeat region) may be sufficient for inducing the structural changes that lead to the production of PrP^{Sc}, they may not be necessary for the transmissibility or progression of disease.

Although the octapeptide-repeat region has no direct homology with other proteins in the protein sequence database, glycine- or proline-rich repetitive sequences do exist in other proteins (Table 7.1). PrP is not strictly speaking a 'proline-rich protein' but the similarity of the octapeptide-repeat to the proline-rich repeating sequences is none the less striking. Where structural information exists for these sequences they are not seen as integral to a protein fold. Rather they form a distinct extended domain and precise three-dimensional information is often not available due to the flexibility of these regions. But in the case of the seed storage protein C hordein (Tatham *et al.* 1989), circular dichroism data of peptides to the repeat motif

Table 7.1 Examples of proline-rich repetitive sequences

Protein	Source	Sequence	Function
Salivary PRP	Man, mouse	(PQGPPQQGG)$_n$	Polyphenol binding
Gluten	Wheat	GYYPTSPQQ, PGQGQQ (many repeats)	Cereal storage protein
C-hordein	Barley	(PQQPFPQQ)$_n$	Cereal storage protein
Rhodopsin	Squid	(PPQGY)$_{10}$	Vision
Synapsin I	Man	(PQPAGPPAQ QVPPPQQG)$_n$	May regulate vesicle release

suggest that they adopt a poly-l-proline type II left-handed extended helix at low temperatures. Recently we have shown that synthetic peptides corresponding to the octapeptide-repeat region of PrP give similar circular dichroism spectra at room temperature. This implies that the N-terminal octapeptide-repeat region could form an extended, flexible domain in the poly-l-proline type II conformation. This is a 'stretched out' helical structure with three residues per turn. Since in the mature protein lacking the amino-terminal signal sequences the octapeptide-repeat region is very close to the amino terminus, it is possible that this domain sticks out of the molecule carrying the six positively charged amino acids away from the rest of the protein.

One possible function of proline-rich repetitive sequences is to act as a low-specificity binding domain, the length and flexibility of which would allow rapid assembly of proteins into a complex (Williamson 1994). Since it has been shown that PrP may play a role in normal synaptic function (see Chapter 6) it is interesting to observe that a number of other proline-rich proteins are associated with the synapse. For some of these, more is known about the mechanism of their function. In the case of synapsin I, phosphorylation of the serines in the proline-rich region (Benfanati *et al.* 1992) reduces its binding to a second vesicle-associated protein (as yet incompletely characterized). At least two other synaptic proteins—synaptophysin and vesicle-associated membrane protein-1—contain proline-rich regions and it seems likely that these domains facilitate the interaction of synaptic proteins to form a system by which synaptic vesicles are activated for release (Trimble and Scheller 1988). It remains to be established whether the PrP octapeptide-repeat domain facilitates the interaction of PrP^C with other proteins.

Hydrophobic region

Synthetic peptides have again been used to examine the properties of the hydrophobic domain discussed above. The peptide which we have used for our own studies contains the hydrophobic domain (underlined) flanked by an additional eight amino acids:

KTNMKH<u>MAGAAAAGAVVGGLGGYVLGSAM</u>SR.

In the absence of detergent or membrane mimetic solvents, the peptide adopts a predominantly random coil and β-sheet conformation, as determined by circular dichroism. However, in detergents such as sodium dodecyl sulphate (SDS) or the solvent trifluoroethanol (TFE), the predominant conformation is that of an α-helix (see Fig. 7.3). Such behaviour is typical of isolated segments of membrane-spanning proteins.

A number of smaller peptides from the hydrophobic region have been generated and their properties studied *in vitro*. One (Forloni *et al.* 1993) has been shown to induce apoptotic cell death in cultural hippocampal neurones and to spontaneously form amyloid fibrils (Gasset *et al.* 1992; Goldfarb *et al.* 1993; Selvaggini *et al.*

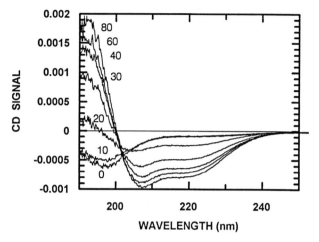

Fig. 7.3 Trifluoroethanol (TFE/water) titration of hydrophobic peptide, valine variant ('TM'-V, valine variant of transmembrane region) monitored by circular dichroism (units are delta epsilon). The concentration of peptide was 0.2 mg/ml and the path length of the cell was 1 mm. The percentage (v/v) of TFE used is shown on each spectrum.

1993). Biophysical studies on this peptide (Selvaggini *et al.* 1993) show it to exist in a number of conformational states depending on the solution conditions used. In 50% TFE or 5% SDS the α-helical conformation predominates, while addition of phosphate buffer at pH 5.0 to the peptide in 50% TFE induces a greater proportion of β-sheet. This sensitivity of peptide conformation to solution conditions, together with the persistence of β-sheet structure even in conditions which strongly induce α-helices, may explain the tendency of this peptide to aggregate into amyloid fibrils and suggests ways by which a pathogenic conformational change could be induced in the cell. It remains to be seen whether these observations are relevant to the properties of the intact prion protein or artefacts of the peptide system.

Secondary structure of PrP

PrP^{Sc}

The method adopted for obtaining secondary structural information from PrP^{Sc} highlights the difficulties involved in studying an insoluble protein. Standard spectroscopic techniques such as circular dichroism are not appropriate because of their requirement for a soluble sample. It has therefore been necessary to use a method which could accommodate a sample in the solid state. Attenuated total reflection fourier transform infra-red spectroscopy (ATR-FTIR) is one such method. Studies carried out on PrP 27–30 (the 27–30 kDa protease-resistant core of PrP^{Sc}) indicated a secondary structure composition of 54% β-sheet, 25% α-helix, 10% turns, and 11% random coil (Gasset *et al.* 1993). Around two-thirds of the β-sheet signal is characteristic of that associated with intermolecular aggregation. This is consistent with the ultrastructural properties of PrP 27–30, which forms rod-shaped amyloid polymers as a result of the treatment with detergents required for its purification. Although the rod-shaped polymers formed by PrP 27–30 are the result of a purification artefact and probably do not exist before extraction, amyloid plaques consisting of PrP are deposited in the brains of most individuals with prion disease. By contrast solubilized PrP^{Sc}, assumed to be closer in conformation to PrP^{C}, was found by ATR-FTIR to have a lower proportion of short wavelength β-sheet structure and therefore a higher overall α content.

PrP^{C}

PrP^{C} is a soluble protein and it might be expected that detailed structural information would be easier to obtain. However, since the principal source of this protein is brain homogenate, and the natural abundance of PrP^{C} is very low even in brain, pure material is both scarce and difficult to produce. This problem can be overcome by the use of expression systems producing normal protein in either bacterial or eukaryotic systems. Those comparative studies made so far suggest that PrP^{C} is rich in α-helix content (42%) and has almost no β-sheet content (3%) (Pan *et al.* 1993).

The differences in β-sheet and α-helix content of PrP^{Sc} and PrP^{C} have suggested that it is conversion of α-helices to β-sheet structure which underlies the production of PrP^{Sc} and strengthens the argument in favour of a conformational difference underlying the disease process.

Proposed tertiary structure of PrP

Based on sequence alignment, secondary structure prediction methods and computational methods for estimating helix–helix packing interactions, Huang *et al.* (1994) have proposed a three-dimensional structure for PrP^{C}. They present four possible arrangements of a four-helix bundle model of PrP^{C} and note that in one arrangement (the X-bundle structure), five of the known pathogenic point mutations occur within its central hydrophobic core. While this is only a hypothetical model it does perhaps allow consideration of strategies to demonstrate whether there are any components of the model which are accurate or which may predict functional properties of the molecule.

NMR solution structure of mouse prion protein domain PrP (121–231) (section added in proof)

Riek *et al.* (1996) have determined the NMR structure of a mouse prion protein domain corresponding to residues 121–231 in the whole protein. This fragment folds independently and cooperatively and is resistant to degradation when expressed in

E. coli. The solution structure of the domain shows it to contain one anti-parallel β-sheet and three α-helices. This is in contrast with the three-dimensional model described (see previous section) by Huang *et al.* of a four-helix bundle for residues 109–218. The approximate positions of the α-helices seen in the NMR structure are from residues 144–154, 179–193, and 200–217. The β-strands are found between residues 128 and 131 and between residues 161 and 164. The domain does not include the distinctive N-terminal octa-repeat region and includes only a part of the hydrophobic region between 106 and 137. Residues 109–121, 129–141, 178–191 and 202–218 were predicted to form α-helices by Huang *et al.* Of these, the helices proposed at 178–191 and 202–218 accord with the α-helices observed via NMR but residues 121–137 in the solution structure contain only a short β-strand. This difference may be due to the absence of residues prior to 121 in PrP (121–231) or, alternatively, to the effect of the folding of this domain. Whether or not β-sheet will feature in the structure of the entire protein, it is interesting to note its presence in this folded fragment of the prion protein and the possibility suggested by Riek *et al.* that it may help initiate the conversion of PrP^C to PrP^{Sc}. The authors also note that many of the point mutations which cause the familial forms of prion disease are positioned either within or next to ordered secondary structures. This suggests that such mutations may exert their pathogenic effect by destabilizing the fold of the protein.

Binding of PrP to other proteins

The properties both of normal and infectious PrP argue that it may bind to other proteins either as part of its normal function or during the disease process. Observations which lead to this conclusion include the finding of region-specific prion replication in hamster brain following intraocular injection, possibly by anterograde transport of prions along neuroanatomical pathways (Scott and Fraser 1989), and the stimulation of astrocyte proliferation by PrP^{Sc} (Dearmond *et al.* 1992). Both of these imply a possible receptor for PrP. The identification and characterization of PrP-binding proteins could therefore promote understanding of both the normal and pathogenic function of PrP. Oesch and colleagues used the ligand blot technique to try to identify any major PrP ligands (designated Plis) (Oesch *et al.* 1990; Oesch 1994). Postnuclear supernatant from normal hamster brain homogenates was pelleted at 100 000 G and cytoplasmic proteins released by osmotic shock. Two PrP-binding proteins, of 110 kDa and 125 kDa, were found in this membrane fraction, and named Pli-110 and Pli-125, respectively. An internal peptide hamster of PrP from residues 140–174 (peptide P5) was used as a probe for both of these proteins. Pli-110 and Pli-125 could be released from the membrane fraction by alkaline wash with sodium carbonate (pH 11.5) suggesting that they were not integral membrane proteins. In addition to Pli-110 and Pli-125, a 45 kDa membrane protein was found to bind PrP and subsequently shown to be glial fibrillary acidic protein. More work will be needed to determine whether any of these proteins play a role in PrP function or whether the binding observed was non-specific.

Intracellular processing of chick PrP

Studies on the processing of chicken PrP^C (chPrP) have been facilitated by the capacity to generate region-specific monoclonal antibodies in mice because of its greater sequence divergence from mammalian PrP. Chicken PrP transfected into mouse neuroblastoma cells and in chicken brain and cerebrospinal fluid (CSF) has been shown to undergo at least two cleavages during its normal metabolism—one within the glycosylphosphatidylinositol anchor and one within the protein itself (Harris *et al.* 1993). The site of the latter cleavage is between Thr114 and Met137 which encompasses the stretch of hydrophobic amino acids that is highly conserved between chicken and mammalian PrPs. Fragments relating to these two processing events have been found in the extracellular medium from conditioned medium, brain supernatant and CSF. The likely site of cleavage within the GPI anchor lies between the ethanolamine residue attaching the anchor to the protein and the diacylglycerol moiety. Borchelt *et al.* (1993) have also reported the secretion of a minority of PrP^C molecules from the cell surface of primary cultures of Syrian hamster brain following periods of metabolic labelling, all of which appear to lack the GPI anchor. The absence of a GPI anchor was inferred from the solubility of the secreted protein in the aqueous phase of a triton X-114 extract in the same manner as PIPLC released PrP^C. PrP^C, which remains bound to cells, partitions in the detergent phase.

　　Further studies have revealed that chPrP constitutively cycles between the cell surface and an endocytic compartment in around 60 minutes, with more than 95% of the protein being returned to the surface intact (Shyng *et al.* 1993). During this process about 1% of the protein per hour is proteolytically cleaved within the conserved stretch of hydrophobic amino acids as described in Fig. 7.4. It is believed that this cleavage takes place in an acidified endocytic compartment. The carboxyl-terminal fragment which is produced accumulates at the cell surface for up to 24 hours. Endocytosis of chPrP has now been shown to be mediated by clathrin-coated pits (Shyng *et al.* 1994). ChPrP is seen in coated pits both in transfected mouse neuroblastoma cells and in coated vesicles purified from chicken brain. Treatments which disrupt clathrin lattices and so inhibit endocytosis, reduced internalization of chPrP in neuroblastoma cells by 70%. Interestingly the authors found that deletion of the N-terminal 67 amino acids greatly reduced the efficiency of chPrP endocytosis and reduced its association with clathrin-coated pits. This includes much of the proline–glycine-rich repeat region which is analogous to the octapeptide-repeat region in mammals.

Inhibition of scrapie formation *in vitro*

Studies on scrapie-infected mouse neuroblastoma cells (Caughey and Raymond 1993; Gabizon *et al.* 1993) show that formation of protease-resistant PrP^{Sc} can be prevented by incubating cells in a range of sulphated glycosaminoglycans which include heparin, chondroitin sulphate, hyaluronic acid, and dermatan sulphate. Subsequent studies (Caughey *et al.* 1994) demonstrated binding of extracts containing PrP^C to heparin–agarose. Congo red, a dye which is traditionally used to stain for

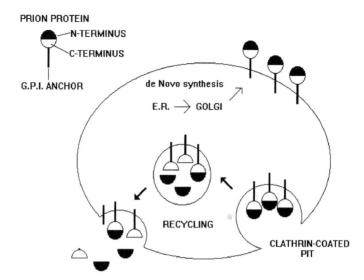

Fig. 7.4 The proteolytic processing and cycling of chPrP. ChPrP is cleaved within the protein in the vesicle and exported to the cell surface. A subsequent cleavage within the GPI anchor results in both N- and C-terminal fragments being released into the extracellular medium.

amyloid, has similar binding properties. The facts that Congo red is able to displace PrP^C from heparin agarose and that PrP^C bound to Congo red glass beads is displaced by heparin suggest that the two compounds share a common binding site. It is suggested that inhibition of PrP^{Sc} accumulation occurs by successfully competing for binding to PrP^C with an endogenous proteoglycan or glycosaminoglycan.

In vitro support for the prion hypothesis

Despite the observation that PrP^{Sc} could be derived from PrP^C in tissue culture, it was not at first clear whether this conversion can only take place in the presence of a cell as a consequence of a complex membrane associated biology, or whether the model of interaction and conversion holds as a purely physical process that could take place between purified molecules *in vitro*. This question has now been answered with respect to the conversion of a proteinase-K susceptible isoform into a resistant isoform. Kocisko and colleagues (1994) have established conditions under which PrP^{Sc}, purified from affected hamster brains, can be denatured in guanidine hydrochloride (GdHCl) and then renatured over a period of 48 hours. Immediately after denaturation the protein was sensitive to proteinase-K digestion, but protease-resistant material reappeared within two minutes and was maximal after two days. Denaturation took place in 3 M GdHCl and refolding occurred after diluting to 0.75 M GdHCl with 130 mM NaCl, 10 mM Tris pH7.0. Since this process of refolding did not occur when PrP^{Sc} was first treated with 6 M GdHCl, it was argued that 6 M GdHCl causes complete denaturation of every molecule while

3 M GdHCl may have resulted in some molecules retaining their native PrP^{Sc} conformation and seeding a conversion event.

To see whether PrP^C is capable of being converted from the denatured state by PrP^{Sc}, radiolabelled PrP^C was immunoprecipitated from tissue culture cells, denatured with 3 M GdHCl and mixed with the unlabelled 3 M GdHCl-denatured PrP^{Sc}. The mixture was again diluted to 0.75 M GdHCl. After two days, radiolabelled material was found that was resistant to proteinase-K and other proteases, indicating that a conversion of conformation had taken place. To test for the specificity of this conversion a mixture of ^{35}S-labelled proteins was added to the PrP^{Sc} renaturation reaction. All of these remained proteolytically sensitive after two days.

This *in vitro* conversion assay has been used to address further questions about both species and strain specificity. The protocol was used to demonstrate that mouse PrP^C could be converted by mouse PrP^{Sc}, while the hamster PrP^{Sc} could not convert this mouse PrP^C (Kocisko *et al.* 1995). This suggests that the species barrier to conversion is at the level of the protein interaction and mimics the situation seen in animal studies. By contrast the reciprocal conversion of hamster PrP^C by mouse PrP^{Sc} was permissible. However, the products showed a different molecular mass following proteinase-K digestion than was generated by conversion with hamster PrP^{Sc} (18 kDa compared with 25 kDa). Increasing the concentration of GdHCl concentration in the refolding reaction showed a species sensitivity. Conversion of mouse PrP^C to PrP^{Sc} was efficient up to 2 M GdHCl, while the efficiency of conversion of hamster PrP^C by the mouse PrP^{Sc} was reduced as the concentration increased.

One requirement of the protein-only hypothesis for prion propagation is that the transfer of strain properties must be mediated by stable variations in PrP^{Sc} structure. To test this, advantage was made of the molecular weight differences of the PrP^{Sc} of two hamster strains, drowsy and hyper. After proteinase-K digestion, hyper PrP^{Sc} is about 1 kDa higher molecular weight than drowsy PrP^{Sc}. When PrP^{Sc} from either strain was mixed with normal hamster PrP^C the conversion product was of the same size as the seeding strain. This demonstrates that the site available for proteinase-K digestion, which is a property of the individual strain, is exposed during the conversion and that the conversion product must therefore adopt the same conformation as the seeding molecule. Strain differences therefore do not require additional information from a nucleic acid or other molecule to account for their presence.

These studies provide some evidence for the selective conversion of PrP^C into PrP^{Sc} in a cell-free system. While this does not rule out the possibility of other molecules being involved as co-factors in the conversion within cells, it does demonstrate that there is no requirement for the biosynthesis of new macromolecules.

Prion homologues

p53

A pathogenic mechanism in which one form of protein induces a conformational change in the other and so confers on it a similar ability to bind and convert other normal molecules may not apply exclusively to the prion diseases. The process by which mutant forms of the tumour-suppressor protein p53 cause tumour progression has similar characteristics. Mutations within conserved domains of the p53 gene cause loss of tumour-suppressor activity and can also cause activation of p53 as an oncogene. Co-translation of wild-typed and activated mutant p53 *in vitro* results in the conversion by mutant p53 of wild-type p53 to the mutant conformation. *In vivo*, such a process would result in the removal of the tumour-suppressor effect of wild-type p53 and this may explain the dominant negative effect of activating p53 mutations on tumour progression (Milner and Medcalf 1991).

Yeast prions

The proposal of the protein recruitment model for prion replication has resulted in the suggestion by Wickner (1994) that a prion-like mechanism may exist in yeast as well as mammals. In one strain of yeast the phenotype is defined by a cytoplasmically inherited element, termed [URE3]. This enables a strain of yeast to use ureidosuccinate despite the presence of ammonium ions (which inhibit its uptake). [URE3] is related to the *URE2* gene and its product, Ure2p, in a number of ways. First, the same phenotype can be induced by chromosomal mutations in the *URE2* gene. Second, propagation of the factor [URE3] depends on the presence of Ure2p. Third, the frequency with which a strain adopted the [URE3] phenotype could be increased greatly by overproduction of Ure2p. The phenotype can be cured by growing yeast strains in the presence of guanidine hydrochloride. However, growth of a cured strain under conditions selective for [URE3] resulted in reappearance of the phenotype without the need to introduce it from other cells. The explanation for this behaviour proposed by Wickner draws on the prion hypothesis in that [URE3] could be an alternative inactive form of Ure2p which is able to convert normal Ure2p to the inactive form.

Wickner also proposed that a second yeast phenotype, [*psi*], which allows efficient t-RNA-mediated nonsense suppression, may have a prion-like determinant. The candidate protein is the product of the *SUP35* gene (Sup35p) (Ter-Avanesyan *et al.* 1994). Interestingly, Sup35p contains a series of several tandem nonapeptide repeats at its N-terminal domain. The repeats are not exact but the consensus sequence is PQGGYQQYN. This sequence is similar to the prion octapeptide-repeat domain in its amino acid composition, although technically it has negligible sequence homology. In yeast, deletion mutations in this region result in a genetically recessive loss of the nonsense-suppression function which may be corrected by overexpression of the N-terminal 114 amino acids of sup35p in *trans*. Furthermore, a single mutation in the second repeat of glycine to aspartate results in loss of the [*psi*⁺] phenotype, a fact which emphasizes the specificity of the sequence required for its maintenance. This demonstration of a functional role for a series of repeats so similar to the prion octapeptide-repeat region is clearly worthy of note, especially in a protein which may be able to transmit is functional properties via a prion-like mechanism.

Relationship of prion structure to function

It is clear that a three-dimensional structure for PrP is needed for full characterization of its structure–function properties. However, the studies outlined in this chapter do provide information concerning the role of some regions of primary structure in both the normal and pathogenic properties of PrP.

Role of the N-terminal repeat region

Studies both on a peptide to the octapeptide-repeat region and on chPrP *in vivo* suggest that the N-terminal repeats have a functional role within the protein. In yeast the repeat region seems to play a crucial role in the characteristics of a strain phenotype, to the extent that a point mutation in one repeat removes the phenotype. The requirement in chicken for the N-terminal repeat region for cycling suggests that it may be involved in binding to a receptor on clathrin-coated vesicles. If this region is involved in non-specific binding of other proteins then it may be required to 'catch' the receptor to allow specific binding at other sites to take place.

Hydrophobic region is cleaved in chPrP and fully conserved

Data concerning the role of the conserved hydrophobic region for normal PrP function is still scarce. One processing event in chPrP involves cleavage within this region but this has not been shown in human PrP. There are more clues concerning the pathogenic function of PrP. The fact that heterozygosity at codon 129 confers some degree of protection from human iatrogenic and sporadic prion disease (Collinge *et al.* 1991; Palmer *et al.* 1991) implies that a highly specific protein–protein interaction at this site is involved in pathogenesis. The strong tendency of peptides to this region to form amyloid fibrils in solution also suggests that it has a role in disease. Finally the demonstration *in vitro* that PrP adopts a transiently membrane-inserted form under some conditions shows how a conformational change might arise and be dictated by the hydrophobic domain and its stop transfer effector. The studies conducted on the 106–126 peptide indicate that the conformation of the hydrophobic domain is very sensitive to solution conditions and prone to aggregate into amyloid fibrils. A region of ambiguous conformation with the potential to alter membrane topology is intriguing. It seems likely that the hydrophobic domain plays a significant part in both the normal and pathogenic role of PrP.

Does PrP bind to the extracellular matrix?

The discovery that sulphated glycosaminoglycans can inhibit scrapie formation has generated speculation that PrP may bind to a proteoglycan *in vivo*. It could be that the pathogenic form is able to bind a proteoglycan which may act as a receptor while the normal form does not. This could result in abnormal transport and processing of PrP which, given the tendency of some of its peptides to form amyloid, could prove detrimental to the cell. One other possibility is that PrP binds reversibly to a proteoglycan (perhaps the extracellular matrix) in its normal form and some change increases the tightness of its binding such that the normal interactions and processing of PrP are disrupted. Irreversible binding to a proteoglycan could render PrP protease resistant. It is possible that a proteoglycan could bind more than one PrP molecule and so promote association of abnormal PrP molecules.

Why is PrP^{Sc} pathogenic?

The answer to this question is still not fully known. PrP^{Sc} is resistant to proteolysis and accumulates within affected cells. It could be that the inability of a cell to regulate build-up of this protein results in disruption of processes vital to its survival. On the other hand, the electrophysiology of PrP-null mice indicates that symptoms such as epilepsy experienced by patients with CJD may be explained by the loss of functional PrP^{C} rather than the acquisition of a new pathogenic 'function' by PrP^{Sc}. It is possible then that the acquisition of protease-resistance and consequent accumulation of PrP may not be the primary cause of the disease symptoms. Although it may prove useful to investigate therapy which could inhibit the formation of protease-resistance PrP, success in this area may not be sufficient to cure the disease. Prevention of accumulation of protease-resistant PrP may well be of therapeutic benefit in that it may limit progression of the disease and reduce infectivity. However if the disease is due to a loss of normal PrP function then the initial causes also become important.

References

Baldwin, M. A., Stahl, N., Reinders, L. G., Gibson, B. W., Prusiner, S. B., and Burlingame, A. L. (1990). Permethylation and tandem mass spectrometry of oligosaccharides having free hexosamine: analysis of the glycoinositol phospholipid anchor glycan from the scrapie prion protein. *Analytical Biochemistry*, **191**, 174–182.

Benfanati, F., Valtorta, F., Rubenstain, J., Gorelick, F., Greegard, P., and Czernik, A. (1992) Synaptic vesicle-associated Ca^{2+}/calmodulin-dependent protein kinase II is a binding protein form synapsin I. *Nature*, **359**, 417–420.

Borchelt, D. R., Rogers, M., Stahl, N., Telling, G., and Prusiner, S. B. (1993). Release of the cellular prion protein from cultured cells after loss of its glycoinositol phospholipid anchor. *Glycobiology*, **3**, 319–329.

Caughey, B. and Raymond, G. J. (1993). Sulfated polyanion inhibition of scrapie-associated PrP accumulation in cultured-cells. *Journal of Virology*, **67**, 643–650.

Caughey, B., Brown, K., Raymond, G. J., Katzenstein, G. E., and Thresher, W. (1994). Binding of the protease-sensitive form of prion protein PrP to sulfated glycosaminoglycan and congo red. *Journal of Virology*, **68**, 2135–2141.

Collinge, J. and Palmer, M. (1994). Human prion diseases. In *Genetics in neurology* (ed. A. Harding), pp. 241–257. Bailliére Tindall, London.

Collinge, J., Palmer, M. S., and Dryden, A. J. (1991). Genetic predisposition to iatrogenic Creutzfeldt–Jakob disease. *Lancet*, **337**, 1441–1442.

De Fea, K., Nakahara, D., Calayag, M., Yost, C. S., Mirels, L. F., Prusiner, S. B., and Lingappa, V. R. (1994). Determinants of carboxyl-terminal domain translocation during prion protein biogenesis. *Journal of Biological Chemistry*, **269**, 16810–16820.

Dearmond, S. J., Kristensson, K., and Bowler, R. P. (1992). PrP^{Sc} causes nerve-cell death and stimulates astrocyte proliferation—a paradox. *Progress in Brain Research*, **94**, 437–446.

Endo, T., Groth, D., Prusiner, S. B., and Kobata, A. (1989). Diversity of oligosaccharide structures linked to asparagines of the scrapie prion protein. *Biochemistry*, **28**, 8380–8388.

Forloni, G., Angeretti, N., Chielsa, R., Monzani, E., Salmona, M., Bugiani, O., and Tagliavini, F. (1993). Neurotoxicity of a prion protein fragment. *Nature*, **362**, 543–546.

Gabizon, R., Meiner, Z., Halimi, M., and Ben, S. S. (1993). Heparin-like molecules bind differentially to prion-proteins and change their intracellular metabolic fate. *Journal of Cellular Physiology*, **157**, 319–325.

Gasset, M., Baldwin, M. A., Lloyd, D. H., Gabriel, J. -M., Holtzman, D. M., Cohen, F., *et al.* (1992). Predicted α-helical regions of the prion protein when synthesized as peptides form amyloid. *Proceedings of the National Academy of Sciences of the USA*, **89**, 10940–10944.

Gasset, M., Baldwin, M. A., Fletterick, R. J., and Prusiner, S. B. (1993). Perturbation of the secondary structure of the scrapie prion protein under conditions that alter infectivity. *Proceedings of the National Academy of Sciences of the USA*, **90**, 1–5.

Goldfarb, L. G., Brown, P., Haltia, M., Ghiso, J., Frangione, B., and Gajdusek, D. C. (1993). Synthetic peptides corresponding to different mutated regions of the amyloid gene in familial Creutzfeldt–Jakob disease show enhanced *in vitro* formation of morphologically different amyloid fibrils. *Proceedings of the National Academy of Sciences of the USA*, **90**, 4451–4454.

Griffiths, J. (1967). Self replication and scrapie. *Nature*, **215**, 1043–1044.

Harris, D. A., Falls, D. L., Johnson, F. A., and Fischbach, G. D. (1991). A prion-like protein from chicken brain copurifies with an acetylcholine receptor-inducing activity. *Proceedings of the National Academy of Sciences of the USA*, **88**, 7664–7668.

Harris, D. A., Huber, M. T., Vandijken, P., Shyng, S. L., Chait, B. T., and Wang, R. (1993). Processing of a cellular prion protein—identification of N-terminal and C-terminal cleavage sites. *Biochemistry*, **32**, 1009–1016.

Huang, Z., Gabriel, J. -M., Baldwin, M., Fletterick, R., Prusiner, S., and Cohen, F. (1994). Proposed three-dimensional structure for the cellular prion protein. *Proceedings of the National Academy of Sciences of the USA*, **91**, 7139–7143.

Kellings, K., Prusiner, S., and Reisner, D. (1994). Nucleic acids in prion preparations: unspecific background or essential component? *Philosophical Transactions of the Royal Society of London*, **343**, 425–430.

Kocisko, D., Come, J., Priola, S., Chesebro, B., Raymond, G., Lansbury, P., *et al.* (1994). Cell-free formation of protease-resistant prion protein. *Nature*, **370**, 471–474.

Kocisko. D., Priola, S., Raymond, G., Chesebro, B., Lansbury, P., and Caughey, B. (1995). Species specificity in the cell-free conversion of prion protein to protease-resistant forms: a model for the scrapie species barrier. *Proceedings of the National Academy of Sciences of the USA*, **92**, 3923–3927.

Lopez, C. D., Yost, C. S., Prusiner, S. B., Myers, R. M., and Lingappa, V. R. (1990). Unusual topogenic sequence directs prion protein biogenesis. *Science*, **248**, 226–229.

Milner, J. and Medcalf, E. A. (1991). Cotranslation of activated mutant p53 with wild type drives the wild type p53 protein into the mutant conformation. *Cell*, **65**, 765–774.

Oesch, B. (1994). Characterization of PrP binding proteins. *Philosophical Transactions of the Royal Society of London*, **343**, 443–445.

Oesch, B., Westaway, D., Walchli, M., McKinley, M. P., Kent, S. B., Aebersold, R., *et al.* (1985). A cellular gene encodes scrapie PrP 27-30 protein. *Cell*, **40**, 735–746.

Oesch, B., Teplow, D. B., Stahl, N., Serban, D., Hood, L. E., and Prusiner, S. B. (1990). Identification of cellular proteins binding to the scrapie prion protein. *Biochemistry*, **29**, 5848–5855.

Palmer, M. S., Dryden, A. J., Hughes, J. T., and Collinge, J. (1991). Homozygous prion protein genotype predisposes to sporadic Creutzfeldt–Jakob disease. *Nature*, **352**, 340–342.

Pan, K. M., Baldwin, M., Nguyen, J., Gasset, M., Serban, A., Groth, D., *et al.* (1993). Conversion of alpha-helices into beta-sheets features in the formation of the scrapie prion proteins. *Proceedings of the National Academy of Sciences of the USA*, **90**, 10962–10966.

Prusiner, S. B. (1982). Novel proteinaceous infectious particles cause scrapie. *Science*, **216**, 136–144.

Riek, R., Hornemann, S., Wider, G., Billeter, M., Glockshuber, R. and Würthrich, K. (1996). NMR structure of the mouse prion protein domain PrP(121–231). *Nature*, **382**, 180–182.

Scott, J. R. and Fraser, H. (1989). Transport and targeting of scrapie infectivity and pathology in the optic nerve projections following intraocular infection. *Progress in Clinical and Biological Research*, **317**, 645–652.

Selvaggini, C., De, G. L., Cantu, L., Ghibaudi, E., Diomede, L., Passerini, F., *et al.* (1993). Molecular characteristics of a protease-resistant, amyloidogenic and neurotoxic peptide homologous to residues 106–126 of the prion protein. *Biochemical and Biophysical Research Communications*, **194**, 1380–1386.

Shyng, S.-L., Huber, M. T., and Harris, D. A. (1993). A prion protein cycles between the cell surface and an endocytic compartment in cultured neuroblastoma cells. *Journal of Biological Chemistry*, **268**, 15922–15928.

Shyng, S.-L., Heuser, J., and Harris, D. (1994). A glycolipid-anchored prion protein is endocytosed via clathrin coated pits. *Journal of Cell Biology,* **125**, 1239–1250.

Somerville, R. A. and Ritchie, L. A. (1990). Differential glycosylation of the protein (PrP) forming scrapie-associated fibrils. *Journal of General Virology*, **71**, 833–839.

Stahl, N., Borchelt, D. R., Hsiao, K., and Prusiner, S. B. (1987). Scrapie prion protein contains a phosphatidylinositol glycolipid. *Cell*, **51**, 229–240.

Stahl, N., Borchelt, D. R., and Prusiner, S. B. (1990). Differential release of cellular and scrapie prion proteins from cellular membranes by phosphatidylinositol-specific phospholipase C. *Biochemistry*, **29**, 5405–5412.

Stahl, N., Baldwin, M. A., Hecker, R., Pan, K. M., Burlingame, A. L. and Prusiner, S. B. (1992). Glycosylinositol phospholipid anchors of the scrapie and cellular prion proteins contain sialic-acid. *Biochemistry*, **31**, 5043–5053.

Stahl, N., Baldwin, M. A., Teplow, D. B., Hood, L., Gibson, B. W., Burlingame, A. L., *et al.* (1993). Structural studies of the scrapie prion protein using mass-spectrometry and amino-acid sequencing. *Biochemistry*, **32**, 1991–2002.

Taraboulos, A., Rogers, M., Borchelt, D. R., McKinley, M. P., Scott, M., Serban, D., *et al.* (1990). Acquisition of protease resistance by prion proteins in scrapie-infected cells does not require asparagine-linked glycosylation. *Proceedings of the National Academy of Sciences of the USA*, **87**, 8262–8266.

Tatham, A. S., Drake, A. F. and Shewry, P. R. (1989). Conformational studies of a synthetic peptide corresponding to the repeat domain of C-hordein. *Biochemical Journal*, **259**, 471–476.

Ter-Avanesyan, M., Dagkesamanskaya, A., Kushnirov, V., and Smirnov, V. (1994). The *SUP35* omnipotent suppressor gene is involved in the maintenance of the non-mendelian determinant [*psi*+] in the yeast *Saccharomyces cerevisiae*. *Genetics*, **137**, 671–676.

Trimble, W. and Scheller, R. (1988). Molecular biology of synaptic vesicle-associated proteins. *Trends in Neurosciences*, **11**, 241–242.

Wickner, R. B. (1994). [URE3] as an altered URE2 protein: evidence for a prion analog in *Saccharomyces cerevisiae*. *Science*, **264**, 566–569.

Williamson, M. (1994). The structure and function of proline-rich regions in proteins. *Journal of Biochemistry*, **297**, 249–260.

Yost, C. S., Lopez, C. D., Prusiner, S. B., Myers, R. M., and Lingappa, V. R. (1990). Non-hydrophobic extracytoplasmic determinant of stop transfer in the prion protein. *Nature*, **343**, 669–672.

Appendix: Alignment of amino acids of the prion protein from eleven species

Numbering of amino acids is based on the human sequence in the first row. All sequences are taken from data submitted to the EMBL database. The mouse sequence corresponds to that of the NZW short incubation time allele and differs from the long incubation allele at positions indicated here as 109 (Leu/Phe) and 190 (Thr/Val). Because of the absence of glycine at position 55 in the mice these residues are 108 and 189 in the mouse sequence. The cow allele is shown as having six octapeptide repeats between residues 51 and 92, but bovine PrP contains either five or six repeats. The final repeat of mink, sheep and goat contain nine amino acids rather than usual eight and are shown displaced from the final octapeptide of the human sequence (between 91–92) aligned with the sixth repeat of cow which also contains nine amino acids. Amino acids which are identical in all species shown are outlined.

	1	2	3	4	5	6	7	8	9	10	11	12	13	14	15	16	17	18	19	20	21	22	23	24	25	26	27	28	29	30	31	32	33	34	35	36	37
Human	M	A	N	L	G	C	W	M	L	V	L	F	V	A	T	W	S	D	L	G	L	C	K	K	R	P	K	P	G	G	W	N	T	G	G	S	R
Gorilla	M	A	N	L	G	C	W	M	L	V	L	F	V	A	T	W	S	D	L	G	L	C	K	K	R	P	K	P	G	G	W	N	T	G	G	S	R
Chimpanzee	M	A	N	L	G	C	W	M	L	V	L	F	V	A	T	W	S	D	L	G	L	C	K	K	R	P	K	P	G	G	W	N	T	G	G	S	R
Mouse	M	A	N	L	G	Y	W	L	L	A	L	F	V	T	M	W	T	D	V	G	L	C	K	K	R	P	K	P	G	G	W	N	T	G	G	S	R
Rat																															W	N	T	G	G	S	R
Syrian Hamster	M	A	N	L	G	S	W	L	L	L								D				C	K	K	R	P	K	P	G	G	W	N	T	G	G	S	R
Mink	M	V	K	S	H	I	G	S	W	L		L	F	V		M	W	S	D	V	G	L	C	K	K	R	P	K	P	G	G	G	W	N	T	G	G	S	R
Sheep	M	V	K	S	H	I	G	S	W	I		L	F	V		M	W	S	D	V	G	L	C	K	K	R	P	K	P	G	G	G	W	N	T	G	G	S	R
Goat	M	V	K	S	H		G	S	W	I		L	F	V		M	W	S	D	V	G	L	C	K	K	R	P	K	P	G	G	G	W	N	T	G	G	S	R
Cow	M	V	K	S	H	I	G	S	W			L	F	V		M	W	S	D	V	A	L	C	K	K	R	P	K	P	G	G	G	W	N	T	G	G	S	R
Greater Kudu	M	V	K	S	H	I	G	S	W	I		L	F	V		M	W	S	D	V	A	L	C	K	K	R	P	K	P	G	G	G	W	N	T	G	G	S	R

	38	39	40	41	42	43	44	45	46	47	48	49	50	51	52	53	54	55	56	57	58	59	60	61	62	63	64	65	66	67	68	69	70	71	72	73	74	75	76	77
Human	Y	P	G	Q	G	S	P	G	G	N	R	Y	P	P	Q	G	G	G	W	G	Q	P	H	G	G	G	W	G	Q	P	H	G	G	G	G	W	G	Q	P	H
Gorilla	Y	P	G	Q	G	S	P	G	G	N	R	Y	P	P	Q	G	G	G	W	G	Q	P	H	G	G	G	W	G	Q	P	H	G	G	G	G	W	G	Q	P	H
Chimpanzee	Y	P	G	Q	G	S	P	G	G	N	R	Y	P	P	Q	G	G	G	W	G	Q	P	H	G	G	G	W	G	Q	P	H	G	G	G	G	W	G	Q	P	H
Mouse	Y	P	G	Q	G	G	G	T	H	N	Q	W	N	K	P	S	K	P	K	T	N	G	Q	P	H	G	G	S	W	G	Q	P	H	G	G	S	W	G	Q	P
Rat	Y	P	G	Q	G	G	G	T	H	N	Q	W	N	K	P	S	K	P	K	T	N	G	Q	P	H	G	G	G	W	G	Q	P	H	G	G	G	W	G	Q	P
Syrian Hamster	Y	P	G	Q	G	S	P	G	G	N	R	Y	P	P	Q	G	G	G	W	G	Q	P	H	G	G	G	W	G	Q	P	H	G	G	G	W	G	Q	P	H	
Mink	Y	P	G	Q	G	S	P	G	G	N	R	Y	P	P	Q	G	G	G	W	G	Q	P	H	G	G	G	W	G	Q	P	H	G	G	G	W	G	Q	P	H	
Sheep	Y	P	G	Q	G	S	P	G	G	N	R	Y	P	P	Q	G	G	G	W	G	Q	P	H	G	G	G	W	G	Q	P	H	G	G	G	W	G	Q	P	H	
Goat	Y	P	G	Q	G	S	P	G	G	N	R	Y	P	P	Q	G	G	G	W	G	Q	P	H	G	G	G	W	G	Q	P	H	G	G	G	W	G	Q	P	H	
Cow	Y	P	G	Q	G	S	P	G	G	S	R	Y	P	S	P	Q	G	G	G	W	G	Q	P	H	G	G	G	W	G	Q	P	H	G	G	G	W	G	Q	P	H
Greater Kudu	Y	P	G	Q	G	S	P	G	G	N	R	Y	P	P	Q	G	G	G	W	G	Q	P	H	G	G	G	W	G	Q	P	H	G	G	G	W	G	Q	P	H	

Protein sequence alignment (residues 78–188) across species.

Residues 78–108

	78	79	80	81	82	83	84	85	86	87	88	89	90	91	92	93	94	95	96	97	98	99	100	101	102	103	104	105	106	107	108
Human	G	G	G	W	G	Q	P	H	G	G	G	W	G	Q	G	G	G	T	H	S	Q	W	N	K	P	S	K	P	K	T	N
Gorilla	G	G	G	W	G	Q	P	H	G	G	G	W	G	Q	G	G	G	T	H	S	Q	W	N	K	P	S	K	P	K	T	N
Chimpanzee	G	G	G	W	G	Q	P	H	G	G	G	W	G	Q	G	G	G	T	H	S	Q	W	N	K	P	S	K	P	K	T	N
Mouse	G	G	G	W	G	Q	P	H	G	G	G	W	G	Q	G	G	G	T	H	N	Q	W	N	K	P	S	K	P	K	T	N
Rat	G	G	G	W	G	Q	P	H	G	G	G	W	G	Q	G	G	G	T	H	N	Q	W	N	K	P	S	K	P	K	T	N
Syrian Hamster	G	G	G	W	G	Q	P	H	G	G	G	W	G	Q	G	G	G	T	H	G	Q	W	N	K	P	S	K	P	K	T	N
Mink	G	G	G	W	G	Q	P	H	G	G	G	W	G	Q	G	G	G	T	H	G	Q	W	N	K	P	S	K	P	K	T	N
Sheep	G	G	G	W	G	Q	P	H	G	G	G	W	G	Q	G	G	G	S	H	S	Q	W	N	K	P	S	K	P	K	T	N
Goat	G	G	G	W	G	Q	P	H	G	G	G	W	G	Q	G	G	G	S	H	S	Q	W	N	K	P	S	K	P	K	T	N
Cow	G	G	G	W	G	Q	P	H	G	G	G	W	G	Q	G	G	G	T	H	G	Q	W	N	K	P	S	K	P	K	T	N
Greater Kudu	G	G	G	W	G	Q	P	H	G	G	G	W	G	Q	G	G	G	T	H	G	Q	W	N	K	P	S	K	P	K	T	N

Residues 109–148

	109	110	111	112	113	114	115	116	117	118	119	120	121	122	123	124	125	126	127	128	129	130	131	132	133	134	135	136	137	138	139	140	141	142	143	144	145	146	147	148
Human	M	K	H	M	A	G	A	A	A	A	G	A	V	V	G	G	L	G	G	Y	M	L	G	S	A	M	S	R	P	I	I	H	F	G	S	D	Y	E	D	R
Gorilla	M	K	H	M	A	G	A	A	A	A	G	A	V	V	G	G	L	G	G	Y	M	L	G	S	A	M	S	R	P	I	I	H	F	G	S	D	Y	E	D	R
Chimpanzee	M	K	H	M	A	G	A	A	A	A	G	A	V	V	G	G	L	G	G	Y	M	L	G	S	A	M	S	R	P	I	I	H	F	G	S	D	Y	E	D	R
Mouse	L	K	H	V	A	G	A	A	A	A	G	A	V	V	G	G	L	G	G	Y	M	L	G	S	A	M	S	R	P	M	M	H	F	G	N	D	W	E	D	R
Rat	L	K	H	V	A	G	A	A	A	A	G	A	V	V	G	G	L	G	G	Y	M	L	G	S	A	M	S	R	P	M	M	H	F	G	N	D	W	E	D	R
Syrian Hamster	M	K	H	M	A	G	A	A	A	A	G	A	V	V	G	G	L	G	G	Y	M	L	G	S	A	M	S	R	P	M	M	H	F	G	N	D	W	E	D	R
Mink	M	K	H	M	A	G	A	A	A	A	G	A	V	V	G	G	L	G	G	Y	M	L	G	S	A	M	S	R	P	M	M	H	F	G	N	D	Y	E	D	R
Sheep	M	K	H	V	A	G	A	A	A	A	G	A	V	V	G	G	L	G	G	Y	M	L	G	S	A	M	S	R	P	L	L	H	F	G	S	D	Y	E	D	R
Goat	M	K	H	V	A	G	A	A	A	A	G	A	V	V	G	G	L	G	G	Y	M	L	G	S	A	M	S	R	P	L	L	H	F	G	S	D	Y	E	D	R
Cow	M	K	H	V	A	G	A	A	A	A	G	A	V	V	G	G	L	G	G	Y	M	L	G	S	A	M	S	R	P	I	I	H	F	G	S	D	Y	E	D	R
Greater Kudu	M	K	H	V	A	G	A	A	A	A	G	A	V	V	G	G	L	G	G	Y	M	L	G	S	A	M	S	R	P	I	I	H	F	G	S	D	Y	E	D	R

Residues 149–188

	149	150	151	152	153	154	155	156	157	158	159	160	161	162	163	164	165	166	167	168	169	170	171	172	173	174	175	176	177	178	179	180	181	182	183	184	185	186	187	188
Human	Y	Y	R	E	N	M	H	R	Y	P	N	Q	V	Y	Y	R	P	M	D	E	Y	S	N	Q	N	N	F	V	H	D	C	V	N	I	T	–	K	Q	H	T
Gorilla	Y	Y	R	E	N	M	H	R	Y	P	N	Q	V	Y	Y	R	P	M	D	Q	Y	S	N	Q	N	N	F	V	H	D	C	V	N	I	T	–	K	Q	H	T
Chimpanzee	Y	Y	R	E	N	M	H	R	Y	P	N	Q	V	Y	Y	R	P	M	D	Q	Y	S	N	Q	N	N	F	V	H	D	C	V	N	I	T	–	K	Q	H	T
Mouse	Y	Y	R	E	N	M	Y	R	Y	P	N	Q	V	Y	Y	R	P	M	D	Q	Y	S	N	Q	N	N	F	V	H	D	C	V	N	I	T	–	K	Q	H	T
Rat	Y	Y	R	E	N	M	Y	R	Y	P	N	Q	V	Y	Y	R	P	M	D	Q	Y	S	N	Q	N	N	F	V	H	D	C	V	N	I	T	–	K	Q	H	T
Syrian Hamster	Y	Y	R	E	N	M	N	R	Y	P	N	Q	V	Y	Y	R	P	M	D	Q	Y	S	N	Q	N	N	F	V	H	D	C	V	N	I	T	–	K	Q	H	T
Mink	Y	Y	R	E	N	M	N	R	Y	P	N	Q	V	Y	Y	R	P	M	D	Q	Y	S	N	Q	N	N	F	V	H	D	C	V	N	I	T	–	K	Q	H	T
Sheep	Y	Y	R	E	N	M	H	R	Y	P	N	Q	V	Y	Y	R	P	M	D	Q	Y	S	N	Q	N	N	F	V	H	D	C	V	N	I	T	V	K	Q	H	T
Goat	Y	Y	R	E	N	M	H	R	Y	P	N	Q	V	Y	Y	R	P	M	D	Q	Y	S	N	Q	N	N	F	V	H	D	C	V	N	I	T	V	K	Q	H	T
Cow	Y	Y	R	E	N	M	H	R	Y	P	N	Q	V	Y	Y	R	P	M	D	R	Y	S	N	Q	N	N	F	V	H	D	C	V	N	I	T	V	K	E	H	T
Greater Kudu	Y	Y	R	E	N	M	Y	R	Y	P	N	Q	V	Y	Y	R	P	V	D	Q	Y	S	N	Q	N	N	F	V	H	D	C	V	N	I	T	V	K	Q	H	T

Amino acid sequence alignment (single-letter code) of prion protein across species. Residue positions are numbered along the top; a dash (–) denotes a gap/identity marker in the alignment.

Positions 189–227

Species	189	190	191	192	193	194	195	196	197	198	199	200	201	202	203	204	205	206	207	208	209	210	211	212	213	214	215	216	217	218	219	220	221	222	223	224	225	226	227
Human	V	T	T	T	T	K	G	E	N	F	T	E	T	D	V	K	M	M	E	R	V	V	E	Q	M	C	I	T	Q	Y	E	R	E	S	Q	A	Y	Y	Q
Gorilla	V	T	T	T	T	K	G	E	N	F	T	E	T	D	V	K	M	M	E	R	V	V	E	Q	M	C	–	T	Q	Y	E	R	E	S	Q	A	Y	Y	Q
Chimpanzee	V	T	T	T	T	K	G	E	N	F	T	E	T	D	V	K	M	M	E	R	V	V	E	Q	M	C	–	T	Q	Y	Q	R	E	S	Q	A	Y	Y	G
Mouse	V	T	T	T	T	K	G	E	N	F	T	E	T	D	V	K	M	M	E	R	V	V	E	Q	M	C	V	T	Q	Y	Q	K	E	S	Q	A	Y	Y	G
Rat	V	T	T	T	T	K	G	E	N	F	T	E	T	D	V	K	–	M	E	R	V	V	E	Q	M	C	T	T	Q	Y	Q	K	E	S	Q	A	Y	Y	G
Syrian Hamster	V	T	T	T	T	K	G	E	N	F	T	E	T	D	M	K	M	M	E	R	V	V	E	Q	M	C	V	T	Q	Y	Q	Q	E	S	Q	A	Y	Y	G
Mink	V	T	T	T	T	K	G	E	N	F	T	E	T	D	V	K	–	M	E	R	V	V	E	Q	M	C	–	T	Q	Y	Q	R	E	S	Q	A	Y	Y	G
Sheep	V	T	T	T	T	K	G	E	N	F	T	E	T	D	V	K	M	M	E	R	V	V	E	Q	M	C	–	T	Q	Y	Q	R	E	S	E	A	Y	Y	G
Goat	V	T	T	T	T	K	G	E	N	F	T	E	T	D	V	K	M	M	E	R	V	V	E	Q	M	C	–	T	Q	Y	Q	R	E	S	Q	A	Y	Y	G
Cow	V	T	T	T	T	K	G	E	N	F	T	E	T	D	V	K	M	M	E	R	V	V	E	Q	M	C	–	T	Q	Y	Q	R	E	S	Q	A	Y	Y	G
Greater Kudu	V	T	T	T	T	K	G	E	N	F	T	E	T	D	V	K	–	M	E	R	V	V	E	Q	M	C	–	T	Q	Y	Q	R	E	S	E	A	Y	Y	G

(Annotation "D" appears above position 226 for Mouse, Rat and Syrian Hamster.)

Positions 228–253

Species	228	229	230	231	232	233	234	235	236	237	238	239	240	241	242	243	244	245	246	247	248	249	250	251	252	253
Human	R	G	S	S	M	V	L	F	S	S	P	P	V	I	L	L	I	S	F	L	I	F	L	I	V	G
Gorilla	R	G	S	S	V	V	L	F	S	S	P	P	V	I	L	L	I	S	F	L	I	F	L	I	V	G
Chimpanzee	R	G	S	S	M	V	L	F	S	S	P	P	V	I	L	L	I	S	F	L	I	F	L	I	V	G
Mouse	R	R	S	S	V	V	L	F	S	S	P	P	V	I	L	L	I	S	F	L	I	F	L	I	V	G
Rat	R	R	S	S	T	V	L	F	S	P	P	P	V	I	L	L	I	S	F	L	I	F	L	I	V	G
Syrian Hamster	R	G	S	S	A	–	L	F	S	S	P	P	V	I	L	L	I	S	F	L	I	F	L	I	V	G
Mink	R	G	A	S	A	–	L	F	S	P	P	P	V	I	L	L	I	S	F	L	I	F	L	I	V	G
Sheep	R	G	G	S	V	–	L	F	S	S	P	P	V	I	L	L	I	S	F	L	I	F	L	I	V	G
Goat	R	G	A	S	V	–	L	F	S	S	P	P	V	I	L	L	I	S	F	L	I	F	L	I	V	G
Cow	R	G	A	S	V	–	L	F	S	S	P	P	V	I	L	L	I	S	F	L	I	F	L	I	V	G
Greater Kudu	R	G	A	S	V	–	L	F	S	S	P	P	V	I	L	L	I	S	F	L	I	F	L	I	V	G

(Annotation "S" appears above position 231 for Syrian Hamster; position 251 is annotated "M" for Mink.)

Index